GASTROINTESTINAL CANCER
CURRENT APPROACHES TO DIAGNOSIS
AND TREATMENT

The University of Texas
M. D. Anderson Hospital and Tumor Institute at Houston
Thirtieth Annual Clinical Conference on Cancer

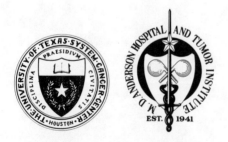

Published for
The University of Texas
M. D. Anderson Hospital and Tumor Institute at Houston
Houston, Texas, by the University of Texas Press, Austin

The University of Texas
M. D. Anderson Hospital and Tumor Institute at Houston
Thirtieth Annual Clinical Conference on Cancer

GASTROINTESTINAL CANCER
Current Approaches to Diagnosis and Treatment

Edited by

Bernard Levin, M.D.

University of Texas Press, Austin

REBECCA TEAFF: Supervising Editor

BARBARA RESCHKE, SUZANNE SIMPSON: Editors

Department of Scientific Publications
The University of Texas M. D. Anderson Hospital
and Tumor Institute at Houston
Houston, Texas

Copyright © 1988 by the University of Texas System Cancer Center

Printed in the United States of America

First Edition, 1988

Requests for permission to reproduce material from this work should be sent to
Permissions, University of Texas Press, Box 7819, Austin, Texas 78713-7819.

Library of Congress Cataloging-in-Publication Data

Clinical Conference on Cancer (30th : 1986 : M. D.
  Anderson Hospital and Tumor Institute at Houston)
  Gastrointestinal cancer.

  Held November 11–15, 1986.

  Includes bibliographies and index.
    1. Digestive organs—Cancer—Congresses.
I. Levin, Bernard, 1942– . II. M. D. Anderson
Hospital and Tumor Institute. III. Title.
[DNLM: 1. Gastrointestinal Neoplasms—diagnosis—
congresses. 2. Gastrointestinal Neoplasms—
therapy—congresses. W3 C162H 30th 1986g /
WI 149 C641 1986g]
RC280.D5C56 1986   616.99′433   87-25501
ISBN 0-292-72735-6

This volume is a compilation of the proceedings of The University of Texas
M. D. Anderson Hospital and Tumor Institute at Houston's 30th Annual
Clinical Conference on Cancer, held November 11–15, 1986, in Houston,
Texas.

The material contained in this volume was submitted as previously unpublished material, except in instances in which credit has been given to the source
from which some of the illustrative material was derived.

Great care has been taken to maintain the accuracy of the information contained in the volume. However, the editorial staff, The University of Texas,
and the University of Texas Press cannot be held responsible for errors or for
any consequences arising from the use of the information contained herein.

To my parents, Simon and Minnie Levin
To Ronnie, Adam, and Katie
and
In memory of my mentor and friend, Dr. Paul Sherlock

Contents

Preface

This volume is dedicated to exploring the latest developments in clinical and basic research as well as clinical management of malignancies of the digestive system, which account for the greatest number of deaths from cancer in the United States. National and international experts provide valuable information regarding the etiology, pathogenesis, biology, and management of tumors of the large bowel, esophagus, pancreas, liver, biliary tract, and stomach.

Much of the discussion here is focused on colorectal cancer, which will afflict an estimated 140,000 people in the U.S. this year, leading to 60,000 deaths. Although when detected in the early stages large bowel cancer can be successfully managed by surgery and increasingly used adjuvant treatment including chemotherapy, radiation therapy, and immunotherapy, this disease is often only diagnosed in late stages, when only palliative treatment is possible. Thus, early diagnosis and prevention of the disease are important and immediate goals.

One promising trend in prevention is the development of special risk clinics to monitor patients at high risk of developing colorectal cancer, particularly those people with a genetic predisposition to the disease. Recent molecular genetic studies have described specific abnormalities of chromosome 5 in patients with familial polyposis and sporadic colorectal cancer. These data provide important clues for future clinical investigations. Innovative attempts to influence the natural history of large bowel cancer by the use of dietary anticarcinogens, improvements in early detection, and the systematic study of patients from whom the precursor lesions for cancer (viz., adenomas) have been resected have also recently been made.

Other important prevention studies are aimed at an attempt to inhibit abnormal development of gastrointestinal cells and subsequent evolution of tumors. Recent studies have shown that modifications of epithelial cell proliferation and differentiation occur in diseases that predispose individuals to gastrointestinal cancer. By using "intermediate biomarkers" of cell proliferation and differentiation in studies of nutritional intervention, it is now possible to evaluate whether the appearance of these biomarkers associated with increased risk of neoplasia can be inhibited.

Striking epidemiological features have stimulated investigations seeking to identify dietary, cultural, and environmental pathogenic factors for cancer of the esophagus, a disease for which mortality rate and incidence are nearly identical. Autopsy studies have shown that in most patients with esophageal cancer, tumor is already disseminated at or shortly after diagnosis; and thus, therapy that is limited to the primary tumor and periesophageal tissue is likely to fail. This has influenced investigators to combine local treatment with systemic chemotherapy to control subclinical metastases. Preoperative chemotherapy has been shown to be useful in that it reduces the size of the tumor, allowing for complete resection, and also may reduce the probability for development of drug-resistant cells. For patients with lesions that are unresectable, endoscopic laser therapy also has been successful in relieving dysphagia, malnutrition, and chest pain.

This volume contains a comprehensive evaluation of the advances of treatment of endocrine gastrointestinal cancer, hepatocellular cancer, and gastric adenocarcinoma. Pathological definition of precursor lesions and their correlation with epidemiological studies have advanced our understanding of the biology of human stomach cancer. Applications and limitations of chemotherapy for the management of gastric cancer are lucidly presented.

As chairman of the 30th Annual Clinical Conference and editor of this book, I was privileged to have the cooperation of outstanding authorities who participated in the proceedings and contributed to this text. All worked together to achieve our conference objective—to gain a better understanding of the basic biologic mechanisms underlying gastrointestinal cancer and to reexamine current approaches and seek to identify better methodologies for its diagnosis and treatment. I believe this volume captures the spirit of our forum and will cause the reader also to view these formidable clinical and research challenges in new and exciting ways.

BERNARD LEVIN, M.D.

Acknowledgments

The 30th Annual Clinical Conference was made possible by the continued support of the American Cancer Society, Texas Division, Inc. We also appreciate the generous contributions of Adria Laboratories, Bristol-Myers, Fujinon, Haynes Radiation Limited, Hoffmann-La Roche, Knoll Pharmaceuticals, Lederle Laboratories, Marion Laboratories, Mead Johnson Oncology, Nucletron, Olympus, Pentax Precision Instrument Corporation, Roerig-Pfizer, Schering Laboratories, Smith Kline & French Laboratories, Triton Biosciences, and Wilson-Cook Medical.

Special thanks go to members of the program committee, including Charles M. Balch, M.D.; Karen R. Cleary, M.D.; Gerald D. Dodd, Jr., M.D.; Isaiah J. Fidler, D.V.M., Ph.D.; Rosemary W. Mackey; Anthony J. Mastromarino, Ph.D.; and Tyvin A. Rich, M.D., as well as those who chaired segments of the program, David M. Ota, M.D.; John M. Jessup, M.D.; Leor D. Roubein, M.D.; Jack A. Roth, M.D.; Clifton M. Mountain, M.D.; Frank Moody, M.D.; Lester J. Peters, M.D.; Guy R. Newell, M.D.; James L. Abbruzzese, M.D.; and Irwin H. Krakoff, M.D. We also wish to thank the following representatives of UT M. D. Anderson Hospital who assisted in planning and preparation for this conference: Jeffrey W. Rasco, Shirley A. Roy, and Carol D. Knight of the Department of Conference Services; James M. Bowen, Ph.D.; Thomas Gee; Charles A. LeMaistre, M.D.; Walter J. Pagel; Steven C. Schultz; and Stephen C. Stuyck; and the editors of this volume, Rebecca Teaff, Suzanne Simpson, and Barbara Reschke of the Department of Scientific Publications for their invaluable support.

HEATH MEMORIAL AWARD LECTURE

Annual Clinical Conference on Cancer, Vol. 30
Gastrointestinal Cancer: Current Approaches to Diagnosis and Treatment
© 1988 by The University of Texas System Cancer Center

1. Trials, Errors, and Glimmers of Success in the Surgical Adjuvant Treatment of Colorectal Cancer

Charles G. Moertel

Cancer originating in the colon and rectum will afflict 140,000 people in this country this year and will lead to 60,000 cancer deaths (Silverberg 1986). As a cause of cancer mortality, it is exceeded in frequency only by lung cancer. Although most large bowel cancers are surgically approachable and can be surgically cured at early stages, we must reluctantly admit that too often the patient presents at a stage at which cure is not possible. National end results statistics still show that well over half of these patients die of their disease (Silverberg 1986). Early diagnosis and prevention are laudable goals, but there is no reasonable evidence indicating that they will be substantially attained in the near future. Our most immediate and tangible hope lies in improved treatment methodologies. Although enormous resources and great efforts have been devoted to chemotherapy or immunotherapy of patients with advanced colorectal cancer, there has been little evidence of success. We have yet to see any suggestion of extension of life, much less of cure. We do know, however, that true antineoplastic effect can be demonstrated with nonsurgical treatment—occasionally with chemotherapy and very frequently with radiation therapy. Animal model studies show us that each of these treatment modalities holds its highest potential for cure when the tumor burden is minimal. In colorectal cancer this circumstance frequently occurs. Usually the patient has had resection of all surgically visible malignant disease but pathology staging has shown a strong likelihood of microscopic residual disease that will eventually lead to recurrence and death. Such a circumstance would seem to be ideal for application of currently available antineoplastic modalities as adjuvants to surgical treatment. Research in this area holds the most realistic hope in the years immediately ahead for improvement of survival of patients with gastrointestinal cancer. The purpose of this chapter is to reflect on our past efforts in surgical adjuvant therapy of colorectal cancer, to consider some of the methodological problems that have clouded our interpretation of results, and to discuss some recent studies that seem to show that early progress is being made.

CONSIDERATIONS OF METHODOLOGY IN SURGICAL ADJUVANT TRIALS

The randomized and controlled method is a sine qua non for establishing that any surgical adjuvant approach is of true value for the patient with cancer. The oncology literature overflows with flamboyant testimonials for treatment breakthroughs that could not be validated when tested with such sound scientific methodology. Certainly, however, the randomized trial is laborious and time-consuming, and a number of maneuvers have been used to circumvent difficulties. Probably the most frequent has been the use of the historically controlled trial. Here it is assumed that a retrospectively selected group of patients treated in some bygone era is prognostically equivalent to a group of patients selected for a new treatment approach today. Obviously, there would be innumerable sources of hidden bias in such comparisons, and differences demonstrated in such a study may just as well be related to differences in patient populations rather than to differences in therapeutic effect. A justification used by those electing to use historical controls in colorectal cancer surgical adjuvant trials is that surgical methodology has not substantively changed over the past 30 years and that surgical results have essentially been at a plateau over this period. As we consider surgical adjuvant therapy, I think it is important that we scrutinize such assumptions to be sure that they really apply to large bowel cancer today. Table 1.1 shows our national end result statistics for colorectal cancer with five-year survival rates related to stage. We see that within each potentially resectable stage there has, in fact, been a steady improvement in survival rates over a 40-year-period—from 53% to 78% in localized disease and from 27% to 45% in regional disease. This, however, could be more illusion than reality. For example, what we see here could simply represent improved pathology staging, not improved surgery. If the pathologist looks more carefully and screens more lymph nodes, many of the localized disease patients will be moved into the regional column, which will improve the survival results for each group. It would seem apparent that if we apply any type of colorectal cancer surgical adjuvant intervention to patients today, and just compare our results, stage for stage, to the results we achieved yesterday, we are going to have positive results, whether the adjuvant treatment is effective or not. The total lack of reliability of claims for positive results made in historically controlled studies of gastrointestinal cancer is evidenced by the fact that in essentially all instances in which subsequent randomized trials have been conducted the claims have not been validated.

Table 1.1. *National End Results Statistics for Colorectal Cancer—Five-Year Survival Rates*

Years	Five-Year Survival Rate (%)	
	Localized	Regional
1940–1949	53	27
1950–1954	62	34
1955–1959	69	36
1960–1964	69	37
1965–1969	71	44
1977–1981	78	45

Source: National Cancer Institute 1981.

It has been argued by some that historically controlled trials could be made more valid if the same eligibility criteria were used for selecting the historical control patients as were used for treatment patients, if the historical controls were recently treated, and if they were treated by the same group of investigators. It has also been argued that correction could be made for any biases in historically controlled studies by utilizing known prognostic parameters and by conducting multivariate analyses. Two recent studies are pertinent to this debate. The first was conducted by Pocock (1977) who utilized data of the Eastern Cooperative Oncology Group in instances in which the same investigating group conducted consecutive studies of the same treatment regimen for the same stage and type of malignant disease utilizing essentially the same eligibility criteria. In 21% of 19 such comparisons the therapeutic results achieved by the same regimen differed at a significant level ($p < .02$). In other words, a false difference was obtained at 10 times the frequency that chance alone would allow, even though no biases could be identified. The futility of trying to ferret out and correct for hidden biases was clearly demonstrated in the Coronary Drug Project. In this study, patients in the control arm who took at least 80% of their prescribed doses of placebo lived significantly longer than patients who took less than 80% of their placebo dose (Canner 1977). The p value for this comparison was less than 10^{-15}. Attempts to adjust away this difference by correcting for the influence of more than 40 potential prognostic variables only succeeded in changing the significance level to less than 10^{-8}, and placebo therapy remained better than placebo therapy.

If there is any substitute for the randomized controlled study in obtaining valid clinical trial results it is yet to be discovered. Even though the randomized controlled study remains the gold standard in clinical research, the fact that a study is so conducted by no means assures validity of results. Error and bias in conducting or interpreting the randomized trial can produce very damaging misinformation, particularly in view of the credibility generally accorded such trials. Certainly a major problem will be produced if the quality of the therapeutic procedure is inadequate. This problem has been particularly evident in large-scale trials using radiation as a surgical adjuvant. In some recently reported studies, major treatment deviations—wrong dose, wrong field—have been recorded in up to 39% of patients assigned to a radiation protocol arm. Similar major protocol compliance problems have been documented in chemotherapy and immunotherapy trials. Under these circumstances one must have serious concern that a treatment regimen may be labeled as worthless, whereas it could have been demonstrated to be of substantive value if it had been properly applied.

A major problem can be introduced to a randomized trial if a large proportion of patients originally randomized are withdrawn either because they are considered not to meet eligibility criteria or because patients withdrew themselves from the study after being assigned to a treatment arm. These eligibility and cancellation problems have been particularly prevalent in large national or international cooperative group studies. In these, up to 30% of patients originally entered on study are later withdrawn from analysis because of ineligibility, cancellation, or major protocol violations. The biases associated with such withdrawals are usually impossible to discern, but clearly they can produce major distortions of results of studies in which a difference between treatment arms of 10% to 15% would constitute a positive result. A striking example of this phenomenon recently occurred when two large American cooperative groups reported the use of the same regimen of combined fluorouracil and methyl CCNU in the surgical adjuvant chemotherapy of gastric cancer. The Gastrointestinal Tumor Study Group (GITSG) achieved a 15% improvement of five-year survivorship in the treated patients and this difference was statistically significant (GITSG 1982). On the other hand, the Eastern Cooperative Oncology Group (ECOG) study showed survival curves to be completely overlapping (Engstrom and Lavin 1983). The GITSG study lost 16% of its patients to analysis because of such problems as ineligibility and cancellations. The ECOG lost 15% of its patients to analysis because of similar quality problems. The difference between the two arms demonstrated in the GITSG study and not demonstrated in the ECOG study was 15%. Unfortunately, neither study gives us convincing evidence of the value or lack of value of this particular treatment regimen.

Another prevalent problem in surgical adjuvant studies has been the frequent reporting of results while the study is in progress, authors often aborting the study and reporting results before all planned patients have been entered. This generally occurs when the interim progression or survival curves spread wide enough to make a $p < .05$ difference. To quantitate the effect of such an action, Dr. Thomas Fleming at our institution simulated with a computer program a hypothetical surgical adjuvant program in which the treatment was totally ineffective (Fleming, Green, and Harrington 1984). The number of patients entered as well as the variability of their survival was such that after two years of patient entry and three years of observation there would only be 1 chance in 20 of a spurious result showing a $p < .05$ difference between the treatment and control arms. He then determined the potential of a false-positive result occurring if repeated interim analyses were performed with the study stopped and results reported as soon as a $p < .05$ difference was observed. The probability of false-positive results rose from 5% to 17% if the study was analyzed at yearly intervals, to 21% if it was analyzed every six months, and to 26% if it was analyzed every three months. In short, the possibility of reporting false differences between treatment arms may be increased up to fivefold.

Another common practice in the analysis of colorectal cancer surgical adjuvant trials is the tendency of some investigators to take a study whose results were totally negative as it was originally designed and attempt to find positive results by performing separate analyses of various subsets of the study population (e.g., by stage, by type of surgical procedure, by age group, by sex). This is clearly data manipulation and massage, since by chance alone one can always find a significant difference within a study if enough subsets are analyzed. Subset analyses can only be considered of value for the development of hypotheses, which must then be prospectively evaluated by separate and independent studies. In the discussion to follow, a number of examples will be presented in which highly significant differences were claimed within subsets of a study population by initial investigators, but for which subsequent confirmatory trials demonstrated no difference whatsoever within the same subsets. In short, when the reader explores the colorectal cancer surgical adjuvant treatment literature, he must carefully scrutinize the experimental and analytic methodology employed and the study quality before accepting any claimed results as truth.

RESULTS OF SURGICAL ADJUVANT TRIALS IN COLON CANCER

Initially surgical adjuvant therapy for colorectal cancer was attempted using thiotepa, a drug with little or no antineoplastic activity in advanced disease. The University Surgeon's Group study results were completely negative (Dixon, Longman, and Holden 1971). The Veterans Administration study illustrated the potential hazards of ineffective surgical adjuvant treatment (Veterans Administration Surgical Adjuvant Cancer Chemotherapy Group 1965). Their five-year survivorship was significantly better in the controls than in the treated patients. Subsequent interest centered around the fluorinated pyrimidines, 5-fluorouracil (5-FU) and floxuridine, which do at least have some advanced disease activity. As is usually the case, there were historically controlled trials that claimed an advantage for therapy. In table 1.2, however, I show the results of all published randomized studies, which have in-

Table 1.2. *Systemic 5-Fluorouracil or Floxuridine as Adjuvant to Potentially Curative Colorectal Cancer Surgery: Randomized Studies with Untreated Controls*

Study	Surgical Adjuvant Regimen	No. of Patients Studied	Survival Comparison
Higgins et al. 1976	5-FU 12 mg/kg/d i.v. × 5 every 2 weeks and 8 to 10 weeks postop	308	No significant difference
Higgins et al. 1976	5-FU 12 mg/kg/d i.v. × 5 every 6 weeks for 1.5 years	522	No significant difference
Dwight et al. 1973	5-FUDR 20 mg/kg i.v. on postop days 1, 2, and 3; 30 mg/kg/d × 5 plus 15 mg/kg every other day × 4 started 5–6 weeks postop	548	No significant difference
Grage and Moss 1981	5-FU 12 mg/kg/d i.v. × 4 plus 6 mg/kg every other day × 5, then 12 mg/kg weekly for 1 year	189	No significant difference
Blokhina et al. 1974	5-FU 15 mg/kg i.v. every other day × 4 at 1 mo and 3 mo postop	265	No significant difference
Hafstrom et al. 1985	5-FU 5 mg/kg/d orally for 3 mo	421	No significant difference
Lawrence et al. 1975	5-FU 30 mg/kg intraluminally at surgery; 10 mg/kg i.v. on postop days 1 and 2; oral 5-FU 12 mg/kg/d × 4 and 6 mg/kg every other day × 7. Courses repeated every 2 mo × 5	156	No significant difference
Grossi et al. 1977	5-FU 30 mg/kg intraluminally at surgery; 10 mg/kg i.v. on postop days 1 and 2	478	No significant difference

Abbreviations: 5-FU, 5-fluorouracil; 5-FUDR, floxuridine.

volved a total of almost 3,000 patients. The first study was stimulated by the report of Li and Ross (1976), who used just two courses of intravenous 5-FU given soon after surgery and claimed a highly significant improvement in both Dukes B and C lesions. This, however, was a historically controlled study. The Veterans Administration Surgical Oncology Group (VASOG) used the same method but in a randomized trial and showed no difference (Higgins et al. 1976). This same group then used intravenous 5-FU over a full year, but again there was no significant difference between treated patients and randomized controls. Earlier this group had shown no advantage for patients receiving floxuridine, the nucleoside derivative of 5-FU (Dwight et al. 1976). Actually, in this study the control patients did slightly better than the treated patients. The Central Oncology Group used a more toxic dose of 5-FU (Grage and Moss 1981). Although their treated group showed a slight advantage, it was not statistically significant. A study was conducted in the Soviet Union using a very gentle dosage schedule of 5-FU over just a three-month period, and the controls did somewhat better than the treated patients (Blokhina, Garin, and Lipstov 1974). A tightly designed placebo controlled study conducted in Sweden with orally administered 5-FU produced survival curves that were virtually identical (Hafstrom, Rudenstam, and Damellof 1985). Rousselot and associates (1972) devised a new method in which they injected a 5-FU solution into the tied-off tumor-containing section of the colon with the expectation that the drug would be disseminated in a high concentration along the routes of vascular and lymphatic tumor cell spread. They claimed a highly significant survival advantage after comparing their results to those from historical controls recorded in national tumor registries. Dr. Walter Lawrence and associates (1975) utilized this same method in a randomized controlled study and demonstrated no survival difference whatsoever. Dr. Rousselot's group attempted to validate their results by conducting a randomized controlled study, and they came up with a completely negative result as well (Grossi et al. 1977). Certainly there is no more vivid example of the total inadequacy of using historical controls.

There are those who try to milk something positive out of these fluorinated pyrimidine studies by analyzing various subsets of their study population or by adding up the results of individual studies—the so-called meta analysis—but this type of data gerrymandering does not produce valid results. We must conclude after randomized studies involving several thousand patients that the fluorinated pyrimidines given systemically are not effective as adjuvants to colorectal cancer surgery.

Nonspecific immunotherapy has periodically been a glamour area, and of course, it has been claimed to be effective in historically controlled studies. *Corynebacterium parvum,* however, when compared to no treatment did not improve survival rates in a study conducted in the United Kingdom (Souter, Gill, and Morris 1982), and bacillus Calmette-Guérin (BCG) has been proved to be similarly ineffective in a large NSABP (National Surgical Adjuvant Breast Program) study (Wolmark et al. 1985).

Single-agent therapy having failed, subsequent adjuvant trials conducted in the United States have involved combination chemotherapy or combined modality chemotherapy plus immunotherapy. There was some animal model support for these studies. A large effort has been devoted to evaluating the combination of 5-FU plus methyl CCNU, which was found to be effective surgical adjuvant treatment for transplanted rodent colon carcinoma lines (Griswold 1975). MER BCG, the methanol extracted residue of BCG, also attracted interest because of similar activity in a transplanted colon carcinoma model (Enker 1978). These results provided a rationale for a GITSG study in which patients were randomized to no adjuvant treatment, to adjuvant immunotherapy with MER BCG, to chemotherapy with 5-FU plus methyl CCNU, and to combined chemotherapy and immunotherapy (GITSG 1984). With all the animal research, however, this study involving over 600 patient entries showed survival curves to completely intertwine. A study with similar negative results on the 5-FU–methyl CCNU combination has been reported by VASOG (Higgins, Amadeo, and McElhinney 1984).

In searching for more productive leads in surgical adjuvant therapy of colon cancer, hopeful notes have been sounded from two interesting European studies. The first emanated from Dr. Irving Taylor and his associates (1984) working in the United Kingdom. They used seven days of portal vein infusion of 5-FU initiated right in the operating theater. This could be expeditiously accomplished because all treatment is completed during initial hospitalization and toxicity is mild. There is some rationale for this approach because the liver is the most frequent site of metastasis from colon cancer. After studying over 200 patients, these investigators claimed an impressive and highly significant survival advantage for the treated group in terms of overall survival and most specifically in terms of the rate of hepatic metastasis. Disturbing features with regard to this report, however, were a very high rate of postoperative complications in both the treatment and control groups and the fact that the five-year survivorship stage for stage was really very low in comparison to contemporary experience—just over 50% for Dukes B lesions and less than 15% with Dukes C lesions. Both the North Central Cancer Treatment Group and the NSABP currently have confirmatory randomized studies that are well under way. It would seem appropriate that this approach not be considered as routine surgical practice until these confirmatory studies are completed.

The second study with positive results has involved levamisole. This is an interesting drug that has been used for many years to treat parasitic infections in humans in the Third World and in domestic animals in our country. It has some nonspecific immunomodulatory effects, and over the past decade it has probably been involved in more randomized studies with positive results than any other investigational agent. The problem has been, though, that these results have not held up in confirmatory studies. Probably the latest trial involving levamisole was reported by the National Cancer Institute of Canada (Quirt et al. 1986). These researchers found that levamisole was significantly superior to controls in both recurrence-free time and survival for surgical adjuvant therapy in poor-risk malignant melanoma. The very fragile nature of this result, however, was demonstrated in the same study when a combination of levamisole and BCG failed to demonstrate any therapeutic advantage at all. Interest in levamisole by my colleagues and me was stimulated by the report of Verhagen (1977) who compared levamisole to a placebo in a small group of patients with resected large bowel cancer and demonstrated a dramatic and statistically significant survival rate improvement (Quirt et al. 1986). We believed this interesting result in a refractory therapeutic setting demanded further exploration, and for purely empiric reasons we also elected to evaluate the combination of levamisole plus 5-FU with the hope that perhaps we could achieve some additive therapeutic effect (Laurie et al. 1986). Four hundred eight patients were entered into this trial. The study quality was very high, and only 2.7% of patients either cancelled or were declared ineligible. Therapy was, in the main, very tolerable, and therefore treatment compliance was excellent. Prognostic factors were well balanced among the three treatment arms. Preliminary results of this study were reported early in 1986 when the median follow-up was 56 months and the minimum 20 months. Both the levamisole and levamisole plus 5-FU arms showed a significant advantage over surgery alone in time to progression for all patients ($p \simeq .04$ and $.02$, respectively). These advantages were most striking for Dukes stage C ($p \simeq .015$ and $.004$). Less mature survival observations were suggestive of treatment advantage (levamisole, $p \simeq .04$; levamisole plus 5-FU, $p \simeq .16$). Again survival advantages were most impressive in Dukes stage C ($p \simeq .02$ and $.04$). Certainly these results are of interest, and it may be that at long last we do have moderately effective surgical adjuvant treatment for colorectal cancer with poor prognosis. Nevertheless, there have been a large number of adjuvant studies conducted in this disease. Our p values are not all that strong, and this just could be the study that turned up with a positive result by chance alone. We believed it was essential that a confirmatory trial be conducted involving a considerably larger number of patients. This trial is already under way and involves three large cooperative groups. The planned patient entry of 1200 will be complete in 1987. We do not believe these approaches should be adapted into standard practice until our results are confirmed by this larger trial.

SURGICAL ADJUVANT TREATMENT OF RECTAL CARCINOMA

The rectal segment of the large bowel presents a specific challenge and opportunity for surgical adjuvant therapy. Here we have had effective nonsurgical treatment of advanced disease for many years. In reviewing our Mayo Clinic results among 157 patients treated with radiation alone for locally unresectable or recurrent carcinoma of the rectum, we found that symptomatic relief was excellent and seemed dose related because it increased from 50% to over 90% as doses escalated from 3,500 to 5,000 cGy. Survival in these patients was quite long with a median of 20 months at the 5,000 cGy dose. There was a small proportion of patients achieving long-term survival, about 8% at five years, and some of these were apparent cures. Our results are quite comparable to those reported by others. Such observations led to consideration of radiation as a surgical adjuvant for resectable rectal carcinoma. As is true for medical oncologists, some radiation oncologists have a penchant for making extravagant claims based on small uncontrolled studies, and we have had those for both preoperative and postoperative radiation. They're just as believable as the uncontrolled chemotherapy studies. There have, however, been a number of randomized studies with substantive case entries providing perspective (table 1.3). The

Table 1.3. *Radiation Therapy as a Surgical Adjuvant for Rectal Carcinoma: Randomized Studies with Untreated Controls*

Study	Regimen Dose (cGy)	Regimen Fractions	Patients Entered	Curative Resections	Survival	Local Recurrence	Comment
			Preoperative Irradiation				
Roswitt et al. 1970 (VASOG)	2,000–2,500	10	700	453	No significant difference	No significant difference	Irradiation significantly superior in survival of anteroposterior resection subset
Stearns et al. 1974 (New York Memorial)	2,000	8	Not stated	790	No significant difference	Not stated	Higher operative mortality in treated patients
Higgins et al. 1986 (VASOG)	3,150	18	361	320	No significant difference	Not stated	Study confined to patients requiring anteroposterior resections
Rider et al. 1977 (Princess Margaret Hospital)	500	1	125	106	No significant difference	Not stated	Irradiation significantly superior in survival of Dukes C subset
Duncan et al. 1984 (Medical Research Council)	2,000 500	10 1	824	578	No significant difference	No significant difference	No significant difference in Dukes C subset
Gerard et al. 1985 (EORTC)	3,450	15	410	318	No significant difference	Significant reduction with radiation	Time to progression improved by irradiation at borderline significance ($p = .054$)
			Postoperative Irradiation				
GITSG 1985	4,000–4,800	23–28	103	103	No significant difference	No significant difference	Slight but not significant improvements in recurrence-free survival, survival, and local recurrence rates
Balslev et al. 1986 (Danish Consortium)	5,000 (Split course)	25	494	494	No significant difference	No significant difference	Delayed local recurrence in Dukes C subset

first was a Veterans Administration study involving preoperative radiation at 2,000 to 2,500 cGy (Roswitt, Higgins, and Keehn 1970). Seven hundred patients were randomized to treatment or control, and resectability was equal in both groups. Among the 453 patients who had curative resections, the five-year survivorship for preoperative radiation was 48% and for untreated controls, 39%. This difference approached statistical significance but did not reach it. The authors, however, did claim a significant advantage in their subset of patients who had abdominal perineal resections. On the other hand, a similar study performed at New York Memorial Hospital had a higher operative mortality rate with radiation with no survival advantage (Stearns et al. 1974). The Veterans Administration Group then performed a second trial using a larger dose of radiation (3,150 cGy) and confining their patient entries to those requiring anteroposterior resection—their predicted favorable subset (Higgins et al. 1986). They observed no difference in either recurrence or survival rates.

Rider and associates (1977), working at the Princess Margaret Hospital, triggered a similar series of events when they gave just a single 500-cGy dose immediately before surgery and compared this treatment with sham radiation. The study, as originally designed, showed no treatment effect. They did, however, claim a highly significant survival advantage for patients with Dukes C lesions. A recently reported Medical Research Council study involving over 800 patients examined this method, and these researchers also again examined the method employed in the original Veterans Administration study of 2,000 cGy preoperatively (Duncan, Smith, and Freedman 1984). They found the survival curves for both treated groups overlapped with untreated controls. They reported only a trivial difference in local recurrence, and when they examined the subset of patients with Dukes C lesions, they again found no survival or recurrence advantage for either preoperative radiation method.

When the European Organization for Research on Treatment of Cancer (EORTC) studied preoperative radiation they moved up the dose to 3,450 cGy (Gerard et al. 1985). They found only a minor survival difference overall in their group of over 400 patients. In their 317 patients who had curative resections, radiation produced a somewhat more favorable survival rate, but this was not significant. With regard to time to progression, however, radiation produced a more impressive advantage that just edged statistical significance. The reduction in local recurrences with radiation was very dramatic—only 17 patients compared with 42 patients in the surgery-only arm.

If one would change sequence and radiate postoperatively, there would be an obvious advantage. The surgical staging would avoid unnecessary radiation for patients with early-stage lesions as well as those who already have distant metastasis that isn't recognized until the abdomen is open. Also, postponing radiation produces a much cleaner study analysis because the diluting effect such patients have on therapeutic comparisons can be avoided. The disadvantage of postoperative radiation is greater risk of severe radiation enteritis. Recent studies, however, would indicate that this complication can be minimized with careful treatment planning. The

GITSG evaluated postoperative radiation as a part of a larger study (see below) using a dose of 4,000 to 4,800 cGy (GITSG 1985). They found a small but not significant delay in recurrence and a slight reduction in local recurrence. A larger study conducted by a consortium of Danish investigators has been reported in preliminary form (Balslev et al. 1986). They randomized 494 patients to either surgery alone or surgery plus postoperative radiation with 5,000 cGy given in a split course. They found no difference in survival rate and no difference in overall recurrence rates. They observed only a small reduction in local recurrences. Within their Dukes C subset, however, they did report a significant delay in local recurrence. An overview of all of these studies, which now involve several thousand patients, would make it appear that radiation alone given either preoperatively or postoperatively at doses of 3,450 to 5,000 cGy possibly delays overall recurrences and probably reduces local recurrence rate, but does not improve survival rates.

In considering radiation as an adjuvant to surgery, one hope of enhancement of antitumor effect derives from a wealth of in vitro and animal studies showing that 5-FU adds to the effect of radiation and may be a true radiation sensitizer. Several years ago, we designed a regimen of rapid injection 5-FU and radiation therapy to the pelvis (Moertel et al. 1969). We compared this to placebo plus radiation in a prospective double-blind study. In duration of symptom control, interval to progression, and, most important, survival, the group receiving 5-FU showed a substantial and significant advantage over those receiving radiation alone. These findings, plus the hope for chemotherapy with combined 5-FU and methyl CCNU raised in animal model studies (see above), formed the background for a recently completed GITSG study (1985). Patients with resectable Dukes B2 and C rectal carcinoma were randomized to no further treatment, to chemotherapy alone, to postoperative radiation therapy alone, or to a regimen of postoperative radiation combined with simultaneous 5-FU and followed by 5-FU and methyl CCNU chemotherapy, all given over a total of 18 months. This study had several problems. There were a substantial number of ineligible and cancelled patients. The rate of major radiation therapy deviations was quite high (39%). In addition, this study was aborted with less than half of the planned patients entered because on repeated interim analyses the recurrence curves were spreading. Nevertheless, the results were interesting. The combined modality arm showed a significant advantage over the untreated controls in recurrence-free time ($p = .009$) and in survival ($p = .005$). There was also a substantial reduction in local recurrence rates for the combined modality arm. Combined modality treatment, however, was not significantly superior to either radiation alone or chemotherapy alone.

When we developed the combined modality arm for the GITSG study, we still had hope that postoperative radiation might be much more effective than what it actually proved to be. In retrospect one might ask whether the combined modality arm was appropriately designed. In this arm, methyl CCNU and 5-FU chemotherapy was not initiated until three to four months after the surgical procedure and was not given full dose until five or six months after surgery. Furthermore, a number of patients never received combination chemotherapy at all because their disease recurred early or they had persistent leukopenia after radiation. This is perhaps not the most ideal setting for surgical adjuvant chemotherapy. These are the considerations we addressed in a recently completed North Central Cancer Treatment Group (NCCTG) study in which we randomized patients with rectal cancer with poor prognosis to postoperative radiation alone or to an entirely new combined modality regimen (Krook et al. 1986). We elected to use radiation alone as our control arm because we believed previous studies had positively established that radiation-treated patients do no worse than untreated patients; and perhaps there is some small advantage, at least in terms of delaying local recurrence. We also did not wish to leave open the question that our new regimen was no better than well-delivered radiation of adequate dose. We believed that 5,000 cGy was close to the highest dose that could reasonably be employed in a cooperative group study. For our combined modality arm we elected to move combination chemotherapy with 5-FU and methyl CCNU to initial treatment and give a full cycle at full dose before beginning radiation and 5-FU. We hoped that this nine-week delay in radiation would not impair local effectiveness. Following radiation we gave only one additional cycle of 5-FU and methyl CCNU. We know of no evidence that longer treatment is more effective, and we believed it was highly likely that this substantial reduction in total methyl CCNU dose would reduce its leukemogenic potential. Indeed, we have not yet seen a case of leukemia. Our study was designed for 200 eligible and evaluable patients. We entered 209. Our study quality was excellent; we lost only five patients to analysis because of ineligibility or cancellation. Patient characteristics were very well balanced between the two treatment arms as were pathology characteristics. With the combination regimen we observed definite but clinically tolerable toxicity, which was primarily hematologic. There were no drug-related deaths. Severe radiation enteritis occurred in only seven of our patients and resulted in only one death. This problem was not increased by the addition of chemotherapy. In preliminary analysis our combined modality arm shows a striking and highly significant superiority in recurrence-free time ($p = .005$). If we look at major subgroups within our study, we find that treatment effect is unrelated to stage. It is interesting, however, that in our patients undergoing anteroposterior resection, recurrence-free survival curves overlap. Our entire treatment advantage is in anterior resection. The combination is markedly superior at a very high level of significance ($p = .00025$). As we look at sites of recurrence, we find that the combination has reduced local failure by almost 50%, and we have a comparable reduction in distant metastasis. In each instance, these differences are significant. The survival curves are just beginning to separate, and we can't predict our final result. It would seem likely, however, that they will follow the same pattern as our recurrence curves (15 of our patients treated with radiation alone have recurrent disease but are not yet dead compared with only six in our combined modality arm).

We believe the evidence is convincing that combined chemotherapy and postoperative radiation given according to the methods we have employed significantly reduce recurrence rates and probably improve survival rates in patients who have rectal cancer with poor prognosis. With careful treatment planning and execution this improvement can be accomplished with a minimum of treatment-related morbidity. One serious question that can be raised about our GITSG study and about our most recent NCCTG study is whether methyl CCNU really contributed to our favorable results or if this same result could be accomplished with 5-FU alone completely avoiding the leukemia hazard. It can be pointed out that 5-FU alone has been used repeatedly in controlled trials for large bowel cancer and has never demonstrated significant advantage. On the other hand, it is of interest that subset analysis in the Veterans Administration study showed the most favorable effect for 5-FU in rectal carcinoma (Higgins et al. 1976). In the Central Oncology Group trial, 5-FU showed a highly significant advantage in the rectal carcinoma subset (Grage and Moss 1981). An even more important question is whether we can improve the favorable results we have already obtained. The concurrent use of 5-FU and radiation seems to be a crucial element in both of our studies. One possible means of improving the efficacy of 5-FU radiation sensitization is to prolong the duration of 5-FU exposure. There is laboratory evidence supporting this approach. Constant infusion 5-FU has been added to radiation in a number of uncontrolled pilot studies with tolerable toxicity and with the opinion expressed by investigators that therapeutic results were very favorable. We believe, however, that any claimed advantage of constant infusion 5-FU must be proven by controlled trial. In our current protocol therefore, we are using a 2-by-2 design in which the chemotherapy elements are either 5-FU alone or 5-FU plus methyl CCNU. Patients are further randomized to receive the 5-FU given concurrently with radiation either by bolus injection or by constant infusion.

It does appear that in rectal carcinoma we have significant therapeutic accomplishment, and it is probably the first instance in which chemotherapy has been clearly proved effective in surgical adjuvant treatment of large bowel cancer.

PROSPECTUS

As we plan further research in surgical adjuvant treatment of gastrointestinal cancer, I believe it is evident that neither surgeon, radiation oncologist, or medical oncologist will produce any substantive accomplishment by working alone. If, however, we can offer our patients the best of all concerned clinical disciplines—working together, in concert, communicating—then we have taken the first step toward optimizing our treatment approaches. I also believe that today we must begin to bring basic scientists into our multidisciplinary clinical team—the pharmacologist, the immunologist, the cellular biologist, the radiation biologist. We have reached the point at which the fruits of basic cancer research should be brought to the bedside of the cancer patient and, indeed, directly into the operating theater. Certainly today the biostatistician should be a full member of the research team from beginning to end of any study. If today we can regard every patient who has colorectal cancer with poor prognosis as a candidate for treatment in a clinical research setting and if we conduct our clinical studies with sound scientific methodology and impeccable quality, then we can confidently anticipate significant improvement in surgical adjuvant treatment for tomorrow's patient with colorectal cancer.

REFERENCES

Balslev IB, Pedersen M, Teglbjaerg PS, et al. 1986. Postoperative radiotherapy in Dukes' B and C carcinoma of the rectum and rectosigmoid. A randomized multicenter study. *Cancer* 58:22–28.

Blokhina NG, Garin AM, Lipstov AM. 1974. Results of 5-year observation after radical surgery for carcinoma of colon and rectum. *Proceedings of the Second All-Union Cancer Chemotherapy Conference.* Kiev. p. 243–244.

Canner, P. 1977. Monitoring clinical trial data for evidence of adverse or beneficial treatment effects. *Multicenter Controlled Trials* 76:131–149.

Dixon WJ, Longmire WP Jr, Holden WD. 1971. Use of triethylenethiophosphoramide as an adjuvant to surgical treatment of gastric and colorectal carcinoma. *Ann Surg* 173:26–39.

Duncan W, Smith AN, Freedman LS. 1984. The evaluation of low dose preoperative x-ray therapy in the management of operable rectal cancer. *Br J Surg* 71:21–25.

Dwight RW, Humphrey EW, Higgins GA, et al. 1973. FUDR as an adjuvant to surgery in cancer of the large bowel. *J Surg Oncol* 5:243–249.

Engstrom P, Lavin P. 1983. Postoperative adjuvant therapy for gastric cancer patients (abstract). *Proceedings of the American Society of Clinical Oncology* 2:114.

Enker WE. 1978. Adjuvant immunotherapy for large bowel cancer. In *Carcinoma of the Colon and Rectum,* WE Enker, ed., pp. 259–282. Chicago: Year Book Medical.

Fleming TR, Green SJ, Harrington DP. 1984. Considerations for monitoring and evaluating treatment effects in clinical trials. *Controlled Clinical Trials* 5:55–66.

Gastrointestinal Tumor Study Group. 1982. Controlled trial of adjuvant chemotherapy following curative resection for gastric cancer. *Cancer* 49:1116–1122.

Gastrointestinal Tumor Study Group. 1984. Adjuvant therapy of colon cancer—Results of a prospectively randomized trial. *N Engl J Med* 310:737–742.

Gastrointestinal Tumor Study Group. 1985. Prolongation of the disease-free interval in surgically treated rectal carcinoma. *N Engl J Med* 312:1465–1472.

Gerard A, Berrod J, Pene F, et al. 1985. Interim analysis of a phase III study of preoperative radiation therapy in resectable rectal carcinoma. *Cancer* 55:2373–2379.

Grage TB, Moss SE. 1981. Adjuvant chemotherapy in cancer of the colon and rectum. *Surg Clin North Am* 61:1321–1329.

Griswold DP. 1975. The potential for murine tumor models in surgical adjuvant chemotherapy. *Cancer Chemother Rep* 5:187–204.

Grossi CE, Wolff WI, Nealon TF Jr, et al. 1977. Intraluminal fluorouracil chemotherapy adjuvant to surgical procedures for resectable carcinoma of the colon and rectum. *Surg Gynecol Obstet* 145:549–554.

Hafstrom L, Rudenstam CM, Damellof L. 1985. A randomized trial of oral 5-fluorouracil versus placebo as adjuvant therapy in colorectal cancer Dukes B and C. *Br J Surg* 72:138–141.

Higgins GA Jr, Amadeo JH, McElhinney J. 1984. Efficacy of prolonged intermittent therapy with combined 5-fluorouracil and methyl CCNU following resection for carcinoma of the large bowel. *Cancer* 53:1–8.

Higgins GA Jr, Humphrey EW, Dwight RW, et al. 1986. Preoperative radiation and surgery for cancer of the rectum. *Cancer* 58:352–359.

Higgins GA Jr, Humphrey EW, Juler GL, et al. 1976. Adjuvant chemotherapy in the surgical treatment of colorectal cancer. *Cancer* 38:1461–1467.

Krook J, Moertel C, Wieand H, et al. 1986. Radiation vs. sequential chemotherapy: Radiation-chemotherapy as surgical adjuvants for rectal carcinoma (abstract). *Proceedings of the American Society of Clinical Oncology* 5:82.

Laurie J, Moertel C, Fleming T, et al. 1986. Surgical adjuvant therapy of poor prognosis colorectal cancer with levamisole alone or combined levamisole and 5-fluorouracil (abstract). *Proceedings of the American Society of Clinical Oncology* 5:81.

Lawrence W Jr, Terz JJ, Horsley S, et al. 1975. Chemotherapy as an adjuvant to surgery for colorectal cancer. *Ann Surg* 181:616–623.

Li MC, Ross ST. 1976. Chemoprophylaxis for patients with colorectal cancer. *JAMA* 235: 2825–2827.

Moertel CG, Childs DS, Reitemeier RJ, et al. 1969. Combined 5-fluorouracil and supervoltage radiation therapy of locally unresectable gastrointestinal cancer. *Lancet* 2:865–867.

National Cancer Institute. *Surveillance, Epidemiology and End Results.* 1981. Washington, D.C.: NCI.

Pocock SJ. 1977. Randomized clinical trials. *Br Med J* 1:1161.

Quirt I, Shelley W, Bodurtha A, et al. 1986. Adjuvant levamisole improves survival and disease-free survival in patients with poor prognosis malignant melanoma (abstract). *Proceedings of the American Society of Clinical Oncology* 5:130.

Rider WD, Palmer JA, Mahoney LJ, et al. 1977. Preoperative irradiation in operable cancer of the rectum. *Can J Surg* 20:335–338.

Roswitt B, Higgins GA Jr, Keehn RJ. 1970. A controlled study of preoperative radiation in cancer of the sigmoid colon and rectum. *Radiology* 97:133–140.

Rousselot LM, Cole DR, Grossi CE, et al. 1972. Adjuvant chemotherapy with 5-fluorouracil in surgery for colorectal cancer. *Dis Colon Rectum* 15:169–174.

Silverberg E. 1986. Cancer statistics 1986. *CA* 36:9–25.

Souter RG, Gill PG, Morris PJ. 1982. A trial of non-specific immunotherapy using systemic *C. parvum* treated patients with Dukes B and C colorectal cancer. *Br J Cancer* 45: 506–512.

Stearns MW, Deddish MR, Quan SHQ, et al. 1974. Preoperative roentgen therapy for cancer of the rectum and rectosigmoid. *Surg Gynecol Obstet* 138:584–586.

Taylor I, Machin D, Mulleet M, et al. 1984. A randomized controlled study of adjuvant portal vein cytotoxic perfusion in colorectal cancer. *Br J Surg* 72:359–363.

Verhagen H. 1977. Postoperative levamisole in colorectal cancer. *Proceedings of the Symposium on Immunotherapy of Malignant Diseases.* Vienna.

Veterans Administration Surgical Adjuvant Cancer Chemotherapy Group. 1965. Adjuvant use of HN2 (NSC-762) and Thio-TEPA (NSC-6396). *Cancer Chemother Rep* 44:27–30.

Wolmark N, Fisher B, Wieand H, et al. 1985. Adjuvant chemotherapy in carcinoma of the colon (abstract). *Proceedings of the American Society of Clinical Oncology* 4:86.

LARGE BOWEL CANCER

Annual Clinical Conference on Cancer, Vol. 30
Gastrointestinal Cancer: Current Approaches to Diagnosis and Treatment
© 1988 by The University of Texas System Cancer Center

2. The Natural History of Colorectal Cancer: Opportunities for Intervention

Sidney J. Winawer

We have made considerable progress in recent years in our understanding of the natural history of colorectal cancer. Together with advances in laboratory investigation and clinical techniques, this progress has provided the basis for new and exciting approaches to the control of this disease. The natural history of colorectal cancer can now be viewed backward from outcome to inception—from adenocarcinoma to adenoma with dysplasia, mucosal phenotypic abnormalities, and finally to the abnormal genotype and susceptibility locus. These points offer opportunities for intervention, and they are the focus of much current research.

DETECTING EARLY ADENOCARCINOMA

The first opportunity for intervention is with adenocarcinoma. Early detection with stool blood testing and sigmoidoscopy in asymptomatic individuals may provide the opportunity for prolonging survival of individuals with colorectal cancer and reducing mortality from this disease in the screened population (Winawer et al. 1982). The usefulness of the stool blood test in screening for colorectal cancer is being evaluated in four controlled trials (Miller in press; Chait et al. 1986; Gilbertsen et al. 1980; Hardcastle et al. 1986). The results of these trials can be categorized under measures of feasibility of this approach and measures of validity or effectiveness. Feasibility parameters include patient compliance; rate of positive tests; the tests' predictive value, sensitivity, and specificity; and results of diagnostic tests. Measures of validity or effectiveness are cancer stage, survival of patients in whom cancer is detected, mortality among the screened population, and cost-effectiveness.

The four controlled trials demonstrated a compliance range of 39% to 80% for initial use of the stool blood test (table 2.1), with higher compliance the result of more patient education or direct contact. The rate of positive tests in the four programs ranged from 1.7% to 4.0% with the use of unhydrated slides. Rehydration of the slides increased the rate of positives to a range of 5.4% to 9.8% in the four programs. The increased rate of positivity was accompanied by increased sensitivity to more acceptable levels, but there was an unacceptable reduction of specificity.

Attempts are being made to provide a more sensitive slide test without loss of specificity. Immunochemical tests have been under evaluation for years, but so far these tests have not been widely applied to screening. The recently introduced Hemoquant test (Ahlquist et al. 1985) is a sophisticated, quantitative test that has

Table 2.1. *Preliminary Long-Term Controlled Trial Results of Fecal Occult Blood Testing*

	Population	Initial Compliance (%)	Rate of Slide Positivity[a] (%)	PV Cancer & Adenoma (%)	Dukes Stages A & B	
					Screen (%)	Control (%)
U.S. (New York)	22,000	70–80	1.7	30	65	33
U.S. (Minnesota)	45,000	77	2.4	31	78	NR
England	20,000	39	4.0	40	90	40
Sweden	27,000	66	1.9	22	65	33

Source: Miller in press.
Abbreviations: PV, predictive value; NR, not reported.
[a] Nonhydrated slide.

not yet been evaluated in a large screening trial. The rate of positivity of the guaiac slide test has been shown to be directly related to the age of the patients being screened and to whether it is a first test, which will uncover a high frequency of prevalent disease, or a subsequent test for which the incidence of disease found will be lower (Winawer and Sherlock 1982).

Screening Validity

Measurements of the validity or effectiveness of screening include the stage of cancers detected by the test compared with that of cancers detected in symptomatic patients, survival of patients relative to the method of detection, and mortality from colorectal cancer in the entire screened population compared with the unscreened population (Winawer, Schottenfeld, and Sherlock 1980).

Early results from the four controlled trials have demonstrated a higher percentage of early-stage (Dukes A and B) cancers in the screened groups—from 65% to 90%—compared with control groups in whom the rate of early-stage cancers ranged from 33% to 40% (data from three of the four trials) (Miller in press; Chait et al. 1986; Gilbertsen et al. 1980; Hardcastle et al. 1986). The national average for patients with early-stage cancers coming to surgery is 44% (Guidelines 1980). We would expect improved survival based on this, and indeed this has been observed in the Memorial Sloan-Kettering Cancer Center (MSKCC)—Strang Clinic trial. Since stage shifts and survival improvement could, however, be a reflection of length and lead-time bias, a reduction in mortality from the disease needs to be seen to validate the earlier measurements of effectiveness. This requires long-term, complete follow-up of all patients and accurate ascertainment of cause of death. The data will begin to come from the various programs over the next few years, provided that follow-up continues to be complete and accurate (Winawer, Schottenfeld, and Sherlock 1985). In the interim, the American Cancer Society guidelines for screening (1984) appear to be reasonable. They encourage people to seek general examinations, and they recommend detailed diagnostic evaluations of people who have symptoms, evaluations of risk factors, screening of asymptomatic people over age 50 with stool-blood testing and sigmoidoscopy at periodic intervals, and complete assessments of persons with positive test results.

Screening with fecal occult blood testing is feasible in a well-motivated population when they come to a health facility for checkups. In our clinic, compliance with preparation of the smears was up to 80%, and the rate of positive test results was low enough to be manageable in terms of patients needing diagnostic assessments. The predictive value for neoplastic lesions, including adenomas and cancers, was high in patients who had a positive screening test; the false-positive rate was acceptable. The false-negative rate is approximately 30%. Data resulting from comparable programs at the University of Minnesota, the University of Nottingham, and the University of Gutenburg, utilizing similar approaches, seem to be in general agreement with data from our program.

The long-term evaluation of screening results will be important. The proximate measure of outcome, Dukes staging, has been encouraging so far, but the long-term survival will be important in partly determining the effectiveness of the screening method. Dukes staging and survival are, however, only preliminary parameters of effectiveness. If screening is to be valid, mortality from colorectal cancer must be lower in the study group than in the control group. This reduces the lead time and length bias that could influence stage and survival.

The question of the value of adenoma detection and removal must be answered because this lesion is found more commonly than cancer. Whether identification of colon adenomas and their removal is associated with a reduced incidence of colon cancer in these patients will be important to learn. Unfortunately, in the entire screened population, the percentage of patients with colon adenomas detected by stool occult blood testing may be small.

Compliance is important in any screening program. In a separate study in our program, patient compliance was further examined by analyzing a random sample of 1,100 patients. It became clear that the issue of compliance was related to socioeconomic status, past medical experience, perceived susceptibility, understanding of asymptomatic disease, and knowledge of colorectal cancer. Compliance was related much less to the use of a restricted diet during the test or the preparation of the smears. The high rate of initial compliance in our program reflected the high motivation of a population that voluntarily sought medical care at the Preventive Medicine Institute. However, compliance for subsequent rescreening was not as good. It appears that sustained interest in screening by asymptomatic individuals is difficult to maintain (Hardcastle et al. 1986).

Methods Change

During a screening program it is apparent that any change in materials or methods may have an important effect on results. This was observed when we changed from the initial Hemoccult (HO) slide to the HO II slide and when slide rehydration was introduced. Laboratory data had indicated that slides stored with blood smeared on them may revert to negative. Rehydration enhanced the slides' sensitivity, allowed

them to be read more easily, and eliminated the storage-produced false-negative results. Observations in the screening programs indicated, however, that rehydration
made the slides too sensitive and sharply increased false positivity, reducing the
value of this approach. To lower the false-positive rate as much as possible would
require making the fecal occult blood test more specific. This could result from
elimination of the effect of peroxidase activity occurring from nonhuman hemoglobin and from dietary and bacterial peroxidases. One such approach is to use an
immunochemical test, which is specific for human hemoglobin. This test is more
complex than the simple biochemical fecal blood test, and its applicability has been
under investigation. Use of this test would not, however, reduce the false positivity
resulting from such nonneoplastic bleeding as physiologic blood loss, angiodys-
plasia, diverticular disease, and hemorrhoids. The extent to which false positivity is
related to nonneoplastic human hemoglobin, compared with nonhemoglobin peroxidase activity, remains to be determined. Other approaches are to use a peroxidase
inhibitor or a non–peroxidase-based test such as the Hemoquant test.

We need to work on false negativity. This would require increasing the sensitivity
of tests without reducing specificity. This does not seem possible with the present
widely used peroxidase-based guaiac tests. The immunochemical and quantitative
tests currently under investigation represent attempts to solve this problem, but they
will have to be widely applicable and cost-effective.

Any screening program for colorectal cancer has two major immediate goals.
First, a higher percentage of patients with localized colorectal cancers without
lymph node metastases and without distant metastases should undergo surgery,
which would result in better long-term survival. Second, asymptomatic patients
harboring significant adenomas of the colon should be identified so that these could
be removed and the future risk of colorectal cancer development reduced.

FOLLOW-UP OF PATIENTS WITH ADENOMAS

Adenomas are the next point of opportunity for intervention. Patients with adenomas
are known to be at a higher risk of developing colon cancer than the general population. The prevalence of adenomas varies among groups, but it is known to be high in
North America and Europe. Autopsy studies show that up to half of the adults over
age 40 in the population of the United States harbor at least one adenoma in the
colon. There is a strong age relationship. Patients with multiple adenomas are at
greater risk of developing colorectal cancer than are patients with single adenomas.
About half of the patients believed to have a single, index adenoma are found to
have a second, synchronous one. Because of the high rate of synchronous adenomas,
initial treatment should include a complete colonoscopy with removal of all polyps.

Once an adenoma has been removed, follow-up is critical because the metachronous rate is reported to be 30% to 50%. There is controversy regarding the appropriate time for follow-up examination once an index polyp has been removed
and whether follow-up should consist of both colonoscopy and barium enema. This
uncertainty arises from several factors. A barium enema may have different results
in the hands of different radiologists; experience and skill in performing an air-

contrast barium enema determine its accuracy. There is a greater sensitivity of the double-contrast barium enema compared with a single-column study in detecting polyps. Another factor important in the accuracy of the barium enema is the preparation the patient self-administers. Several studies have suggested that colonoscopy is more sensitive than barium enema for a follow-up exam after the removal of a polyp (Winawer and Sherlock 1982). Colonoscopy also provides the advantage of biopsy and polypectomy but is more invasive and most costly.

National Polyp Study

The National Polyp Study (NPS) is a multicenter trial with eight participating centers and MSKCC as the headquarters (Winawer et al. 1986). Participating centers are Mount Sinai Hospital, New York; Veterans Administration Medical Center, Minneapolis; Medical College of Wisconsin, Milwaukee; St. Luke's Hospital, Racine; Massachusetts General Hospital, Boston; Cedars-Sinai Medical Center, Los Angeles; Valley Presbyterian Hospital, Van Nuys; and Mallory Institute of Pathology, Boston. To be eligible, patients must have had one or more adenomas removed at the time of enrollment, have had no previous polypectomy, and have had a complete colonoscopy. Patients are stratified and then randomized into a more frequent and a less frequent follow-up arm (fig. 2.1). The age distribution at enrollment demonstrates a five-year mean age difference among NPS adenoma patients and those of the Surveillance, Epidemiology and End Results Program (SEER) with adenocarcinoma of the colon. There is a male predominance. About 45% of the patients have

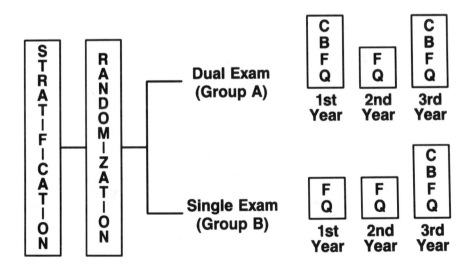

Fig. 2.1. Randomization scheme of National Polyp Study: Treatment arms after stratification of participating medical center, histology, and number of adenomas. *C,* colonoscopy; *B,* barium enema; *F,* fecal occult blood test; *Q,* interval history questionnaire.

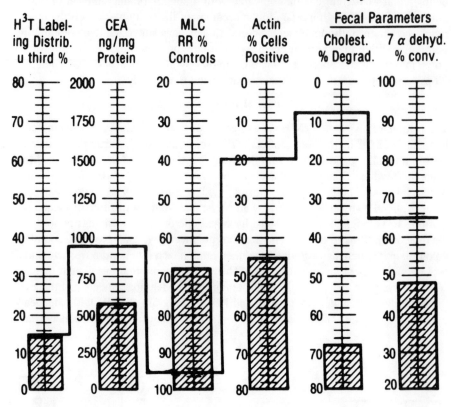

Fig. 2.2. A portion of the colorectal cancer risk profile currently being developed to quantitate phenotypic attributes in subjects at varying degrees of susceptibility to colorectal neoplasia. Column 1, percentage of thymidine ³H-labeled epithelial cells in upper and middle thirds of colonic crypts, in random biopsy specimens of flat colonic mucosa; Column 2, amount of carcinoembryonic antigen in colonic lavage specimens (ng/mg protein); Column 3, mixed leukocyte response, RR (relative response as percentage of control group); Column 4, percentage of cutaneous fibroblasts with normal pattern of actin. Fecal parameters are given in columns 5 to 6: undegraded cholesterol (mg/g of dry feces); 7α dehydroxylase (percentage of cholic acid converted to deoxycholic acid). Shaded areas show tentative normal ranges, with upper limits at two standard deviations from mean values in control groups. Horizontal lines show test results of an individual with symptomatic familial polyposis. Reprinted with permission from *Am J Med* 1980; 68:917–931.

more than one adenoma on enrollment. First-year follow-up to date demonstrates rapid reconstitution of adenoma in the colon, but most of the new adenomas are small and tubular with little significant dysplasia and with a more proximal distribution. Early three-year follow-up data demonstrate a slightly higher recurrence rate of adenomas, but these are also small and tubular. At this time, however, the distribution is more uniform throughout the colon. Significant dysplasia in adenomas correlates with the patients' ages and with histological characteristics, size, and multiplicity of the adenomas. Recurrence rate is also correlated with histological type and multiplicity of adenomas.

The NPS was designed to address several basic issues (fig. 2.2). One goal is to establish guidelines for the interval between follow-up surveillance examinations after polypectomy. The study will also compare barium enema and colonoscopy for sensitivity, complications, and patient compliance. In these follow-up examinations, the barium enema is done before colonoscopy. The NPS local coordinator knows the results of the barium enema and is present in the procedure room during colonoscopy. The endoscopist then advances the colonoscope to the cecum. During withdrawal of the colonoscope, the endoscopist reexamines each segment of colon and reports the findings to the NPS coordinator. If there is a discrepancy between the endoscopic findings and those of the barium enema, the endoscopist reevaluates the area in question. The NPS coordinator then records the reported results of the endoscopist's examination.

The NPS is collecting data on patient characteristics (age, sex, race, family history), number of index adenomas, size of adenomas removed, anatomic location, histology, and degree of dysplasia in search of patterns that would indicate high risk of developing metachronous adenomas or colon cancer or both (tables 2.2 and 2.3).

Table 2.2. *National Polyp Study: Relative Frequency of Patient Characteristics (N = 710)*

	Randomized Patients (N = 348)		Eligible, Nonrandomized Patients (N = 134)		Ineligible Patients (N = 228)	
	No.	(%)	No.	(%)	No.	(%)
Sex						
Male	242	(70)	77	(57)	140	(61)
Female	106	(30)	57	(43)	88	(39)
Age, mean ± SD	61 ± 11		63 ± 12		59 ± 12	
Race						
White	317	(91)	103	(75)	188	(82)
Nonwhite	31	(9)	33	(25)	40	(18)
History of cancer	32	(9)	15	(11)	24	(11)
Family history						
Colon cancer	64	(18)	19	(14)	32	(14)
Polyps	34	(10)	11	(8)	14	(6)
Other cancer	171	(49)	46	(34)	83	(36)
Number of adenomas, mean ± SD	1.9 ± 1.4		1.8 ± 1.3		0.7 ± 1.4	

Source: Data Base Summary, January 1, 1983.

Table 2.3. *Pathological and Other Characteristics of Individual Polyps*

Variables	Randomized Patients (N = 782)		Eligible, Nonrandomized Patients (N = 283)		Ineligible Patients (N = 440)	
	No.	(%)	No.	(%)	No.	(%)
Location						
Rectum	76	(10)	33	(12)	86	(20)
Sigmoid colon	329	(42)	123	(43)	167	(38)
Descending colon	110	(14)	28	(10)	61	(14)
Splenic flexure	16	(2)	5	(2)	17	(4)
Transverse colon	86	(1)	28	(10)	30	(7)
Hepatic flexure	35	(4)	17	(6)	19	(4)
Ascending colon	70	(9)	25	(9)	25	(6)
Cecum	60	(8)	24	(8)	35	(8)
Shape						
Sessile	484	(62)	175	(62)	354	(80)
Pedunculated	294	(38)	108	(38)	83	(19)
Removal status						
Biopsy fulguration	246	(31)	88	(31)	210	(48)
Cautery snare	484	(62)	186	(66)	187	(43)
Size (cm), mean ± SD	0.8 ± 0.7		0.8 ± 0.6		0.8 ± 0.8	

Source: Data Base Summary, January 1, 1983.
N = 1,505 polyps; infiltrating carcinomas excluded.

The prevalence of adenomatous polyps increases with advancing age; larger size, more severe grades of dysplasia, and a greater likelihood of multiple adenomas are seen in older patients. If an index adenoma is more than 2 cm in diameter, the risk of developing metachronous lesions is higher than for smaller adenomas. Several studies have shown that numbers of index adenomas are predictive for increased risk of metachronous adenomas. When a single index adenoma is removed, the rate of metachronous lesions is 35% to 38%, compared with a rate of 55% to 63% for multiple index adenomas. Whether an increase in dysplasia is associated with a greater incidence of recurrent adenomas is the subject of conflicting reports (Winawer, Ritchie, and Diaz 1986).

Another NPS goal is to integrate data collected on family history. Patients are given a detailed questionnaire concerning the medical histories, occurrences of cancer, and, where pertinent, cause of death of their first- and second-degree relatives. The NPS is addressing the question of the most effective patient surveillance after polypectomy for the control of large bowel cancer. This is an opportunity for interrupting the adenoma-carcinoma sequence.

ABNORMAL PHENOTYPE

Another opportunity for intervention is based on the current understanding that adenomas and adenocarcinomas arise within the mucosa that has phenotypic abnormalities, which can be identified by laboratory assay of biopsy samples obtained endoscopically (Sherlock, Lipkin, and Newmark 1985). These abnormalities have been used as intermediate markers to determine the influence of such dietary supplements as calcium on the mucosal risk of neoplasia (Lipkin and Newmark 1985). Phenotypic abnormalities include cell proliferation and differentiation, gene expression, physiological cell response, cell repair, and others. In our studies of cell proliferation over the years, it has become clear that, once a neoplastic lesion occurs, the entire colonic mucosa is transformed into a premalignant state. The proliferation characteristics of epithelial cells in the colon correlate with risk of adenomas and cancer. Low-risk individuals—Seventh Day Adventists, for example— have a quiescent pattern consisting of a small number of proliferating cells located deep in the crypts. In contrast, high-risk individuals—such as those with a strong family history of colon cancer—have an increased number of proliferating cells with extension to the surface of the crypts (fig. 2.2). Associated with these changes are abnormalities in colon cellular differentiation and in cell repair of circulating mononuclear cells. These abnormalities have been used recently to determine the influence of nutritional intervention on the state of the colon lining. Calcium supplementation was shown to decrease cell proliferation, improving the risk pattern of the mucosa in a small group of patients. The calcium study suggested that this phenotypic abnormality, which may be genetically determined, may be modulated by environmental manipulation. This is the focus of further study.

GENETICS

Finally, a genetic basis for colorectal cancer has been suggested, possibly providing a susceptibility for the expression of environmental factors (Burt et al. 1985). Rare genetic syndromes such as familial polyposis, Gardner's syndrome, and the non-polyposis inherited colon cancer syndrome (site-specific colon cancer, family cancer syndrome) are now known to account for only a small percentage of the cases of colon cancer seen today, perhaps in up to 5,000 patients annually (Lynch, Rozen, and Schuelke 1983). The "sporadic cases" previously thought to be nongenetic to a large extent are now believed to be genetically determined, perhaps as an autosomal dominant trait also but with very low expression. The studies from Utah (Burt et al. 1985) support this thesis, which needs to be further examined. If individuals at risk could be identified, nutritional intervention and screening strategies could be more effective, with better cost-effectiveness and improved patient compliance.

CONCLUSION

In the future, our insight into the natural history of colorectal cancer will increase, and we hope this will lead to more feasible and effective approaches for the control of this cancer and to a greater understanding of its biology. We have made much progress in recent years in understanding the natural history of colorectal cancer. Active research is helping us to determine whether the natural history of the disease can be modified to provide a better outcome for individuals at risk. Conceptually, we have learned much; we now have extremely effective clinical diagnostic tools that can also be used to obtain samples for laboratory study; we have exciting laboratory research in progress; and we have under evaluation potentially beneficial strategies for nutritional intervention, for control of premalignant adenomas, and for early detection of cancer.

REFERENCES

Ahlquist DA, McGill DB, Schwartz S, et al. 1985. Fecal blood levels in health and disease. *N Engl J Med* 312:1422–1428.

American Cancer Society 1987. Cancer facts and figures, 1987. New York: ACS.

Burt RW, Bishop DT, Cannon LA, et al. 1985. Dominant inheritance of adenomatous colonic polyps and colorectal cancer. *N Engl J Med* 312:1540–1544.

Chait M, Herbert E, Guthrie M, et al. 1986. The Memorial Sloan-Kettering Cancer Center-Strang Clinic program: A progress report. In *Frontiers of Gastrointestinal Research*, vol. 10, *Secondary Prevention of Colorectal Cancer: An International Perspective*, P Rozen, SJ Winawer, eds., pp. 102–110. Basel: S Karger.

Gilbertsen VA, McHugh R, Schuman L, et al. 1980. The earlier detection of colorectal cancers: A preliminary report of the results of the occult blood study. *Cancer* 45:2899–2901.

Guidelines for the cancer-related checkup: Recommendations and rationale. 1980. *CA* 30:194–240.

Hardcastle JD, Armitage NC, Chamberlain J, et al. 1986. Fecal occult blood screening for colorectal cancer in the general population: Results of a controlled trial. *Cancer* 58:397–403.

Lipkin M, Newmark H. 1985. Effect of added dietary calcium on colonic epithelial-proliferation in subjects at high risk for familial colonic cancer. *N Engl J Med* 313:1381–1384.

Lynch HT, Rozen P, Schuelke GS. 1983. Hereditary colon cancer: Polyposis and non-polyposis variants. In *Third International Symposium on Colorectal Cancer*. ACS Professional Education Publication, pp. 53–73.

Miller A., ed. In press. *Proceedings of the UICC Conference on Screening*. Geneva: International Union Against Cancer.

Sherlock P, Lipkin M, Winawer SJ. 1980. The prevention of colon cancer. A combined clinical and basic science seminar. *Am J Med* 68:917–931.

Winawer SJ, Fleisher M, Baldwin M, et al. 1982. Current status of fecal occult blood testing in screening for colorectal cancer. *CA* 32:100–112.

Winawer SJ, Ritchie M, Diaz B. 1986. The National Polyp Study: Aims and organization. In *Frontiers of Gastrointestinal Research*, vol. 10, *Secondary Prevention of Colorectal Cancer: An International Perspective*. P Rozen, SJ Winawer, eds., pp. 216–225. Basel: S Karger.

Winawer SJ, Schottenfeld D, Sherlock P. 1985. Screening for colorectal cancer: The issues. Editorial. *Gastroenterology* 88:841–844.

Winawer SJ, Sherlock P. 1982. Surveillance for colorectal cancer in average-risk patients, familial high-risk groups, and patients with adenomas. *Cancer* 50:2609–2614.

Annual Clinical Conference on Cancer, Vol. 30
Gastrointestinal Cancer: Current Approaches to Diagnosis and Treatment
© 1988 by The University of Texas System Cancer Center

3. Fecal Blood Testing: Demystifying the Occult

David A. Ahlquist

Carcinoma of the colorectum satisfies features of a disease in which screening is useful. First, it is very common: approximately 1 in 20 North Americans develop colon cancer (Silverberg and Lubera 1983), and colon cancer is the second most common internal malignancy in the United States. Second, it is serious: if untreated, this cancer kills most patients. Third, its presymptomatic course appears to be long in most cases: patients may harbor premalignant adenomas and early-stage lesions for years without symptoms. Finally, early detection and treatment likely confer a favorable prognosis: five-year survival after surgery is over 90% in patients whose disease is screen detected but less than 50% in those who present because of symptoms (Axtell, Asire, and Myers 1976).

Yet, to screen or not to screen is the question in colorectal cancer control as 1990 draws near. On the one hand, the increasing focus on early detection seems warranted because therapeutic advances have failed to reduce the death toll from colorectal cancer in industrialized nations over recent decades. On the other, a fully satisfactory screening tool for colorectal cancer has not yet been established. To date, no screening approach to this malignancy has been of proven benefit.

Although various screening techniques, including serological and cytological ones, have fallen by the wayside because of poor patient compliance and the tests' cost ineffectiveness or insensitivity, measurement of blood in the feces continues to be advocated and utilized. Routine fecal blood testing is taught as a compulsory component of the patient medical examinations at many institutions. Manufacturers now widely market the many available fecal blood tests directly to the public through multimedia advertisements and community promotions. Fueled by the highly visible diagnosis and treatment of Ronald Reagan's cecal cancer during his presidency, the popularity of fecal blood screening is at an all-time high. The American Cancer Society has infused the screening effort with legitimacy by encouraging annual fecal blood testing for anyone 50 years old or older. However, there are problems with each step of the screening process, which remains unsystematized.

Recent extensive reviews on fecal blood testing for colorectal cancer (Frank 1985a, 1985b, 1985c; Simon 1985) have cautioned that it may be premature to recommend screening with currently used methods, as efficacy has not been established. Numerous uncontrolled screening trials that used guaiac-impregnated pads (Hastings 1974; Glober and Peskoe 1974; Bralow and Kopel 1979; Larkin 1980; Shigin 1980; Miller and Knight 1977; Gnauck 1977; Rose et al. 1981) have suggested that cancers may be detected at an early stage, but such studies are subject to inescapable biases (Cole and Morrison 1980; Chuong 1983), which prevent firm conclusions. The few controlled screening trials under way (Gilbertsen 1979, 1980a, 1980b; Winawer 1983; Winawer et al. 1980; Hardcastle et al. 1983), two for nearly 10 years, have not shown that fecal blood screening reduces colon cancer–specific mortality. This ineffectiveness of the screening might be due to the enormous logistic complexities of mass screening, to a limited knowledge of bleeding patterns in asymptomatic colorectal neoplasia, or to major technical problems with the tests themselves.

To reliably detect bleeding from colorectal neoplasms, fecal occult blood tests must first reliably measure blood. Until recently, the only tests available to most physicians have been based on guaiac or other leuco-dyes. These qualitative, non-specific tests have changed little over past decades and are hampered by frequent false-positive and false-negative reactions. False-positive results create patient anxiety and often launch a cascade of unnecessary, uncomfortable, time-consuming, and potentially harmful diagnostic tests: the low unit price of these seemingly simple tests belies the large costs accrued because of biochemical error (Elwood, Erickson, and Liberman 1978; Frank 1985b; Neuhauser 1980). False-negative results lead to missed diagnoses and thus to false reassurance.

Refinements in the application of guaiac tests have offered some clinical improvement, but it is the emergence of radically different tests that promises needed advances in measurement sensitivity and specificity. These newer approaches include immunochemical techniques and the HemoQuant test, which is a quantitative test based on the fluorescence of heme-derived porphyrin. Direct comparative studies with these more accurate tests, especially with the HemoQuant test, have pointed out serious biochemical deficiencies inherent in guaiac tests.

This chapter examines the performance of available fecal blood tests, identifies problems with stool sampling and patient compliance, and discusses the assumptions about cancer bleeding upon which fecal blood screening is based. It is an updated and expanded version of a previous review (Ahlquist and Beart 1985).

THE TESTS

Guaiac Tests

Guaiac has been used to detect blood for well over a century. In Sir Arthur Conan Doyle's novel *A Study in Scarlet,* Sherlock Holmes comments upon the "old guaiacum test . . . very clumsy and uncertain" as he works in the laboratory. Holmes then asks about brownish stains, "Are they blood stains, or mud stains, or rust stains, or fruit stains, or what are they? That is the question that has puzzled many an expert, and why? Because there was no reliable test." The same specificity and sensitivity problems of guaiac tests persist to this day.

Guaiac was first used to indicate fecal blood in 1864 (VanDeen 1864), and Boas employed it in 1901 to detect gastrointestinal malignancies (Boas 1901). However, the familiar tests that use guaiac-impregnated pads to specifically screen for asymptomatic colorectal cancer were not developed until 1967 (Greegor 1971).

LEUCO-DYE TESTS: CHEMICAL BASIS

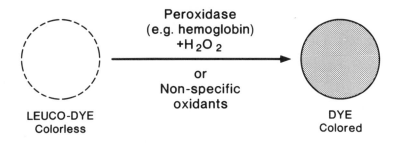

Fig. 3.1. Chemical basis of leuco-dye (guaiac) tests.

Guaiac is an impure, colorless compound that, like other leuco-dyes, becomes colored in the presence of adequate concentrations of peroxidase and hydrogen peroxide (fig. 3.1). Numerous constituents of animals and plants, including constituents of bacteria, exhibit peroxidase activity. Hemoglobin exhibits such activity; accordingly, leuco-dyes have been used to detect it.

Commercially available tests that utilize guaiac-impregnated pads include Hemoccult (SmithKline Diagnostics, Sunnyvale, California), the most widely used of these tests; HemoFec (Boehringer-Mannheim, Mannheim, West Germany); Colo-Screen (Helena Laboratories, Beaumont, Texas); Colo-Rect (Roche Diagnostics, Nutley, New Jersey); Hema-Chek (Miles Laboratories, Elkhart, Indiana); Quick-Cult (Laboratory Diagnostics, Morganville, New Jersey); Haemo-Screen (E. Merck Diagnostics, Darmstadt, West Germany); and several new, over-the-counter tests. These pad tests are easy to use, inexpensive, highly portable, and require no sophisticated laboratory equipment. Although these tests may be readily done at the bedside, some studies suggest that they are more reliable if performed in a laboratory setting (Hoffman et al. 1983). However, several serious technical weaknesses must be taken into account.

The clinical interpretation of guaiac pad tests is confounded by their unpredictable reactivity. There is no consistent fecal hemoglobin level above which guaiac tests become positive and below which they remain negative (Ahlquist et al. 1984; Ostrow et al. 1973; Doran and Hardcastle 1982; Stroehlein et al. 1976b; Bassett and Goulston 1980). Hence, these qualitative tests cannot discriminate normal from abnormal bleeding levels. Further, that their results are reported as "positive" or "negative" has led to the common misconception that fecal blood is simply present

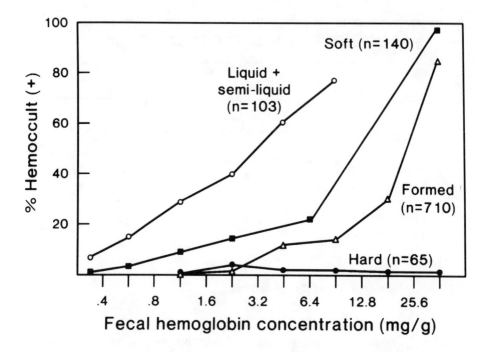

Fig. 3.2. Effect of stool consistency and hemoglobin concentration on Hemoccult reactivity. The HemoQuant assay was used to quantify hemoglobin concentrations; its upper limit for normal hemoglobin levels is 2 mg/g. From Ahlquist et al., reprinted by permission of *Annals of Internal Medicine,* 101; 299, 1984.

or absent. In fact, fecal blood ranges in a continuum from physiological to pathologically elevated values.

Water dramatically influences reactivity in guaiac tests. It is well known that Hemoccult sensitivity can be augmented by hydrating the fecal smear prior to addition of the peroxide catalyst (Macrae and St. John 1982). Positive reactions can be induced in stools that are initially Hemoccult negative simply by progressive aqueous dilution, even in stools with normal hemoglobin levels (Ahlquist et al. 1984). Most important, the natural water content of individual stools varies widely. As shown by figure 3.2, wetter stools tend to be Hemoccult positive, drier stools tend to be Hemoccult negative, and driest stools, graded hard, may remain negative at any hemoglobin concentration (Ahlquist et al. 1984).

Numerous factors besides water content can nonspecifically either trigger or abolish the color reaction. Certain fruits and vegetables, including radishes, broccoli, turnips, cantaloupes, bean sprouts, cauliflower, and grapes, can cause false-positive reactions (Illingworth 1965; Macrae et al. 1982). One study has shown Hemoccult to be positive in over half of healthy volunteers ingesting standard therapeutic doses of iron (Lifton and Kreiser 1982). In addition to the ubiquitous peroxidase compounds other than hemoglobin, halogens (Ahlquist and Schwartz 1975) and certain other drugs such as cimetidine (Schentag 1980) can also cause leuco-dye reactions.

Guaiac tests often remain nonreactive despite increased enteric blood loss. Such false-negative reactions were recognized as early as 1919 (Von Snapper 1919). Hemoccult is relatively insensitive and in one study failed to react with over 80% of stools that contained more than the accepted upper normal limit of 2 mg hemoglobin/g (Ahlquist et al. 1984). Several studies have clearly shown that fecal hemoglobin levels above 10 mg/g (roughly equal to 10 ml daily blood loss) are necessary to ensure that Hemoccult is positive at least half the time in samples known to contain abnormal levels of blood (Ostrow et al. 1974; Doran and Hardcastle 1982; Stroehlein et al. 1976b; Bassett and Goulston 1980). Hemoccult false negatives have been documented with daily fecal blood losses exceeding 80 ml (Heinrich 1980). Proven causes of false negatives in guaiac pad tests include presence in the feces of reducing substances such as ascorbic acid (Jaffe et al. 1975), an acid pH, ingestion of antacids (Layne, Mcllow, and Lipman 1981), defective reagents (Markman 1967), heat, and heme degradation caused by enteric passage (Schwartz and Ellefson 1985; Ahlquist et al. 1985), or fecal storage (Ahlquist et al. 1984; Stroehlein et al. 1976a; Fleisher, Schwartz, and Winawer 1977).

Hemoglobin heme is converted to porphyrin during enterocolic transit (Schwartz and Ellefson 1985; Ahlquist et al. 1985), presumably by bacteria. As guaiac does not react with porphyrin, this conversion is a likely explanation for many Hemoccult false negatives (fig. 3.3). Heme degradation probably accounts for the relative insensitivity of Hemoccult for right colon and more proximal neoplasms (Herzog et al. 1982; Ahlquist et al. 1985) and for the inability of Hemoccult to detect fecal hemoglobin after ingestion of 15 to 30 ml blood per day (Schwartz et al. 1983; Hunt 1981). Conversion of fecal hemoglobin to porphyrin continues during storage, and Hemoccult positivity correspondingly falls: as many as 40% of stools initially Hemoccult positive become negative after storage at room temperature for four to eight days (Ahlquist et al. 1984). This time-dependent heme degradation diminishes the validity of guaiac tests applied to mailed-in or stored specimens. Thus, guaiac and related tests, which require intact hemoglobin for chemical detection, tend to underestimate enteric blood loss.

The biochemical performance of guaiac tests can somewhat be improved by certain test modifications. Methods to increase sensitivity, such as hydrating the smeared fecal aliquot prior to testing, often succeed at the expense of specificity (Macrae and St. John 1982; Winawer and Fleisher 1982). Sensitivity can be improved (i.e., false negatives reduced) without losing specificity by first purifying fecal hemoglobin by solvent extraction (Jaffe and Zierdt 1979) or electrostatic filtration (Graham et al. 1984). However, sensitivity cannot be recovered if conversion of heme to porphyrin has occurred, as peroxidase activity is then irreversibly lost. Guaiac test specificity can be enhanced (i.e., false positives reduced) by placing patients on strict peroxidase-poor diets and by stopping iron administration or ulcerogenic drugs prior to screening (Bassett and Goulston 1980; Macrae et al. 1982).

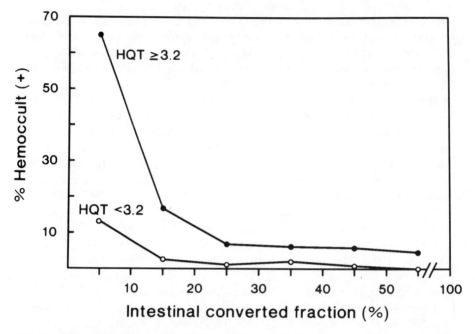

Fig. 3.3. Effect of fecal heme degradation on Hemoccult reactivity. The intestinal converted fraction is that portion of fecal heme converted to porphyrin during luminal transit. Those stools with high hemoglobin levels by HemoQuant (*HQT*) analysis (≥3.2 mg/g) and those with low levels by HemoQuant (<3.2 mg/g) are considered separately. From Ahlquist et al., reprinted by permission of *Annals of Internal Medicine*, 101; 299, 1984.

Clinical false-positive and false-negative rates with guaiac testing vary according to technique used, population screened, and investigative rigor. In the above-cited screening studies, colorectal neoplasms account for a relatively small minority of positive guaiac reactions; the majority of positive reactions are false positives as they are either unexplained or associated with trivial pathology. Data are not available on the false-negative rate for asymptomatic colorectal cancers, as diagnostic colon studies are not performed on subjects with guaiac-negative results in screening programs. However, under optimal test conditions, Hemoccult has been disappointingly insensitive when used in patients with symptomatic, proven cancer. Three series found Hemoccult, tested on three to six fecal aliquots, to be positive in only 40%, 52%, and 67% of patients with proven colorectal cancer (Songster, Barrows, and Jarrett 1980; Crowley et al. 1983; Ahlquist et al. 1985). This low cancer detection rate may reflect guaiac insensitivity for blood rather than nonbleeding lesions.

Immunochemical Tests

Several immunochemical assays specific for the globulin portions of human hemoglobin have been developed over the past decade (Barrows et al. 1978; Adams and Layman 1974; Songster, Barrows, and Jarrett 1980; Yoshida et al. 1986). Antihemoglobin antibodies, used in these tests, do not react with dietary blood, nonhemo-globin peroxidase compounds, or any medications. Accordingly, immunochemical tests represent an advance in specificity over guaiac tests. Human hemoglobino-pathies do not alter the sensitivity of immunochemical assays. A smear punch-disc immunodiffusion test appears to be simple and inexpensive (Barrows et al. 1978). A distinct advantage of immunochemical tests over other tests is the obviation of awkward dietary preparations.

The smear punch-disc immunodiffusion test also appears to be more sensitive than the Hemoccult test. Approximately 0.3 mg hemoglobin/g stool was required to yield a positive immunoassay, compared with 5 to 10 times this amount for a positive Hemoccult test in the same study (Barrows et al. 1978). Further, of 150 patients with proven colorectal cancer, the immunologic test was positive in 65%, compared with only 40% by Hemoccult (Songster, Barrows, and Jarrett 1980).

Enteric degradation of hemoglobin poses a potentially serious obstacle to the im-munologic measurement of fecal blood. As hemoglobin is denatured and digested during intestinal and colonic transit, its antigenic properties are altered. As with guaiac tests, immunoassays are less likely to detect proximal than distal gut lesions despite comparable bleeding rates (Adams and Layman 1974). Immunochemical tests have been uniformly unsuccessful in detecting any fecal hemoglobin following ingestion of 20 ml of autologous blood by volunteers. The effect of fecal storage on these tests has not been established.

Some immunochemical approaches, including various radioimmunoassays and agglutination tests, have been complicated by frequent nonspecific positive reactions due to particulate fecal debris (Barrows et al. 1978). Also, the punch-disc immunodiffusion test requires up to 24 hours of incubation and, like guaiac pad tests, is qualitative. A more recently discussed immunochemical test can be performed in a few minutes and by a laboratory technician (Yoshida et al. 1986).

HemoQuant Test

Our understanding of bleeding patterns in health and disease has been limited by the lack of a simple means to quantify fecal blood. Available quantitative assays, based on the recovery of intravenously injected radiolabeled erythrocytes, are obviously impractical for large-volume, routine use. Measurement of fecal blood has remained among the few nonquantitative routine tests in medicine. Yet quantitation of fecal blood levels provides the clinician with more meaningful diagnostic information.

A recently described assay (Schwartz et al. 1983) called HemoQuant (SmithKline-BioScience, Van Nuys, California) offers clear advantages over existing occult blood tests. It is quantitative, noninvasive, specific for heme, chemically sensitive, and suitable for automation. HemoQuant differs from all other fecal blood tests in its chemical basis: it removes the iron from hemoglobin heme and measures the fluo-rescence of the derived porphyrin (fig. 3.4). Unlike guaiac or immunochemical tests, the HemoQuant assay includes that important fraction of heme already con-verted to porphyrin during fecal transit, referred to as the "intestinal converted fraction."

The HemoQuant test is laboratory based and requires approximately 90 minutes

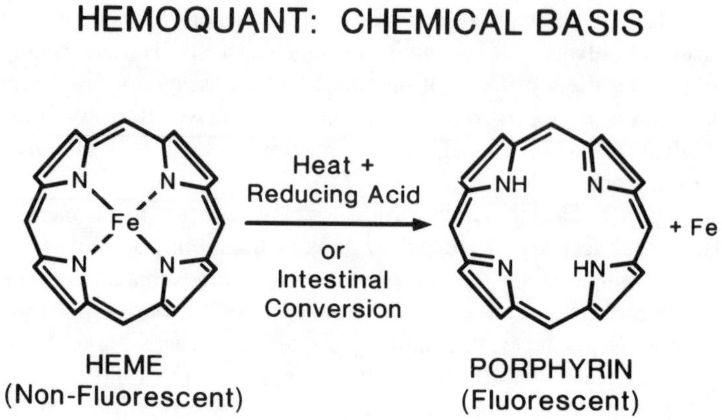

HEMOQUANT: CHEMICAL BASIS

HEME
(Non-Fluorescent)

Heat +
Reducing Acid

or
Intestinal
Conversion

+ Fe

PORPHYRIN
(Fluorescent)

Fig. 3.4. Chemical basis of HemoQuant.

to perform manually. A small amount of feces is heated in a reducing acid to remove heme iron and yield free porphyrin. A solvent purification step then removes contaminating fluorescence compounds but recovers heme-derived porphyrins for fluorometric assay. The test is performed without preliminary concentration or dilution of the sample. Results are calculated as hemoglobin-equivalents and reported as milligrams of hemoglobin per gram of stool. Fecal hemoglobin concentrations from 0.01 to 500 mg/g can be measured, with values below 2 mg/g considered normal values.

HemoQuant has become available to physicians throughout the United States, but in most settings specimens must be sent to the commercial reference laboratory for analysis. The inevitable two- to four-day delay in results is a distinct disincentive for many physicians. HemoQuant testing at the Mayo Clinic is unique, as assays have been performed in our own laboratory for nearly two years using an automated system. This system can accommodate 100 to 150 samples per hour with minimal assistance by technicians. Results are reported to physicians on the same day specimens are submitted. Over 50,000 routine HemoQuant tests are done annually at the Mayo Clinic, and patient compliance has been 97% in this setting.

HemoQuant has been validated by a greater than 99% recovery of blood directly added to stools (fig. 3.5), by an 88% fecal recovery of ingested blood, and by a close correlation with other quantitative assays (Ahlquist et al. 1984; Schwartz and Ellefson 1985; Schwartz et al. 1983). HemoQuant measures heme and heme-derived porphyrins only. It is not affected by iron, cimetidine, ascorbic acid, vegetable peroxidase, antacids, or other substances known to interfere with guaiac tests (Schwartz et al. 1983; Ahlquist et al. 1984). As shown in figure 3.6, HemoQuant, unlike Hemoccult, is not affected by fecal storage (Ahlquist et al. 1984).

It is of major importance that this fluorometric test includes degraded as well as intact hemoglobin in its measurement. This intestinal converted fraction, assayed

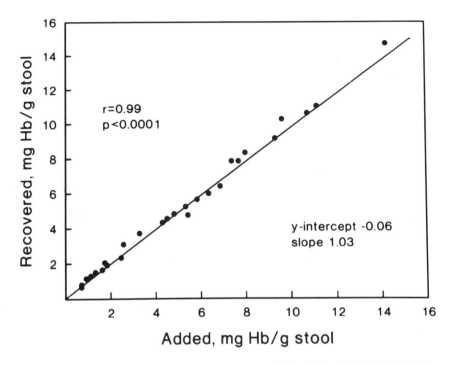

Fig. 3.5. Validation of HemoQuant by recovery of hemoglobin (*Hb*) added to 27 stools. From Ahlquist et al., reprinted by permission of *Annals of Internal Medicine,* 101; 298, 1984.

separately in a parallel determination (Schwartz et al. 1983), may account for nearly all fecal hemoglobin equivalents. In a recent study of stools from over 1,000 patients (Ahlquist et al. 1984), the median intestinal converted fraction was 32% (range, 1%–99%). As mentioned above, guaiac tests such as Hemoccult do not detect the intestinal converted fraction.

Since more heme is converted to porphyrin during intestinal transit from proximal than from distal bleeding sources, separate measurement of the intestinal converted fraction would logically help predict the anatomic site of gastrointestinal lesions (fig. 3.7). Preliminary studies (Ahlquist et al. 1985) have indeed shown that the mean intestinal converted fraction was 6% from rectal cancers, compared with over 26% from more proximal lesions; Hemoccult was positive in 82% of these patients with rectal lesions but in only about 30% of those with the more proximal lesions, despite comparable bleeding rates in these groups. Unfortunately, the large within-site variations of the intestinal converted fraction diminish its clinical predictive value (Goldschmidt et al. 1986).

HemoQuant has been used to quantify fecal hemoglobin in healthy volunteers and in patients undergoing gastrointestinal diagnostic studies because of symptoms (fig. 3.8). Among healthy subjects and patients with a variety of diagnoses, the

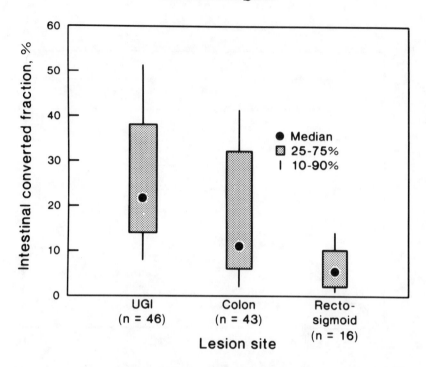

Fig. 3.6. Effect of fecal storage time and temperature on (A) HemoQuant (*HQT*) results, (B) intestinal converted fraction (*IFC*) results, and (C) Hemoccult (*HO*) results. Multiple aliquots from 10 stools, all initially Hemoccult positive, were stored in moisture-tight tubes under the designated conditions. From Ahlquist et al., reprinted by permission of *Annals of Internal Medicine*, 101; 300, 1984.

lowest fecal hemoglobin levels were in healthy volunteers: 98% had values below 2 mg/g. The highest levels were in colorectal cancer patients, 97% of whom had HemoQuant values above 2 mg/g. Thus, HemoQuant measurements highly discriminated patients with symptoms of colorectal cancer from healthy volunteers. Intermediate HemoQuant values were found in patients with large polyps and benign ulcers. Patients in whom diagnostic studies were negative for disease, those with small polyps, and those with only trivial lesions such as hemorrhoids or diverticula had fecal hemoglobin levels similar to those of healthy volunteers.

HemoQuant has been more sensitive than Hemoccult in detecting colorectal neoplasms and other gastrointestinal sources of bleeding. HemoQuant and Hemoccult were used on divided, unstored samples from patients who had histologically proven colorectal carcinoma or adenoma and most of whom had symptoms of the disease (Ahlquist et al. 1985). HemoQuant revealed elevated fecal hemoglobin levels in 97% of colorectal cancer patients and in 58% of those with adenomas 2 cm or more in diameter, compared with Hemoccult positives in 67% and 17%, respectively. In patients with microcytic anemia, HemoQuant yielded hemoglobin values above nor-

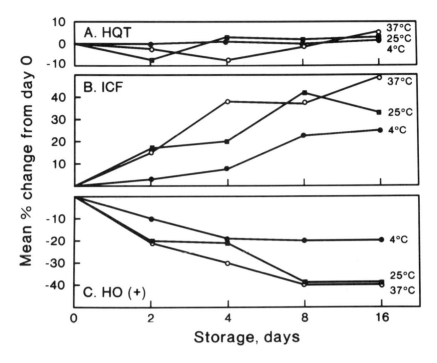

Fig. 3.7. Relation between the intestinal converted fraction and the anatomic site of bleeding. The intestinal converted fraction refers to the portion of fecal hemoglobin-heme degraded to porphyrin during intestinal transit or fecal storage. Only lesions likely to bleed, such as ulcers and cancers, were considered. Upper gastrointestinal (*UGI*) lesions were defined as those proximal to the ileocecal valve. From Ahlquist et al., reprinted by permission of *The New England Journal of Medicine,* 312; 1425, 1985.

mal in 81% of those found to have significant gastrointestinal lesions, compared with 34% Hemoccult positivity (Fleming et al. 1986).

In a large group of subjects without known disease, use of aspirin and ingestion of red meat caused slight increases in fecal hemoglobin measured by HemoQuant: median values were 1.19 mg/g overall, 0.68 mg/g in those taking no aspirin, and only 0.22 mg/g in those ingesting neither red meat nor aspirin (Ahlquist et al. 1985). Ingestion of poultry, fish, or peroxidase-rich vegetables did not influence fecal hemoglobin levels as measured by HemoQuant (Schwartz and Ellefson 1985), nor did moderate alcohol consumption unless aspirin was also taken (Fleming et al. in press). In one study, HemoQuant has been used to show that long-distance running causes enteric bleeding (fig. 3.9): of 24 runners, 88% had increased fecal blood levels after a marathon or similar endurance event, and one runner had a level of 43 mg/g (Stewart et al. 1984). An understanding of such factors must be considered in the clinical interpretation and use of HemoQuant just as in other fecal blood tests.

A multicenter trial currently under way was designed to compare the validity of HemoQuant with that of Hemoccult in a large population that is without symptoms

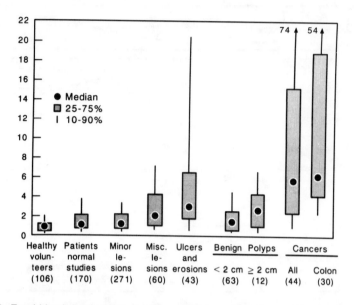

Fig. 3.8. Fecal blood distribution in healthy volunteers and patients with gastrointestinal disease. Data are based on a single HemoQuant measurement per subject. *Misc.* denotes miscellaneous. The healthy volunteers ingested no red meat or medications for one week before study. Neither diet nor medication was controlled in the other groups. From Ahlquist et al., reprinted by permission of *The New England Journal of Medicine,* 312; 1424, 1985.

of colorectal disease but at higher than average risk for developing colorectal cancer. Preliminary results should be reported in 1988.

SPECIMEN COLLECTION AND PATIENT COMPLIANCE

Accurate fecal blood testing requires careful control of each step of the testing process. Yet mobilization of the stool for sampling, the critical first step, has been largely ignored in commercial test kit instructions and in reported screening trials. Patients are usually instructed to smear a sample of stool onto a test pad using a three-inch applicator stick provided in the kit—a difficult task if the stool has sunk. How the stool is gathered and sampled has, surprisingly, been left to the patient's imagination.

Sampling the stool from within the toilet basin is not only technically difficult but introduces major biochemical contamination. An unpredictable portion of fecal blood is lost into the toilet water. Over half of the blood contained in the superficial 3- to 6-mm layer of some stools (the portion usually sampled) leaches into the surrounding toilet water after only four to eight minutes, although other stools retain more blood (Samuel Schwartz, M.D., Minneapolis Medical Research Foundation, personal communication, July 1986). As noted above, fecal hydration also dramati-

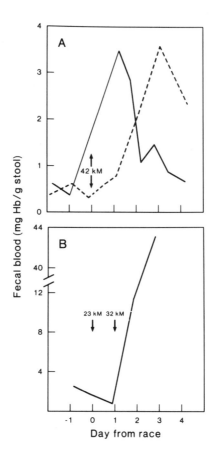

Fig. 3.9. Effect of exercise on fecal blood levels: (A) in two runners before and after a marathon; (B) in one runner after long-distance races on two consecutive days. Hemoglobin (*Hb*) levels measured by HemoQuant assay. From Stewart et al., reprinted by permission of *Annals of Internal Medicine*, 100; 844, 1984.

cally alters the reactivity of guaiac pad tests. Reducing substances excreted in urine, such as ascorbic acid (Jaffe et al. 1975) and naturally occurring compounds (Ahlquist and Schwartz 1975), can inhibit the reaction of guaiac or other leuco-dyes and cause false-negative results. False positives can occur when stool samples are taken from toilet water contaminated by menstrual blood or blood from urine (Dardick 1984).

There are no published data on specific approaches to stool collection taken by patients for occult blood testing. Recent recommendations, such as those by Gnauck, Macrae, and Fleisher (1984), on how to perform fecal blood tests include no mention of techniques to mobilize stools for sampling. My coworkers and I surveyed a group of patients to learn specifically how they had contended with gathering and sampling their stools. Most retrieved their specimens from the toilet water, for instance, by using long-handled spoons, wearing rubber gloves, or rolling up their sleeves. Others described the unpleasant extremes of catching their stool in a frying pan or kitchen bowl, defecating onto newspaper placed on the floor, and so forth. These experiences are offensive to anyone and may understandably prove insurmountable to the more squeamish.

Spector and colleagues' 1981 report on a Hemoccult screening program noted that personal objection to stool handling was more common among subjects whose participation was not voluntary. However, most studies that have analyzed patient compliance in stool testing (Sontag et al. 1984; Hardcastle et al. 1983; Nichols et al. 1986; Morrow et al. 1982; Elwood, Erickson, and Liberman 1978; Hamper et al. 1980) have demonstrated the influence of certain demographic and socioeconomic factors but have not elaborated on the role of patient aversion to the ordeal of stool collection. Patient compliance in these studies has ranged from 19% to 80% and has generally been higher after patients have met with a physician regarding the testing. Compliance to guaiac testing has been as low as 26% (Winchester et al. 1980) or 30% (Sontag et al. 1983), even in patients who agreed or requested to participate in screening. Patient reluctance to labor through the awkward retrieval of stool may in part be responsible for these low compliance rates.

Regardless of which test is used, variability in techniques of stool collection and sampling will confound screening efforts. Failure to develop procedures for these first steps in the screening process results in measurement error, creates an awkward chore for patients, and probably reduces compliance. To avoid these problems, the HemoQuant kit contains a collection device that the patient affixes to the toilet seat. This device is cheap and easy to use, to mail, and to discard.

BLEEDING PATTERNS OF COLORECTAL NEOPLASMS

The major premise upon which colorectal cancer screening is based, that asymptomatic lesions bleed enough and often enough to permit biochemical detection, remains completely unproven. There are no reported data on the natural bleeding history of truly asymptomatic colorectal neoplasms. Available information on colorectal cancer bleeding has been almost entirely obtained from patients with symptomatic and usually advanced disease. Observed fecal blood levels in these patients may have been affected by endoscopic biopsies, barium studies, or cathartic preparations, as the studies on bleeding typically had to be done in a narrow window of time between diagnosis and surgical treatment. Furthermore, because of self-selection biases, screen detection may not actually reflect populations without symptoms; indeed, in one large screening study that used Hemoccult (Gnauck 1977), 72 of the 89 patients in whom colorectal carcinoma was discovered (81%) had previously noted bleeding or other symptoms.

Studies that have used radiochemical methods (Macrae and St. John 1982; Dybdahl et al. 1984; Doran and Hardcastle 1982; Rosenfield et al. 1979) or HemoQuant (Ahlquist et al. 1985) to quantify fecal blood levels in samples from patients with colorectal cancer have shown that the levels vary widely, from normal to elevated;

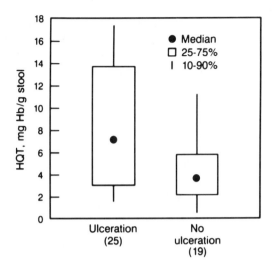

Fig. 3.10. Effect of ulceration in histologically proven colorectal carcinoma on fecal hemoglobin (*Hb*) concentration as measured by HemoQuant (*HQT*). Previously unpublished results from the Mayo Clinic.

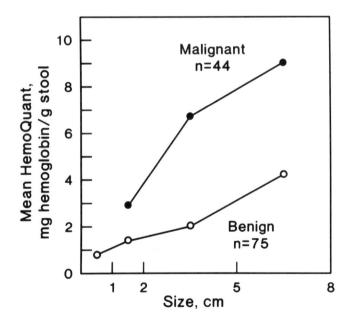

Fig. 3.11. Effect of lesion size on fecal hemoglobin levels. From Ahlquist et al., reprinted by permission of *The New England Journal of Medicine,* 312; 1425, 1985.

that blood within stools is nonuniformly distributed; and that the large majority of stools contain less than 10 mg hemoglobin/g. The last observation is most disturbing given the above-cited findings that more than 10 mg hemoglobin/g stool is required to ensure that Hemoccult reacts half the time. Our analyses utilizing Hemo-Quant (Ahlquist et al. 1985) have shown bleeding from colorectal neoplasms to increase with surface ulceration (fig. 3.10) and greater lesion size (fig. 3.11), supporting pre-HemoQuant findings by Crowley et al. (1983). It is important from a screening standpoint that localized cancers may bleed as much as those with regional extension or distant metastases (Ahlquist et al. 1985), although these data were also obtained largely from patients with symptoms of the disease.

Bleeding from a colorectal lesion varies over time, the level in most cases intermittently falling below the range detectable by fecal blood tests, and accordingly multiple stool testing has been shown to increase detection rates (Farrands and Hardcastle 1983; Macrae and St. John 1982; Doran and Hardcastle 1982). On the other hand, it is possible that too many stool tests per screening interval increase the false-positive rate and compromise patient compliance. The most common practice at present is to test two aliquots from each of three consecutive stools, which does not vary from the original screening recommendations (Greegor 1971). However, even multiple testing with the currently used guaiac tests may fail to detect minimal to moderate elevations in fecal blood from colon cancer lesions (fig. 3.12).

That measurement of fecal blood can detect benign colorectal adenomas is highly questionable. Some reports of polyp bleeding rates, such as Herzog and colleagues' 1982 study, have been based on samples from patients who either presented with bleeding or had large lesions. Most studies that have quantified bleeding from

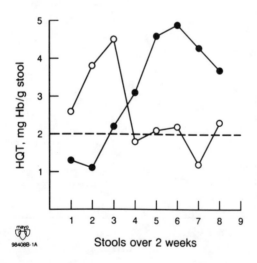

Fig. 3.12. HemoQuant (*HQT*) shows varying levels of hemoglobin (*Hb*) over time in stools from two Mayo Clinic patients with histologically proven, asymptomatic colorectal carcinoma. All stool samples were Hemoccult negative.

patients with colorectal adenomas have shown that fecal blood distribution is indistinguishable between healthy subjects and patients with polyps 2 cm or smaller (Macrae and St. John 1982; Dybdahl et al. 1984; Ahlquist et al. 1985). Discovery of adenomas in screening trials has often been used to explain Hemoccult positivity, despite the fact that most of these polyps have been diminutive and thus unlikely to bleed. The age-dependent prevalence of colorectal adenomas in patients with Hemoccult-positive findings (Winawer 1983; Winawer et al. 1980) does not appear to be different from that in the general population, based on autopsy series (Chapman 1963; Rickert et al. 1979).

The current and widespread practice of colorectal cancer screening is rooted in the assumptions that asymptomatic neoplasms bleed, that available tests detect this bleeding, and that such detection will reduce cancer-specific mortality. The efficacy of this screening approach remains to be established. Accordingly, it is premature to attempt full cost-effectiveness analysis for colorectal cancer screening, as has been pointed out by Frank (1985b), because the "effectiveness" is unknown. It has become increasingly apparent that guaiac tests have serious biochemical deficiencies, and the use of these tests to assess whether fecal blood measurement is a feasible screening approach to colorectal cancer may cripple this massive effort in disease control. Prospective detection studies with the newer, more reliable tests may help provide more definitive answers to these basic screening questions.

REFERENCES

Adams EC, Layman KM. 1974. Immunochemical confirmation of gastrointestinal bleeding. *Ann Clin Lab Sci* 4:343–349.

Ahlquist DA, Beart RW. 1985. Use of fecal occult tests in the detection of colorectal neoplasia. *Problems in General Surgery* 2:200–210.

Ahlquist DA, McGill DB, Schwartz S, et al. 1984. HemoQuant, a new quantitative assay for fecal hemoglobin: Comparison with Hemoccult. *Ann Intern Med* 101:297–302.

Ahlquist DA, McGill DB, Schwartz S, et al. 1985. Fecal blood levels in health and disease. A study using HemoQuant. *N Engl J Med* 312:1422–1428.

Ahlquist DA, Schwartz S. 1975. Use of leuco-dyes in the quantitative colorimetric microdetermination of hemoglobin and other heme compounds. *Clin Chem* 21:362–369.

Axtell LM, Asire JA, Myers MD, eds. 1976. *Cancer Patient Survival*. Report No. 5. DHEW Publication No. (NIH) 77-992. Bethesda, Md.: National Cancer Institute.

Barrows GH, Burton RM, Jarrett DD, et al. 1978. Immunochemical detection of human blood in feces. *Am J Clin Pathol* 69:342–346.

Bassett ML, Goulston KJ. 1980. False positive and negative Hemoccult reactions on a normal diet and effect of diet restriction. *Aust NZ J Med* 10:1–4.

Boas I. 1901. Uber Okkulte Magen Blumtunge. *Dtsch Med Wochenschr* 27:315–321.

Bralow SP, Kopel J. 1979. Hemoccult screening for colorectal cancer. An impact study on Sarasota, Florida. *J Fla Med Assoc* 66:915–919.

Chapman I. 1963. Adenomatous polyps of large intestine: Incidence and distribution. *Ann Surg* 157:223–226.

Chuong JJH. 1983. A screening primer: Basic principles, criteria, and pitfalls of screening, with comments on colorectal carcinoma. *J Clin Gastroenterol* 5:229–233.

Cole P, Morrison AS. 1980. Basic issues in population screening for cancer. *JNCI* 64:1263–1272.

Crowley ML, Freeman LD, Mottet MD, et al. 1983. Sensitivity of guaiac-impregnated cards for the detection of colorectal neoplasia. *J Clin Gastroenterol* 5:127–130.

Dardick KR. 1984. Hematuria and false-positive tests for stool occult blood. *Am Fam Physician* 29:201–202.

Doran J, Hardcastle JD. 1982. Bleeding patterns in colorectal cancer: The effect of aspirin and implications for faecal occult blood testing. *Br J Surg* 69:711–713.

Dybdahl JH, Daae LNW, Larsen S, et al. 1984. Occult faecal blood loss determined by a ^{51}Cr method and chemical tests in patients referred for colonoscopy. *Scand J Gastroenterol* 19:245–254.

Elwood TW, Erickson A, Liberman S. 1978. Comparative education approaches to screening for colorectal cancer. *Am J Public Health* 68:135–138.

Farrands PA, Hardcastle JD. 1983. Accuracy of occult blood tests over a six-day period. *Clinical Oncology* 9:217–225.

Fleisher M, Schwartz MK, Winawer SJ. 1977. The false-negative Hemoccult test. *Gastroenterology* 72:782–784.

Fleming JF, Ahlquist DA, McGill DB, et al. 1986. Fecal blood testing in microcytic anemia: Comparison of HemoQuant with Hemoccult (abstract). *Gastroenterology* 90:1417.

Fleming JF, Ahlquist DA, McGill DB, et al. 1987. Acute effects of ethanol and aspirin on fecal blood levels: A study using HemoQuant. *Mayo Clin Proc* 62:159–163.

Frank JW. 1985a. Occult blood screening for colorectal cancer: The benefits. *American Journal of Preventive Medicine* 1:3–9.

Frank JW. 1985b. Occult blood screening for colorectal cancer: The yield and costs. *American Journal of Preventive Medicine* 1:18–24.

Frank JW. 1985c. Occult blood screening for colorectal cancer: The risks. *American Journal of Preventive Medicine* 1:25–32.

Gilbertsen VA. 1979. The earlier detection of colorectal cancers. In *Screening and Early Detection of Colorectal Cancer,* DR Brodie, ed. NIH Publication No. 211–215. Washington: U.S. Department of Health, Education, and Welfare.

Gilbertsen VA, McHugh RB, Schuman LM, et al. 1980a. Colon cancer control study: An interim report. In *Colorectal Cancer: Prevention, Epidemiology, and Screening,* SJ Winawer, D Schottenfeld, P Sherlock, eds., pp. 261–266. New York: Raven Press.

Gilbertsen VA, McHugh R, Schuman LM, et al. 1980b. The earlier detection of colorectal cancers: A preliminary report of the results of the Occult Blood Study. *Cancer* 45:2899–2901.

Glober GA, Peskoe SM. 1974. Outpatient screening of gastrointestinal lesions using guaiac-impregnated slides. *American Journal of Digestive Diseases* 19:399–403.

Gnauck R. 1977. Dickdarmkarzinom-screening mit Haemoccult. *Leber Magen Darm* 7:32–35.

Gnauck R, Macrae FA, Fleisher M. 1984. How to perform the fecal occult blood test. *CA* 34:134–147.

Goldschmidt M, Ahlquist DA, Taylor WF, et al. 1986. Measurement of degraded fecal hemoglobin by HemoQuant to estimate the gastrointestinal site of occult bleeding (abstract). *Gastroenterology* 90:1431.

Graham DY, Sackman JW, Wallis CH, et al. 1984. The Hemo-matic Analyzer: A new occult blood testing device. *Am J Gastroenterol* 79:117–121.

Greegor DH. 1971. Occult blood testing for detection of asymptomatic colon cancer. *Cancer* 28:131–134.

Hamper MS, Winawer S, Brody RS, et al. 1980. Issues of patient compliance. In *Colorectal Cancer: Prevention, Epidemiology, and Screening,* SJ Winawer, D Schottenfeld, P Sherlock, eds., pp. 299–310. New York: Raven Press.

Hardcastle JD, Farrands PA, Balfour TW, et al. 1983. Controlled trial of faecal occult blood testing in the detection of colorectal cancer. *Lancet* 2:1–4.

Hastings JB. 1974. Mass screening for colorectal cancer. *Am J Surg* 127:228–233.

Heinrich HCL. 1980. Occult blood tests (letter). *Lancet* 1:822–823.

Herzog P, Holtermüller KH, Preiss J, et al. 1982. Fecal blood loss in patients with colonic polyps: A comparison of measurements with ^{51}chromium-labeled erythrocytes and with the Haemoccult test. *Gastroenterology* 83:957–962.

Hoffman A, Young Q, Bright-Asare P, et al. 1983. Early detection of bowel cancer at an urban public hospital: Demonstration project. *CA* 33:344–358.

Hunt RH. 1981. Evaluation of diagnostic techniques for colon cancer. Presented at the Second International Symposium on Colorectal Cancer. Washington, D.C.

Illingworth DG. 1965. Influence of diet on occult blood tests. *Gut* 6:595–598.

Jaffe RM, Kasten B, Young DS, et al. 1975. False-negative stool occult blood tests caused by ingestion of ascorbic acid (vitamin C). *Ann Intern Med* 83:824–826.

Jaffe RM, Zierdt W. 1979. A new occult blood test not subject to false-negative results from reducing substances. *J Lab Clin Med* 93:879–886.

Larkin KK. 1980. Mass screening in colorectal cancer. *Aust NZ J Surg* 50:467–469.

Layne EA, Mellow MH, Lipman TO. 1981. Insensitivity of guaiac slide tests for detection of blood in gastric juice. *Ann Intern Med* 94:774–776.

Lifton LJ, Kreiser J. 1982. False-positive stool occult blood tests caused by iron preparations. A controlled study and review of literature. *Gastroenterology* 83:860–863.

Macrae FA, St. John DJB. 1982. Relationship between patterns of bleeding and Hemoccult sensitivity in patients with colorectal cancers or adenomas. *Gastroenterology* 82:891–898.

Macrae FA, St. John DJB, Caligiore P, et al. 1982. Optimal dietary conditions for Hemoccult testing. *Gastroenterology* 82:899–903.

Markman HD. 1967. Errors in the guaiac test for occult blood (letter). *JAMA* 202:846–847.

Miller SF, Knight AR. 1977. The early detection of colorectal cancer. *Cancer* 40:945–949.

Morrow GR, Way J, Hoagland AC, et al. 1982. Patient compliance with self-directed Hemoccult testing. *Prev Med* 11:512–520.

Neuhauser D. 1980. Cost effectiveness of screening for occult blood in the stool: Another look (letter). *N Engl J Med* 303:1306–1307.

Nichols S, Koch E, Lallermand RC, et al. 1986. Randomized trial of compliance with screening for colorectal cancer. *Br Med J [Clin Res]* 293:107–110.

Ostrow JD, Mulvaeny CA, Hansell JR, et al. 1973. Sensitivity and reproducibility of chemical tests for fecal occult blood with an emphasis on false-positive reactions. *American Journal of Digestive Diseases* 18:930–940.

Rickert RR, Auerbach O, Garfinkel L, et al. 1979. Adenomatous lesions of the large bowel: An autopsy survey. *Cancer* 43:1847–1857.

Rose P, Fireman A, Terdemain R, et al. 1981. Selective screening for colorectal tumors in the Tel-Aviv area: Relevance of epidemiology and family history. *Cancer* 47:827–831.

Rosenfield RE, Kochwa A, Kaczera A, et al. 1979. Nonuniform distribution of occult blood in feces. *Am J Clin Pathol* 71:204–209.

Schentag JJ. 1980. False-positive "Hemoccult" reaction with cimetidine (letter). *N Engl J Med* 303:110.

Schwartz S, Dahl J. Ellefson M, et al. 1983. The "HemoQuant" test: A specific and quantitative determination of heme (hemoglobin) in feces and other materials. *Clin Chem* 29:2061–2067.

Schwartz S, Ellefson M. 1985. Quantitative fecal recovery of ingested hemoglobin-heme in blood: Comparisons by HemoQuant assay with ingested meat and fish. *Gastroenterology* 89:19–26.

Shigin Z. 1980. Screening and prevention of colorectal cancer in Haining count. *Chin Med J [Engl]* 93:843–848.

Silverberg E, Lubera JA. 1983. A review of American Cancer Society estimates of cancer cases and deaths. *CA* 33:2–8.

Simon JB. 1985. Occult blood screening for colorectal carcinoma: A critical review. *Gastroenterology* 88:820–837.

Songster CL, Barrows GH, Jarrett DD. 1980. Immunochemical detection of fecal occult blood—The fecal smear punch-disc test: A new non-invasive screening test for colorectal cancer. *Cancer* 45(Suppl 5):1099–1102.

Sontag SJ, Durczak A, Aranha GV, et al. 1983. Fecal occult blood screening for colorectal cancer in a Veterans Administration Hospital. *Am J Surg* 145:89–94.

Spector MH, Applegate WB, Olmstead SJ, et al. 1981. Assessment of attitudes toward mass screening for colorectal cancer and polyps. *Prev Med* 10:105–109.

Stewart JG, Ahlquist DA, McGill DB, et al. 1984. Gastrointestinal blood loss and anemia in runners. *Ann Intern Med* 100:843–845.

Stroehlein JR, Fairbanks VF, Go VL, et al. 1976a. Hemoccult stool tests: False-negative results due to storage of specimens. *Mayo Clin Proc* 51:548–552.

Stroehlein JR, Fairbanks VF, McGill DS, et al. 1976b. Hemoccult detection of fecal occult blood quantitated by radioassay. *American Journal of Digestive Diseases* 21:841–844.

VanDeen J. 1864. Tincture gaujaci, und ein ozontrague, als reagens auf sehr geringe blutmengen, namentlich in medico-forensischen falen. *Arch Holland Beitr Natura Heilk* 3:228–231.

Von Snapper J. 1919. Uber die notwendigkeit, die spektroskopische methode fuer den nachweis von blut in den faces zu benutzen. *Archiv fuer Verdauungs-Krankheiten* 25:230–240.

Winawer SJ. 1983. Detection and diagnosis of colorectal cancer. *Cancer* 51 (Suppl 12): 2519–2524.

Winawer SJ, Andrews M, Miller CH, et al. 1980. Review of screening for colorectal cancer using fecal occult blood testing. In *Colorectal Cancer: Prevention, Epidemiology, and Screening*, SJ Winawer, D Schottenfeld, P Sherlock, eds., pp. 249–260. New York: Raven Press.

Winawer SJ, Fleisher M. 1982. Sensitivity and specificity of the fecal occult blood test for colorectal neoplasia. *Gastroenterology* 82:986–991.

Winchester DP, Shull JH, Scanlon EF, et al. 1980. A mass screening program for colorectal cancer using chemical testing for occult blood in the stool. *Cancer* 45:2955–2958.

Yoshida Y, Saito H, Tsuchida S, et al. 1986. A simple sensitive immunologic fecal occult blood test suitable for mass screening for colorectal cancer (abstract). *Gastroenterology* 90:1699.

Annual Clinical Conference on Cancer, Vol. 30
Gastrointestinal Cancer: Current Approaches to Diagnosis and Treatment
© 1988 by The University of Texas System Cancer Center

4. Experimental Chemopreventive Agents: Inhibition of Gastrointestinal Cancer in Animals

Michael J. Wargovich

The process of gastrointestinal carcinogenesis has provided a unique challenge to the probing mind of the cell biologist. On the face of the challenge is the central question of how the "jettisonable" cell population that characterizes the mucosal epithelium of the gastrointestinal tract ever develops into cancer. The mucosa has been designed by nature to produce cells quickly to alleviate the normal cell loss due, in part, to the ingestion of a variety of dietary substances that are cytotoxic. Coincidentally, some of these same cytotoxic chemicals provide the essential elements of nutrition and come from the basic food groups. Another seeming paradox is found by comparing the growth rate of normal gastrointestinal epithelial mucosa with that of transformed (i.e., premalignant and cancerous) gastrointestinal epithelium. The former rapidly proliferates in a metronomic rhythm dictated by steady-state kinetics; however, the growth of adenomas and adenocarcinomas is slow and methodical, and only after many years is there eruption so that the underlying serosa spews cells destined for metastatic dissemination to the liver and lung.

Laboratory identification of dietary chemicals responsible for the profound cellular alterations leading to gastrointestinal cancer has proved a difficult task. Though clues have emerged and theories expounded on the dietary origins of cancer, the identification of a single etiologic agent for human gastrointestinal cancer is still beyond the reach of the cell biologist. However, progress has been made in that some dietary factors that have the ability to inhibit carcinogenesis have been discovered. These factors, present in minute amounts and known as chemopreventive agents, have in some cases shown extraordinary promise in their capacity to suppress experimentally induced cancers of the esophagus, liver, stomach, and colon (Wattenberg 1985).

The road to the discovery of chemopreventive agents began with solid leads from controlled epidemiological studies conducted in populations at low risk for major malignancies. The pioneering studies of Hirayama led to the conclusion that consumption of green and yellow vegetables protects against cancers of the stomach and lung (Hirayama 1981). Other epidemiological investigations supported the hypothesis that vegetables and fruits contain anticarcinogens that may inhibit neoplasia (Graham et al. 1978; Haenszel, Locke, and Segi 1980). These population studies have generated laboratory investigations of the dietary factors that accelerate carcinogenesis. It is now thought that tumor-promoting chemicals exist in several dietary sources; many such chemicals seem to play a role in the stimulation of cellular proliferation. It is also thought that antipromoters have the ability to moderate the biologic effects of tumor promoters, and the search for these substances in diet is under way.

This chapter focuses on more recent developments in the isolation of anticarcinogens and antipromoters from the diet, with some emphasis on the laboratory approaches that my colleagues and I use at UT M. D. Anderson Hospital. However, it is instructive to also review the possible mechanisms of action of the experimental chemopreventive agents and the applicability of these agents in the prevention of certain forms of gastrointestinal cancer.

DIETARY ANTICARCINOGENS

Based on epidemiological evidence linking consumption of certain fruits and vegetables with reduced risk for cancer, early experiments involved the feeding of animals with freeze-dried vegetables for the purpose of inhibiting induced forms of cancer. Also, a number of in vitro studies demonstrated antimutagenic properties of extracts of a number of commonly consumed herbs (Abraham, Mahajan, and Kesavan 1986; Ito, Maeda, and Sugiyama 1986). These experiments were performed in an effort to explain some of the anecdotal medicinal effects reported for the consumption of certain herbs.

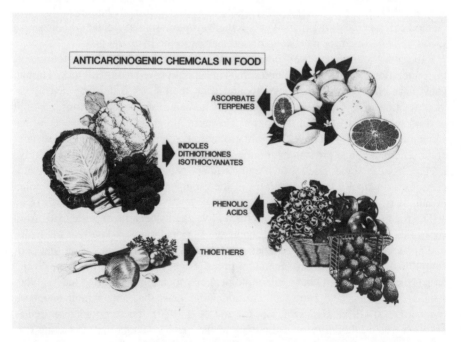

Fig. 4.1. These chemicals from common foods have been shown to have anticarcinogenic properties.

Recognition of the striking ability of cruciferous vegetables to inhibit cancers of the forestomach, liver, and lungs (Wattenberg 1983; Boyd et al. 1982) followed the chemical separation and identification of indoles, coumarins, isothiocyanates, and flavonoids as the inhibitory substances (Wattenberg and Loub 1978; Wattenberg and Leong 1970). Research conducted in the last few years has added considerably to the list of dietary anticarcinogens. Newer examples include dithiothiones found in cruciferous vegetables (Kensler et al. 1985), hydroxylated flavonoids and terpenes in citrus oils (Sparnins and Wattenberg 1985; Elegbede et al. 1986), and thioethers in garlic and onion (Wargovich 1987) (fig. 4.1).

Much has been proposed about the mechanisms of cellular events through which anticarcinogens protect against cancer development. Table 4.1 lists some of the current hypotheses and cites selected studies that support them.

Most newly identified anticarcinogens have been shown to be better antagonists of carcinogens with which they share a structural similarity in chemistry. For instance, the planar configuration of coumarins, flavonoids, and plant phenols is common to polycyclic aromatic hydrocarbons such as benzo[*a*]pyrene, the most ubiquitous carcinogen in the environment. Few of the known anticarcinogens have shown pronounced inhibitory effects on methylating carcinogens that have an aliphatic structure. But the organic thioethers that commonly occur in onion and garlic constitute an exception to these findings (Brodnitz, Pascale, and Vanderslice 1971).

Thioethers, which appear chemically as dialkyl sulfides, are responsible for the characteristic aromas of *Allium* species. Of the dozen thioethers chromatographically isolated from garlic, one in particular, diallyl sulfide (DAS), may hold some

Table 4.1. *Examples of Dietary Anticarcinogens and Proposed Mechanisms of Inhibition of Carcinogenesis*

Dietary Compound	Hypothesized Mechanism	Study
Plant phenolic acids	Nucleophilic substitute for carcinogen binding	Newmark 1984
Dithiothiones, dialkyl thioethers	Induction of glutathione transferases	Ansher, Dolan, and Bueding 1986
Coumarins, flavonoids	Induction of carcinogen-metabolizing enzymes	Wattenberg 1983
Ascorbate, tocopherol	Prevention of chemical carcinogen formation	Newmark and Mergens 1981; Mirvish 1981
Selenium	Induction of glutathione peroxidase	Bergman and Slanina 1986

promise as a new chemopreventive agent. Our laboratory has actively investigated DAS for inhibitory activity against a number of potent methylating carcinogens that also induce colorectal cancer in rodents.

In our initial attempts at screening organic sulfides in garlic for cancer-suppressing activity, we found that DAS strongly inhibited in rodents the generation of nuclear aberrations induced by the colon-specific carcinogen dimethylhydrazine (DMH) (Wargovich and Goldberg 1985). Nuclear aberrations in colon epithelial cells are morphological evidence of interaction of the proliferating mucosal cells with a carcinogen; their detection may herald carcinogenesis in this organ (Wargovich, Medline, and Bruce 1983). DAS was found to substantially reduce the nucleotoxic effects of DMH in mouse intestinal cells, and we predicted from this observation that DAS would prove to be anticarcinogenic as well.

We have subsequently tested DAS in a carcinogenesis protocol in mice for the ability to suppress DMH colon tumorigenesis. DAS was found to inhibit tumor formation by 75% in animals treated prophylactically with the sulfide three hours prior to the administration of the carcinogen (Wargovich 1987). This finding is important in view of the potent alkylating nature of DMH. Second, DAS could inhibit a non-aromatically structured carcinogen. It is possible that DAS and other related sulfides will also prove to be capable of inhibiting carcinogenesis elsewhere in the gastrointestinal tract. Concordant with this hypothesis, experiments are under way in our laboratory to test whether DAS can inhibit esophageal cancer induced in rats.

Because of the possibility that dietary anticarcinogens have a selective specificity for the carcinogenic chemicals they inhibit, it may be necessary to combine several of these agents to achieve practical suppression of tumorigenesis. Few studies of this design have been performed and little is known about the potential for synergistic, competitive, or antagonistic behavior of dietary anticarcinogens given in a combined protocol.

Data from the search for anticarcinogens in foodstuffs will allow stronger public recommendations about changes in diet to take advantage of naturally occurring chemopreventive agents. Yet, the distinct possibility will always remain that cells of the gastrointestinal tract will interact with a carcinogen that has eluded the anticarcinogenic defenses. In the case of the initiated cell, the propensity to transform into the malignant phenotype will greatly increase in a proliferating cell population. To guard against clonal expansion of initiated cells, the action of substances that enhance cellular proliferation must be neutralized. The biologic features of dietary promoters and antipromoters of gastrointestinal cancer are now being recognized in the laboratory.

DIETARY FACTORS THAT PROMOTE CANCER

The process by which tumorigenesis is enhanced by events subsequent to the initial genetic alterations is called *tumor promotion* (Farber 1982), and factors that encourage this process are called *tumor promoters* (Hicks 1983). Tumor promotion has been observed in many organs and cell populations (Farber 1984), but the complex-

Table 4.2. *Effects of Dietary Factors on Tumor Promotion in the Gastrointestinal Tract*

Dietary Factor	Organ Site	Study
Zinc deficiency	Stomach	Newberne 1985
Sodium chloride	Esophagus	Takahashi et al. 1983
Secondary bile acids (e.g., deoxycholate)	Colon	Reddy et al. 1976
Polyunsaturated fats (e.g., corn oil)	Colon	Sakaguchi et al. 1984
Saturated fats (e.g., beef tallow, lard)	Colon	Reddy and Maeura 1984
Nonfermentable fibers (e.g., cellulose)	Colon	Jacobs and Lupton 1986

ity of the biology allows for few generalizations. One feature that is more common to all tumor promoters than not is a general stimulatory effect on the rate of cellular proliferation. Caution must be applied to this simplistic definition of tumor promotion when the gastrointestinal tract is considered, since the epithelial population is naturally proliferative. In this specific case, tumor promoters are considered to be such when the normal kinetic growth rates are greatly exceeded. In many cases in which putative tumor promoters have been identified for gastrointestinal cancer, the ability to increase mucosal proliferation and the ability to enhance tumorigenesis are linked. Dietary substances that share these biologic effects are shown in table 4.2.

What are the consequences of enhanced cellular proliferation? In the lining of the gastrointestinal tract, cells that have undergone initiation by a carcinogen are faced with several outcomes. DNA damage may be routinely repaired if cells are not forced into a proliferative mode by an exogenous stimulus. Initiated cells may also be sloughed off by the normal dynamics of mucosal differentiation. Should the mucosal lining be injured, however, a hyperproliferative response may increase the chances of expression of a cell with fixed genetic lesions.

The foregoing may explain the tumor-promoting effects of dietary lipids. Bile acids and fatty acids in a basic pH environment are topically toxic to the colon epithelium, destroying the pericryptal and cryptal surface structure (Saunders et al. 1975). Loss of cells at the crypt surface—that is, epitheliolysis—may serve as the impetus for the stem cells in the crypt base to enter a hyperproliferative mode. Indeed, several studies have indicated that the detergent effects of ionized lipids have adverse consequences on the cells of the colon epithelium (Chadwick et al. 1976; Vahouny et al. 1984). There are at least two possibilities for remedy of this situation, short of simply removing lipids from the diet (an impractical solution!). The first is to create an acidic environment in which the bile or fatty acids are nonionized and nontoxic. In fact, a study by Rafter et al. (1986) confirms a protective effect of a lower pH; nonionized lipids do not cause epitheliolysis. Coincidentally, lower fecal pH is suggested in several human studies to correlate with lower risk for colon cancer (Thornton 1981; van Dokkum et al. 1983). The second solution is to interdict the effects of the bile and fatty acids with a biologic or chemical agent.

Apart from their known effects on the physiology and morphology of the crypt, ionized fatty acids and bile acids have a strong binding affinity for divalent cations, especially those of calcium (Newmark, Wargovich, and Bruce 1984). Maintenance of calcium levels is extremely important to the mucosal epithelium since this element is required for stabilization of cellular membrane structure and tight junctions, is required for the control of cellular DNA synthesis, and has been implicated in the control of the mitotic process (MacManus, Boynton, and Whitfield 1978; Whitfield et al. 1980). Imbalances in calcium levels or interference with intracellular transport of calicum may trigger the abnormal proliferative response (Hait and Lazo 1986).

Our laboratory has investigated the role of calcium as a potential *antipromoter* of neoplasia. We have found, for example, that adequate intake of dietary calcium can offset the proliferative stimulus of deoxycholic acid or oleic acid in the colons of mice (Wargovich et al. 1983, 1984). We have also observed that phytic acid, a component of certain forms of bran, also stimulates mucosal proliferation, presumably through its ability to tightly bind calcium (Wargovich 1986). The bioavailability of calcium may also be affected by other factors, including phosphates and the binding capacity of certain forms of dietary fiber. The benefit of adequate levels of dietary calcium has found support in an epidemiological study (Garland et al. 1985) and in a small clinical series in which proliferative abnormalities of patients considered at high risk for colon cancer were modified by calcium supplementation (Lipkin and Newmark 1985).

Identification of other dietary antipromoters will certainly follow, and investigations combining highly effective anticarcinogenic chemicals with compounds that suppress tumor promotion will be of interest.

PROSPECTS FOR CHEMOPREVENTION OF GASTROINTESTINAL CANCER IN HUMANS

Clinical trials of the newer chemopreventive agents have not yet been initiated. Conducted clinical trials have focused upon natural and synthetic forms of vitamin A, supplemental vitamin C and vitamin E, and the effects of wheat bran. In most cases, the ongoing trials have used recurrence of the adenomatous polyp as the biologic end point. Much remains to be discovered about the efficacy of the newer chemopreventive agents in humans. Little is known about adverse effects, if any, of these agents when given in purified form. If chemopreventive agents act by the alteration of enzymes responsible for carcinogen metabolism, might drug metabolism also be altered? Will cancer prevention effects be true of only purified compounds, or will consumption of foods containing chemopreventive compounds suffice? Answers to these questions must be found to enable approval for advanced study in populations at increased risk for gastrointestinal cancer or with premalignant lesions. An advantage may reside in the fact that the chemopreventive chemicals are routinely ingested in a moderately varied diet; the chemicals are not xenobiotic substances.

REFERENCES

Abraham SK, Mahajan S, Kesavan PC. 1986. Inhibitory effects of dietary vegetables on the in vivo clastogenicity of cyclophosphamide. *Mutat Res* 172:51–54.

Ansher S, Dolan P, Bueding E. 1986. Biochemical effects of dithiolthiones. *Food Chem Toxicol* 24:405–415.

Bergman K, Slanina P. 1986. Effects of dietary selenium compounds on benzo(a)pyrene-induced forestomach tumours and whole-blood glutathione peroxidase activities in C3H mice. *Anticancer Res* 6:785–790.

Boyd JN, Babish JG, Stoewsand GS, et al. 1982. Modification of beet and cabbage diets of aflatoxin B$_1$-induced rat plasma alpha-foetoprotein elevation, hepatic tumorigenesis, and mutagenicity of urine. *Food Chem Toxicol* 20:47–52.

Brodnitz MH, Pascale JV, Vanderslice L. 1971. Flavor components of garlic extracts. *Journal of Agricultural and Food Chemistry* 19:273–275.

Chadwick VS, Gaginella TS, Debongie JC, et al. 1976. Mucosal epitheliolysis: A mechanism for the increased colonic permeability induced by dihydroxy bile acids (abstract). *Gut* 17:816.

Elegbede JA, Elson CE, Tanner MA, et al. 1986. Regression of rat primary mammary tumors following dietary *d*-limonene. *JNCI* 76:323–325.

Farber E. 1982. Chemical carcinogenesis: A biologic perspective. *Am J Pathol* 106:271–296.

Farber E. 1984. The multistep nature of cancer development. *Cancer Res* 44:4217–4223.

Garland C, Shekelle RB, Barrett-Connor E, et al. 1985. Dietary vitamin D and calcium and risk of colorectal cancer: A 19-year prospective study in men. *Lancet* 1:307–309.

Graham S, Dayal H, Swanson M, et al. 1978. Diet in the epidemiology of cancer of the colon and rectum. *JNCI* 61:709–714.

Haenszel W, Locke FB, Segi M. 1980. A case-control study of large bowel cancer in Japan. *JNCI* 64:17–22.

Hait WN, Lazo JS. 1986. Calmodulin: A potential target for cancer chemotherapeutic agents. *J Clin Oncol* 4:994–1012.

Hicks RM. 1983. Pathological and biochemical aspects of tumour promotion (commentary). *Carcinogenesis* 4:1209–1214.

Hirayama T. 1981. A large scale cohort study on the relationship between diet and selected cancer of the digestive organs. *Banbury Report* 7:409–430.

Ito Y, Maeda S, Sugiyama T. 1986. Suppression of 7,12-dimethylbenz[*a*]anthracene-induced chromosome aberrations in rat bone marrow cells by vegetable juices. *Mutat Res* 172:55–60.

Jacobs LR, Lupton JR. 1986. Relationship between colonic luminal pH, cell proliferation, and colon carcinogenesis in 1,2-dimethylhydrazine treated rats fed high fiber diets. *Cancer Res* 46:1727–1734.

Kensler TW, Egner PA, Trush MA, et al. 1985. Modification of aflatoxin B1 binding to DNA *in vivo* in rats fed phenolic antioxidants, ethoxyquin and a dithiothione. *Carcinogenesis* 6:759–763.

Lipkin M, Newmark H. 1985. Effect of added dietary calcium on colonic epithelial-cell proliferation in subjects at high risk for familial colonic cancer. *N Engl J Med* 313:1381–1384.

MacManus JP, Boynton AL, Whitfield JF. 1978. Cyclic AMP and calcium as intracycle regulators in the control of cell proliferation. *Advances in Cyclic Nucleotide Research* 9:485–491.

Mirvish SS. 1981. Ascorbic acid inhibition of *n*-nitroso compound formation in chemical, food, and biological systems. In *Inhibition of Tumor Formation and Development*, MS Zedeck, M Lipkin, eds., pp. 101–126. New York: Plenum.

Newberne P. 1985. Dietary factors affecting biological responses to esophageal and colon chemical carcinogenesis. In *Xenobiotic Metabolism: Nutritional Effects*, JW Finley, DE Schwass, eds., pp. 163–176. Washington, D.C.: American Chemical Society.

Newmark HL. 1984. A hypothesis for dietary components as blocking agents of chemical carcinogenesis: Plant phenolics and pyrrole pigments. *Nutr Cancer* 6:58–70.

Newmark HL, Mergens WJ. 1981. α-Tocopherol (vitamin E) and its relationship to tumor induction and development. In *Inhibition of Tumor Formation and Development*, MS Zedeck, M Lipkin, eds., pp. 127–168. New York: Plenum.

Newmark HL, Wargovich MJ, Bruce WR. 1984. Colon cancer and dietary fat, phosphate, and calcium: A hypothesis. *JNCI* 72:1323–1325.

Rafter JJ, Eng VWS, Furrer R, et al. 1986. Effects of calcium and pH on the mucosal damage produced by deoxycholic acid in the rat colon. *Gut* 27:1320–1329.

Reddy BS, Maeura Y. 1984. Tumor promotion by dietary fat in azoxymethane-induced colon carcinogenesis in female F344 rats: Influence of amount and source of dietary fat. *JNCI* 72:745–750.

Reddy BS, Narasawa T, Weisburger JH, et al. 1976. Promoting effect of sodium deoxycholate on colon adenocarcinoma in germfree rats (brief communication). *JNCI* 56:441–442.

Sakaguchi M, Hiramatsu Y, Takada H, et al. 1984. Effect of dietary unsaturated and saturated fats on azoxymethane-induced colon carcinogenesis in rats. *Cancer Res* 44:1472–1477.

Saunders DR, Hedges JR, Sillery J, et al. 1975. Morphological and functional effects of bile salts on rat colon. *Gastroenterology* 68:1236–1245.

Sparnins VL, Wattenberg LW. 1985. Effects of citrus fruit oils on glutathione-*s*-transferase (gst) activity and benzo[*a*]pyrene (BP)–induced neoplasia (abstract 487). *Proceedings of the American Association for Cancer Research* 26:123.

Takahashi M, Kokubo T, Furukawa F, et al. 1983. Effect of high salt diet on rat gastric carcinogenesis by *N*-methyl-*N*´-nitro-*N*-nitrosoguanidine. *Gann* 74:28–34.

Thornton JR. 1981. High colonic pH promotes colorectal cancer. *Lancet* 1:1081–1083.

Vahouny GV, Satchithanandam S, Lightfoot F, et al. 1984. Morphological disruption of colonic mucosa by free or cholestyramine-bound bile acids. *Dig Dis Sci* 29:432–442.

van Dokkum W, de Boer BC, van Faassen CJ, et al. 1983. Diet, faecal pH and colorectal cancer. *Br J Cancer* 48:109–110.

Wargovich MJ. 1986. Phytic acid, a major calcium chelator from fiber-rich cereals, stimulates colonic cellular proliferation (abstract). *Gastroenterology* 90:1684.

Wargovich MJ. 1987. Diallyl sulfide, a flavor component of garlic (*Allium sativum*), inhibits dimethylhydrazine-induced colon cancer. *Carcinogenesis* 8:487–489.

Wargovich MJ, Eng VWS, Newmark HL, et al. 1983. Calcium ameliorates the toxic effects of deoxycholic acid on colonic epithelium. *Carcinogenesis* 4:1205–1207.

Wargovich MJ, Eng VWS, Newmark HL, et al. 1984. Calcium modification of the promoting stimulus of fatty acids to the colonic epithelium. *Cancer Lett* 23:256–261.

Wargovich MJ, Goldberg MT. 1985. Diallyl sulfide: A naturally occurring thioether that inhibits carcinogen-induced damage to colon epithelial cells in vivo. *Mutat Res* 143:127–129.

Wargovich MJ, Medline A, Bruce WR. 1983. Early histopathologic events to evolution of colon cancer in C57BL/6 and CF1 mice treated with 1,2-dimethylhydrazine. *JNCI* 71:125–131.

Wattenberg LW. 1983. Inhibition of neoplasia by minor dietary constituents. *Cancer Res* 43(Suppl 5):2448s–2453s.

Wattenberg LW. 1985. Chemoprevention of cancer. *Cancer Res* 45:1–9.

Wattenberg LW, Leong JL. 1970. Inhibition of the carcinogenic action of benzo(a)pyrene by flavones. *Cancer Res* 30:1922–1925.

Wattenberg LW, Loub WD. 1978. Inhibition of polycyclic hydrocarbon-induced neoplasia by naturally occurring indoles. *Cancer Res* 38:1410–1413.

Whitfield JF, Boynton AL, MacManus JP, et al. 1980. The roles of calcium and cyclic AMP in cell proliferation. *Ann NY Acad Sci* 329:216–240.

5. Development of Intermediate Biomarkers and the Primary Prevention of Cancer of the Large Intestine

Martin Lipkin

Recent findings have shown that modifications of epithelial cell proliferation and differentiation occur in diseases that predispose individuals to gastrointestinal cancer. Among early developments is an expansion of cell proliferation within the epithelial lining of the gastrointestinal organ that is affected. In diseases that lead to increased risk of gastrointestinal cancer, a true hyperproliferative state eventually develops in each cancer-prone region of the gastrointestinal tract. This occurs in the esophagus, stomach, and colon of human beings and also in gastrointestinal cells of the same organs in rodents when chemical carcinogens are given.

These findings have aided the development of studies in which there is an attempt to inhibit the abnormal development of gastrointestinal cells and the subsequent evolution of tumors in human beings. By using "intermediate biomarkers" of cell proliferation and differentiation in studies of nutritional intervention, it is now possible to evaluate whether the appearance of early changes in cells associated with increased risk of neoplasia can be inhibited. In this article I will give background information on epithelial cell proliferation and differentiation in gastrointestinal diseases and summarize recent applications of cell proliferation and differentiation to studies of nutritional intervention.

ESOPHAGUS

In precancerous diseases of the esophagus, proliferative abnormalities develop in esophageal epithelial cells that resemble those found in other regions of the gastrointestinal tract. Thus, in a recent study (Muñoz et al. 1985), an expansion of cell proliferation, measured by tritiated thymidine ([^{3}H]dThd) labeling of esophageal epithelial cells, occurred in the epithelial lining of the esophagus in subjects from a geographic region where the population is at high risk of developing esophageal cancer (fig. 5.1). In patients with reflux esophagitis, biopsy specimens also showed more incorporation of [^{3}H]dThd than in normal subjects (Livstone et al. 1977). Mitotic figures also appeared more frequently in the basal zone, thus suggesting that these cells may contribute to a thickened basal layer (Ismail-Beigi, Horton, and Pope 1970; Ismail-Beigi and Pope 1974).

Cell turnover increased in esophageal biopsy specimens from patients with Barrett's epithelium or columnar-lined esophagus (Herbst et al. 1976), and labeled surface cells in noncancerous areas of esophageal tissue were observed. Current

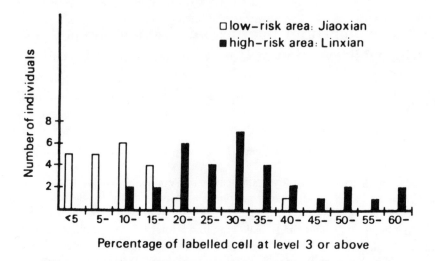

Fig. 5.1. Histogram of percentage of [³H]dThd-labeled cells at esophageal cell level of 3 and above (expansion of proliferative compartment of basal layer cells) in normal and precancerous human esophageal biopsies. Categories of the abscissa refer to percentages up to the following category. Reprinted from Muñoz N, Lipkin M, Crespi M, et al., Proliferative abnormalities of the oesophageal epithelium of Chinese populations at high and low risk for oesophageal cancer. *Int J Cancer* 1987; 36:187–189.

information concerning Barrett's epithelium suggests that the disease is a premalignant condition (Naef, Savary, and Ozzello 1975).

STOMACH

In the stomach, precancerous dysplasia and atrophy occur in populations having modified nutritional intake (Correa et al. 1976). In gastritis, the G_1 phase of the cell cycle appeared to be shortest in the atrophic type and longest in the superficial type of gastritis (Castrup and Fuchs 1974). Synthesis of nucleic acid and protein were abnormal in atrophic gastritis (Deschner, Winawer, and Lipkin 1972). In the normal stomach, synthesis of RNA, protein, and DNA were most active in proliferative areas at the base of the gastric pits; when mild gastritis was present, these activities increased in gastric surface cells of histologically normal mucosa. The same was apparent in atrophic gastritis and in intestinalized gastric mucosa (Winawer and Lipkin 1969; Deschner, Winawer, and Lipkin 1972).

More mitotic activity also occurred in intestinal metaplastic glands of atrophic gastritis than in normal gastric pits. The mitotic index doubled (from 1% to 2.3%) and the labeling index increased as small intestinal cells appeared in the stomach (Hansen, Pedersen, and Larsen 1975).

In a population at increased risk of developing gastric cancer because of chronic atrophic gastritis, an expansion of the proliferative compartment also was observed (fig. 5.2) as well as a subpopulation of hyperproliferating cells that expressed an

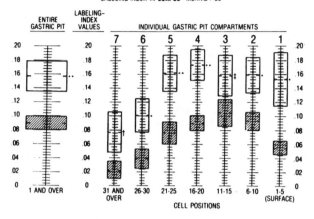

Fig. 5.2. In the mucosa of the corpus of the stomach: comparison of labeling index statistics between a population with chronic atrophic gastritis (light areas) and a normal population (diagonal shading) for individual gastric pit compartments and for the gastric pit as a whole. Symbols:**$p < 0.006$; *$p < 0.02$; † $p < 0.07$ for compartment 7; ‡ $p = 0.12$ for compartment 3; no symbol, 20% < p < 33%. Reprinted from Lipkin M, Correa P, Mikol YB, et al., Proliferative and antigenic modifications in epithelial cells in chronic atrophic gastritis. *JNCI* 1985; 75:613–619.

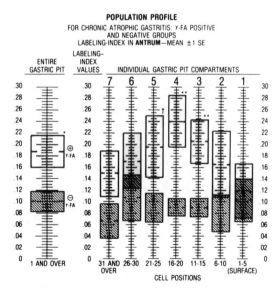

Fig. 5.3. In the mucosa of the antrum of the stomach: comparison of labeling index statistics between chronic atrophic gastritis (CAG) subgroup having positive γ-fetal antigen (FA) reactivity (light areas) and the CAG subgroup having negative γ-FA reactivity (diagonal shading) for individual gastric pit compartments and for the gastric pit as a whole. Symbols:**$p < 0.006$; *$p < 0.02$; † p < 0.07. Reprinted from Lipkin M, Correa P, Mikol YB, et al., Proliferative and antigenic modifications in epithelial cells in chronic atrophic gastritis. *JNCI* 1985; 75:613–619.

abnormal antigen (γ-fetal antigen) not seen in normal gastrointestinal cells (Lipkin et al. 1985b) (fig. 5.3).

LARGE INTESTINE

In the colonic mucosa of patients who have developed adenomas, colon cancer, or familial polyposis—diseases that predispose to the development of colorectal cancer—increased epithelial cell proliferative activity also has been noted. During progressive stages of abnormal development, epithelial cells gain an increased ability to proliferate and to accumulate in the mucosa. Identification of these changes has aided our understanding of early events that occur during neoplastic transformation of colonic cells (e.g., Deschner et al. 1970; Lipkin 1974; Bleiberg, Mainguet, and Galand 1972; Iwana, Utsunomiya, and Sasaki 1977; Lipkin et al. 1985a; Terpstra et al. 1986). The abnormal proliferative changes are similar to those occurring in the colonic epithelial cells of rodents exposed to chemical carcinogens (e.g., Thurnherr et al. 1973; Deschner et al. 1983; Rubio and Lagerlof 1983). In vitro assays that measure the location of cells incorporating [³H]dThd within colonic crypts make it possible to improve the identification of those changes.

Analysis of Proliferative Activity

To facilitate the analysis of abnormal proliferative activity in gastrointestinal epithelial cells, five new analytical methods have recently been developed (Lipkin et al. 1983; Lipkin et al. 1984a). With these analyses, differences in the patterns of [³H]dThd-labeled cells can be measured throughout the gastrointestinal tract, both in normal and cancer-prone persons, as can modifications occurring under different dietary regimens. For each analysis, labeled cells are identified by their height in the gastric pits or intestinal crypt columns or in the basal layer of esophagus in relation to the lumen of the gastrointestinal tract. Applications of these analytical methods to the colon are summarized here.

Measurement of Height-Distribution Patterns of Labeled Cells

The number of labeled cells in an *i*th mucosal-height compartment for all individuals in a population defined a frequency of occurrence of labeled cells (f_i), and the ratio of f_i to group totals over all the compartments were used to identify the distributions of labeled cells in various populations. Measurements in the colon revealed that persons known to be at low risk for colon cancer had smaller occupancy fractions of labeled cells in the upper crypt regions near the luminal surface of the mucosa and a more quiescent proliferative equilibrium than did populations at higher risk (fig. 5.4). Low-risk populations included a group who were consuming a vegetarian diet. Persons at high risk of esophageal and gastric cancer showed similar expansions of the proliferative compartment of cells and impaired maturation of epithelial cells near the luminal surface of the mucosa.

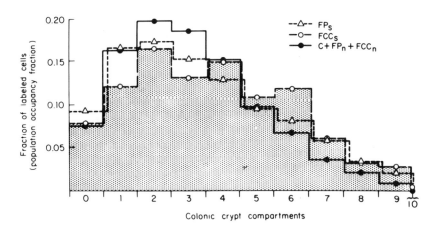

Fig. 5.4. Comparison of population occupancy fractions of [³H]dThd-labeled epithelial cells In the colonic crypt compartments of a high-risk group (FP$_s$) with symptomatic familial polyposis (Δ), a high-risk group (FCC$_s$) previously affected with familial colon cancer (O), and a low-risk group from the general population (●). *Abscissa:* colonic-crypt height compartments. *Ordinate:* fraction of a given population's labeled cells that occupy any specified height compartment in the colonic crypts. Reprinted from Lipkin M, Blattner W, Fraumeni JF, et al., Tritiated thymidine (φ$_p$, φ$_h$) labeling distribution as a marker for hereditary predisposition to colon cancer. *Cancer Res* 1983; 43:1899–1904.

Intermediate Data χ$_i$ in Further Amplifying Crypt-Compartment Frequency Distributions of Labeled Cells between High- and Low-Risk Populations

Recently, χ^2 intermediate data χ_i have been used to further amplify differences between the frequency distributions of labeled cells in high- and low-risk populations. The χ_i values provide a sensitive measure of the polarity of differences between cell-labeling patterns for pairs of high- and low-risk groups. These values showed the proportions of cells labeled with [³H]dThd to be consistently greater in regions of mucosa adjacent to the surfaces of the crypts in the high-risk group (fig. 5.5) (Lipkin et al. 1983). Recently, this analysis revealed that measurements of cell proliferation could be combined with measurements of abnormal antigen expression in colon epithelial cells. In ulcerative colitis, using [³H]dThd labeling of the cells and antibody to a fetal antigen (Lipkin et al. 1985b), it was found that hyperproliferating subpopulations of cells could be identified.

Consolidation of the Upper-Crypt Height Compartments to Facilitate Risk Discrimination

On the basis of the χ_i comparisons in the normal colon noted above, upper-crypt compartments 6 through 10 (the upper 40% of the crypt) were further consolidated and defined as a quantity ϕ_h, computed as $\phi_h = \phi_6 + \phi_7 + \phi_8 + \phi_9 + \phi_{10}$. The fraction of individuals in a group where the value of ϕ_h equaled or exceeded a specific ϕ_h value was denoted by ϕ_p (population fraction) and analyzed as a function of

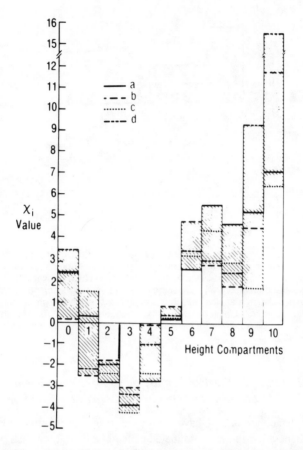

Fig. 5.5. χ_i histograms showing comparisons between four pairs of high-risk and low-risk groups: *a,* the high-risk group (FP$_s$) versus low-risk groups; *b,* the high-risk group (FCC$_s$) versus the same low-risk group; *c,* the high-risk group (FP$_s$) versus its low-risk kindred (FP$_n$); *d,* the high-risk group (FCC$_s$) versus its low-risk kindred (FCC$_n$). Reprinted from Lipkin M, Blattner W, Fraumeni JF, et al., Tritiated thymidine (ϕ_p, ϕ_h) labeling distribution as a marker for hereditary predisposition to colon cancer. *Cancer Res* 1983; 43:1899–1904.

ϕ_h. Graphs of (ϕ_p,ϕ_h) are essentially the complemented integrated probability distributions of the ϕ_h values for the population, with the ordinate defining the fractile axis for the (ϕ_p,ϕ_h) graph. For the colon, (ϕ_p,ϕ_h) graphs clearly separated populations affected by and at risk of familial polyposis and familial colon cancer from populations derived from cancer-free families believed to be at 12% risk and from other low-risk control groups in the general population (figs. 5.6 and 5.7) (Lipkin et al. 1983).

Probabilistic Method of Detecting Individuals at High and Low Risk

A probabilistic analysis was further developed for automatic risk categorization of individuals in both cancer-prone populations and the general population under dif-

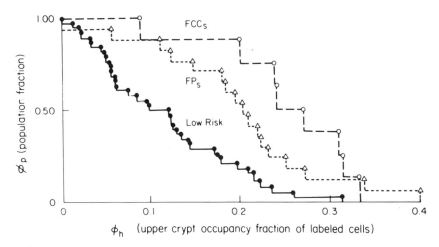

Fig. 5.6. Comparison of fractional distributions of ϕ_h between the high-risk populations (FP$_s$ and FCC$_s$) and the low-risk population. *Abscissa:* ϕ_h, the "high fraction" or upper-crypt occupancy fraction, i.e., the fraction of an individual's [³H]dThd-labeled epithelial cells found in the upper 40% of the crypt, including the luminal surface. *Ordinate:* ϕ_p, the fraction of all individuals in a given population whose ϕ_h values equal or exceed the abscissa value. Reprinted from Lipkin M, Blattner W, Fraumeni JF, et al., Tritiated thymidine (ϕ_p, ϕ_h) labeling distribution as a marker for hereditary predisposition to colon cancer. *Cancer Res* 1983; 43:1899–1904.

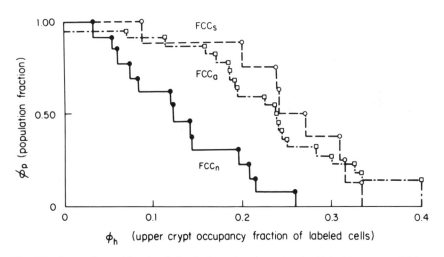

Fig. 5.7. Comparison of fractional distribution of ϕ_h between the high-risk groups (FCC$_s$ and FCC$_a$) previously affected with familial colon cancer and risk of familial colon cancer, respectively, and cancer-free family branches (FCC$_n$). *Abscissa:* ϕ_h, the "high fraction" or upper-crypt occupancy fraction, i.e., the fraction of an individual's [³H]dThd-labeled epithelial cells found in the upper 40% of the crypt, including the luminal surface. *Ordinate:* ϕ_p, the fraction of all individuals in a given population whose measured ϕ_h values equal or exceed the abscissa value. Reprinted from Lipkin M, Blattner W, Fraumeni JF, et al., Tritiated thymidine (ϕ_p, ϕ_h) labeling distribution as a marker for hereditary predisposition to colon cancer. *Cancer Res* 1983; 43: 1899–1904.

ferent dietary and environmental exposures (Lipkin et al. 1984). This analysis is available for further comparison of modifications induced by agents administered to inhibit neoplasia. Using this method, each subject's microautoradiographic epithelial cell–labeling pattern was quantitated for its degree of similarity to the labeling patterns of high- and low-risk reference populations. For each subject, linear scores, a prognostic index, and a relative risk were measured. Application of the method to various diseases of the colon revealed (Lipkin et al. 1984) that 78 individuals who had familial polyposis or were at low risk were classified correctly with 71% sensitivity and 70% specificity; 47 high- and low-risk subjects from nonpolyposis colon cancer kindreds were classified correctly with 92% sensitivity and 88% specificity. Fifty-three subjects at 50% risk were largely bimodally distributed to nearly zero or full risk (fig. 5.8).

Labeling Index Profiles over Colonic Crypt Compartments

This analytical approach was applied to measure the biomarker of cell proliferation during dietary intervention (Lipkin et al. 1985). An increased intake of dietary fat has been associated with increased colon cancer in high-risk geographic regions (Segi and Kurihara 1972; Doll and Peto 1981). In animal studies, dietary fat ap-

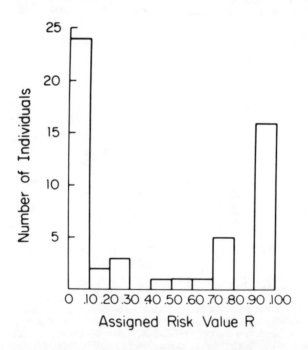

Fig. 5.8. Histogram showing the distribution of assigned risk values (*R*) derived from [³H]dThd cell-labeling patterns of individuals believed to be at 50% risk of familial colon cancer. Reprinted from Lipkin M, Blattner WA, Gardner EJ, et al., Classification and risk assessment of individuals with familial polyposis, Gardner's syndrome, and familial non-polyposis colon cancer from [³H]dThd-labeling patterns in colonic epithelial cells. *Cancer Res* 1984; 44:4201–4207.

peared to act as a promoter of colon carcinogenesis (Newmark, Wargovich, and Bruce 1984). Direct instillation of bile acids (Wargovich et al. 1983) or fatty acids (Wargovich, Eng, and Newmark 1984) into rodents was shown to be irritating and toxic to the colon, resulting in a compensatory increase in the proliferation of colon epithelial cells; these damaging effects were reduced by oral administration of calcium. A mechanism has been proposed to explain the interactions of dietary fat, phosphate, and calcium on colon cancer (Newmark, Wargovich, and Bruce 1984), and it was suggested that putative adverse effects of dietary fat on colon epithelium in humans might be modified by increased dietary intake of calcium.

We recently studied the proliferation of colon epithelial cells in the colonic mucosa of subjects from a population previously identified to be at high risk of familial colon cancer, before and after oral dietary supplementation with calcium carbonate (Lipkin and Newmark 1985). Patterns of cell proliferation were defined by subdividing the colonic crypt into longitudinal compartments and comparing the numbers and fractions of [³H]dThd-labeled epithelial cells in the various compartments. Before dietary supplementation with calcium, the profile of proliferating epithelial cells in the colonic crypts was comparable to that previously observed for individuals affected by familial colon cancer. After calcium supplementation, epithelial cell proliferation was significantly reduced, yielding an altered colonic-crypt profile approaching that previously observed in subjects at low risk of colon cancer. The findings indicated that oral calcium induced a more quiescent proliferative equilibrium in the colonic mucosa of high-risk individuals, similar to that observed for persons at low risk of colon cancer (table 5.1).

Recently, Garland et al. (1985) reported that the risk of colon cancer in humans decreased with increased dietary calcium intake. In our study, the amount of calcium ingested was within the range studied by Garland (Garland et al. 1985) as related to the lowest colon cancer risk. Thus, according to these recent reports, high calcium intake in humans may be associated both with modification of cell proliferation in colonic crypts and the incidence of colon cancer in humans.

CONCLUSION

Current findings thus indicate that increased cell proliferation occurs in diseases of the gastrointestinal tract that are accompanied by increased frequencies of cancer; a more quiescent proliferative equilibrium in the epithelial lining of the gastrointestinal tract is accompanied by decreased risk. Accompanying these changes are other modifications of cell differentiation and maturation that are beginning to be identified.

The possibility of inhibiting the development of human tumors by dietary intervention is an important topic for current studies. Measurements of cell proliferation and differentiation are beginning to be applied to clinical trials with this objective, as illustrated above. Since it is now possible to carry out small pilot studies to measure whether modifications of cell proliferation and differentiation occur as a result of dietary intervention, initial studies of this type are easier to carry out than before. If a particular intervention modality appears to be useful in pilot studies, then mea-

Table 5.1. *Proliferation Patterns of [^{3}H]dThd-Labeled Epithelial Cells in Colonic Crypts for a Group of 10 Subjects Before and After Dietary Calcium Supplementation*

Proliferation Parameter Analyzed	Before Calcium Supplementation	After Calcium Supplementation
Integer cell findings, by crypt compartment (total cells, labeled cells)		
Compartment 1 totals	3,896, 810	3,950, 600[a]
Compartment 2 totals	4,149, 1,105	4,149, 729[a]
Compartment 3 totals	4,107, 816	4,146, 416[a]
Compartment 4 totals	4,149, 487	4,140, 229[a]
Compartment 5 totals	4,324, 184	4,296, 101[a]
Labeling index (fraction of epithelial cells found to be labeled) by crypt compartment (mean [SE])		
Compartment 1 totals	0.2148 (0.03)	0.1526 (0.02)[b]
Compartment 2 totals	0.2661 (0.05)	0.1733 (0.02)[b]
Compartment 3 totals	0.2011 (0.03)	0.0985 (0.01)[c]
Compartment 4 totals	0.1194 (0.02)	0.0565 (0.01)[d]
Compartment 5 totals	0.0429 (0.01)	0.0254 (0.01)
Compartments 4 and 5 Combined	0.0804 (0.01)	0.0407 (0.01)[c]
whole crypt (all compartments combined)	0.1671 (0.02)	0.1003 (0.01)[e]

Source: Lipkin and Newmark 1985.
[a]Significantly reduced after calcium supplementation (χ^2, $p < 0.001$).
[b]Significantly modified after calcium supplementation (t test, $p < 0.10$).
[c]Significantly reduced after calcium supplementation (t test, $p < 0.02$).
[d]Significantly reduced after calcium supplementation (t test, $p < 0.004$).
[e]Significantly reduced after calcium supplementation (t test, $p < 0.04$).

surements in larger numbers of participants for longer durations can be attempted. Further studies involving the application of intermediate biomarkers to measure the effects of nutritional intervention will eventually indicate whether we can improve our ability to inhibit human gastrointestinal tumor development.

ACKNOWLEDGMENTS

The various projects reported here were funded by American Cancer Society Grant SIG-7, Grant R0140876 and Institutional Grant 08748 from the National Cancer Institute, and by a grant from the National Dairy Board administered in cooperation with the National Dairy Council. Ms. Rosemarie Petras, Peggy Monaghan, and Loretta Ayanian assisted in carrying out the projects.

REFERENCES

Bleiberg H, Mainguet P, Galand P. 1972. Cell renewal in familial polyposis: Comparison between polyps and adjacent healthy mucosa. *Gastroenterology* 63:240–245.

Castrup HJ, Fuchs K. 1974. Cell renewal in inflammatory changes of the gastric mucosa. *Dtsch Med Wochenschr* 99:892–895.

Correa P, Cuello C, Duque E, et al. 1976. Gastric cancer in Colombia. I-III. *JNCI* 57: 1015–1035.

Deschner EE, Lipkin M. 1970. Study of human rectal epithelial cells in vitro. III. RNA, protein and DNA synthesis in polyps and adjacent mucosa. *JNCI* 44:175–185.

Deschner EE, Winawer SJ, Lipkin M. 1972. Patterns of nucleic acid and protein synthesis in normal human gastric mucosa and atrophic gastritis. *JNCI* 48:1567–1574.

Deschner EE, Long FC, Hakissian M, et al. 1983. Differential susceptibility of AKR, C57BL/6J, and CF1 mice to 1,2-dimethylhydrazine–induced colonic tumor formation predicted by proliferative characteristics of colonic epithelial cells. *JNCI* 70:279–282.

Doll R, Peto R. 1981. The causes of cancer: Quantitative estimates of avoidable risks of cancer in the United States today. *JNCI* 66:1191–1308.

Garland C, Shekelle RB, Barrett-Conner E. et al. 1985. Dietary vitamin D and calcium risk of colorectal cancer: A 19 year prospective study in men. *Lancet* 1:307–309.

Hansen PH, Pedersen T, Larsen JK. 1975. A method to study cell proliferation kinetics in human gastric mucosa. *Gut* 16:23–27.

Herbst JJ, Berenson MM, Wiser WC, et al. 1976. Cell proliferation in Barrett's esophageal epithelium (abstract). *Clin Res* 24:168A.

Ismail-Beigi F, Horton PF, Pope CE. 1970. Histological consequences of gastroesophageal reflux in man. *Gastroenterology* 58:163–174.

Ismail-Beigi F, Pope CE. 1974. Distribution of the histological changes of gastroesophageal reflux in the distal esophagus of man. *Gastroenterology* 66:1109–1113.

Iwana T, Utsunomiya J, Sasaki J. 1977. Epithelial cell kinetics in the crypts of familial polyposis of colon. *Jpn J Surg* 7:230–234.

Lipkin M. 1974. Phase 1 and phase 2 proliferative lesions of colonic epithelial cells in diseases leading to colonic cancer. *Cancer* 43:878–888.

Lipkin M, Blattner W, Fraumeni JF, et al. 1983. Tritiated thymidine (ϕ_p,ϕ_h) labeling distribution as a marker for hereditary predisposition to colon cancer. *Cancer Res* 43: 1899–1904.

Lipkin M, Blattner WA, Gardner EJ, et al. 1984. Classification and risk assessment of individuals with familial polyposis, Gardner syndrome and familial non-polyposis colon cancer from [^{3}H]dThd-labeling patterns in colonic epithelial cells. *Cancer Res* 44:4201–4207.

Lipkin M, Correa P, Mikol YB, et al. 1985b. Proliferative and antigenic modifications in epithelial cells in chronic atrophic gastritis. *JNCI* 75:613–619.

Lipkin M, Newmark H. 1985. Effect of added dietary calcium on colonic epithelial-cell proliferation in subjects at high risk for familial colonic cancer. *N Engl J Med* 313: 1381–1384.

Lipkin M, Uehara K, Winawer S, et al. 1985a. Seventh-Day Adventist vegetarians have a quiescent proliferative activity in colonic mucosa. *Cancer Lett* 26:139–144.

Livstone EM, Sheahan DG, Behar J. 1977. Studies of esophageal epithelial cell proliferation in patients with reflux esophagitis. *Gastroenterology* 73:1315–1319.

Muñoz N, Lipkin M, Crespi M, et al. 1985. Proliferative abnormalities of the oesophageal epithelium of Chinese populations at high and low risk for oesophageal cancer. *Int J Cancer* 36:187–189.

Newmark HL, Wargovich MJ, Bruce WR. 1984. Colon cancer and dietary fat, phosphate and calcium: A hypothesis. *JNCI* 72:1323–1325.

Naef AP, Savary M, Ozzello L. 1975. Columnar-lined lower esophagus: An acquired lesion with malignant predisposition. Report on 140 cases of Barrett's esophagus with 12 adenocarcinomas. *Thorac Cardiovasc Surg* 70:826–835.

Rubio CA, Lagerlof B. 1983. Epithelial lesions antedating esophageal carcinoma. I. Histological study in mice. *Pathol Res Pract* 176:269–275.

Segi M, Kurihara M. 1972. Cancer mortality for selected sites in 24 countries. No. 6 (1966–67). *Japanese Cancer Society.*

Terpstra OT, van Blankenstein M, Dees J, et al. 1986. Abnormal cell proliferation in the entire colonic mucosa in patients with colon adenomas or colon cancer. *Gastroenterology* 90 (part 2): 1662.

Thurnherr N, Deschner EE, Stonehill EH, et al. 1973. Induction of adenocarcinomas of the colon in mice by weekly injections of 1,2-dimethylhydrazine. *Cancer Res* 33:940–945.

Wargovich MJ, Eng VWS, Newmark HL, et al. 1983. Calcium ameliorates the toxic effect in deoxycholic acid on colonic epithelium. *Carcinogenesis* 4:1205–1207.

Wargovich MJ, Eng VWS, Newmark HL. 1984. Calcium inhibits the damaging and compensating proliferative effects of fatty acids on mouse colon epithelium. *Cancer Lett* 23:253–258.

Winawer SJ, Lipkin M. 1969. Cell proliferation kinetics in the gastrointestinal tract of man. IV. Cell renewal in the intestinalized gastric mucosa. *JNCI* 42:9–17.

Annual Clinical Conference on Cancer, Vol. 30
Gastrointestinal Cancer: Current Approaches to Diagnosis and Treatment
© 1988 by The University of Texas System Cancer Center

6. Growth Factors and Colon Cancer

Bruce M. Boman, Patrice Lointier, and David M. Wildrick

The major factors underlying the uncontrolled growth of cancer appear to be altera-tions in cellular response to growth factors and to hormones. Such alterations can occur at four levels: (1) activation of autologous growth-factor synthesis (autocrine production), (2) resistance to natural growth-inhibitory factors, (3) abnormal syn-thesis/regulation of receptors for circulating hormones or growth factors, or (4) ac-tivation of a growth factor–related signal pathway such as through oncogene ex-pression. In this chapter we examine alterations that can occur at each of these levels (see fig. 6.1).

Specific growth factors that are produced by colon carcinomas include transform-ing growth factor (TGF alpha) and insulin-like growth factor-II. In addition, human chorionic gonadotropin (hCG) is a hormone produced ectopically by some colon carcinomas. The production of these factors may occur in an autocrine-related manner.

At the second level, it has been reported that TGF beta, a different type of trans-forming growth factor, brings about the growth inhibition of several epithelial cell types, including some of those in cultured colon carcinoma cell lines. However, other colon carcinoma lines are resistant to its inhibitory action.

Evidence for abnormal expression of receptors for circulating hormones has come from recent work on steroid hormone receptors. Receptors for estrogen, proges-terone, androgen, and glucocorticoid hormones have been detected in primary colon cancer tissue. Recent studies on the effects of these steroid hormones on a human colon carcinoma cell line suggest that some of them may affect the growth of colon carcinoma cells. Gastrin and insulin receptors also occur in human carcinoma cells, and the growth of such cells is stimulated by both gastrin and insulin.

Finally, recent work on oncogenes has shown increased expression of c-*myc* and c-*ras* in colon carcinomas. Several studies suggest that the expression of these on-cogene protein products may have a role in the normal intracellular growth factor–signal pathway. Therefore, oncogene activation in colon cancer cells may mimic the growth factor–related cellular response. Further molecular studies on the altera-tions in the growth factor–receptor signaling pathway should be helpful in under-standing the pathogenesis of colon cancer.

AUTOCRINE PRODUCTION OF GROWTH FACTORS

Autocrine secretion is defined as the ability of cells to produce their own growth factors and respond to them (see review by Goustin et al. 1986). It has been sug-

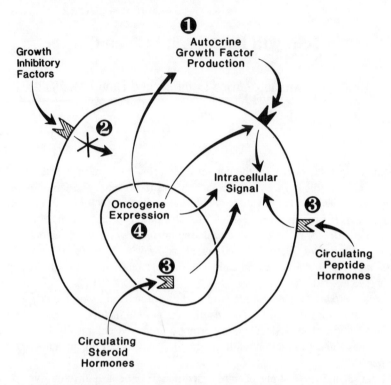

Fig. 6.1. Possible mechanisms that may give cancer cells a selective growth advantage: (1) autocrine production of growth-stimulatory factors, (2) resistance to growth-inhibitory factors, (3) abnormal expression or synthesis of receptors for circulating hormones, or (4) activation of a growth factor–related signal pathway through oncogene expression.

gested that the autonomous nature of cancer cells may be related to their endogenous production of polypeptide growth factors that act on their own functional external surface receptors. Autocrine-type growth factor production was identified by the ability of medium conditioned by cultured malignant cells to stimulate the anchorage-independent growth (in soft agar) in cells that are otherwise anchorage dependent. Initially, murine sarcoma virus–transformed cells were found to secrete such a growth factor, described as sarcoma growth factor (SGF) (DeLarco and Todaro 1978). Further studies showed that SGF is composed of two different growth factors that are now termed TGF alpha and TGF beta (Anzano et al. 1983). The fact that SGF was able to block the binding of a different substance, epidermal growth factor (EGF), to cells (Todaro, DeLarco, and Cohen 1976) suggested that the growth-stimulatory activity of SGF was somehow related to the action of EGF.

EGF was initially identified by Cohen (1962) as a protein important in the maturation of newborn mice. EGF is produced by several normal tissues, including the gastrointestinal tract, and is identical to urogastrone purified from human urine (Gregory 1975). Although tumors have not been found to produce EGF, this substance stimulates the growth of many types of cancer cells in vitro (Rose, Pruss, and Herschman 1975; Shipley et al. 1984; Singletary et al. 1987).

Transforming Growth Factor Alpha

TGF alpha is produced by a variety of malignant cells in vitro. The sequence of TGF alpha shows significant homology with that of EGF, and both factors are synthesized from precursor factors that require processing to become active (Marquardt et al. 1984). Early studies showed TGF alpha to be present only in embryonic tissues and placenta, which suggested that TGF alpha may be the embryonic form of EGF (Stromberg et al. 1982). However, more recent studies have revealed that TGF alpha is present in normal adult tissues, including human keratinocytes (Coffey et al. in press; Derynck et al. 1987). TGF alpha is defined in vitro by its ability to stimulate anchorage-independent growth of cells in soft agar. Both TGF alpha and EGF bind to a common cell-surface receptor and have identical biologic properties in vivo (Tam 1985). Because both EGF and TGF alpha are produced by normal adult tissues and bind to a common receptor, they may be involved in a coordinated regulatory mechanism of normal cell growth control. Cancer cells may gain a selective growth advantage through activation of autologous growth-factor synthesis, leading to enhanced or uncontrolled TGF alpha production.

Recent studies by Coffey, Shipley, and Moses (1986) showed that three poorly differentiated, human colon cancer cell lines—SW480, SW620, and WIDR—produced TGF-alpha-like activity in conditioned culture medium. Two of these cell lines possessed the ability to bind EGF specifically, but SW620 appeared to lack EGF receptors. The addition of exogenous EGF had no significant effect on the soft agar growth of these colon carcinoma cells. The production of TGF-alpha-like activity by colon cancer cell lines suggests that this growth factor may be functioning on the cells in an autocrine manner. The lack of response of these cells to exogenous EGF may be due to receptor occupancy by TGF alpha or to an activated intracellular TGF-alpha signal pathway. Further studies by Heilig et al. (1986) showed that TGF-alpha mRNA is expressed by primary colon cancer tissue but not by normal colonic epithelium. An EGF-related TGF has also been detected in the urine of patients with colon cancer (Sherwin et al. 1983).

Friedman et al. (1981) studied the effects of EGF on the in vitro growth of cultured human colonic epithelial cells from adenomas and found that the growth of cells from tubular adenomas was stimulated by EGF but that cells from villous adenomas were resistant to EGF. Willson et al. (1987) studied adenomatous cell lines in long-term culture and found that tubular, but not villous, adenoma cells require EGF for growth in vitro. These results suggest that cultured villous adenomatous cells are less dependent on EGF. Preliminary studies on primary adenomatous tissue showed TGF-alpha expression in villous adenomas that were analyzed (Heilig et al. 1986).

Brattain, Matthews, and Brattain (1986) and Boyd et al. (in press) studied the effect of EGF on 15 colon cancer cell lines that were classified into three groups on the basis of their biologic properties, including histology of xenografts, growth in soft agar, secretion of carcinoembryonic antigen (CEA), and growth rate in tissue culture. The groups (Brattain et al. 1984) were classified as most aggressive, un-differentiated (group I), least aggressive, well-differentiated (group III), and lines with intermediate properties relative to the other groups (group II). These results showed that the plating efficiency of the least aggressive, well-differentiated colon cancer lines was stimulated by EGF but that the most aggressive, undifferentiated colon cell lines were unaffected. Scatchard analysis by Wan, Brattain, and Yeoman (1986) showed that the number of receptors was greater in the least aggressive colon cancer lines than in the undifferentiated lines. These results suggest that the un-differentiated colon cancer lines have an activated EGF-related intracellular path-way or produce TGF alpha that binds to the EGF receptor in an autocrine manner, overriding the effect of exogenous EGF.

Human Chorionic Gonadotropin

The glycoprotein hormone hCG is composed of two subunits, alpha and beta (see review by Hussa 1981). The alpha subunit is necessary for biologic activity, and the beta subunit confers specificity for cell-surface receptor binding. hCG and the an-cestrally related luteinizing hormone bind to a common cell-surface receptor. Intact hCG has not been detected in active form in normal adult tissues and appears to be produced only by the placenta. Its primary function is to maintain the corpus luteum during pregnancy. hCG has also been found to have immunosuppressive properties (Bartocci et al. 1983). Recent studies show that hCG can also stimulate the in vitro growth of cells (Melmed and Braunstein 1983; Mukherjee and Das 1984).

On immunohistochemical analysis, approximately 40% of primary human colon carcinomas stained positive for beta hCG (Buckley and Fox 1979; Fukayama, Hayashi, and Koike 1987; Campo et al. 1987). Tumors that stained positive were more commonly located in the distal colon (Buckley and Fox 1979; Shousha et al. 1986). A small number of adenomas were studied and found to stain negatively. Recent studies have shown that the endocrine-like cells of normal colon were immunoreactive for alpha hCG but not beta hCG (Fukayama, Hayashi, and Koike 1987). Several other studies have shown that immunoreactive beta hCG is detectable in the sera of approximately 10% of patients with colon cancer (Rosen 1975).

We have studied six colon cancer cell lines and normal colonic epithelial cells (in culture) for the secretion of beta hCG into the conditioned medium (table 6.1). The cultured normal cells did not secrete detectable quantities of hCG, and the LoVo colon carcinoma cells produced only minimal amounts of hCG. However, the five SW colon cancer cell lines secreted detectable quantities of hCG. We have also found that hCG stimulates the growth of the cultured, normal colonic epithelial cells and the LoVo cell line (unpublished data), which suggests that ectopic hCG produc-tion in colon cancer may function in an autocrine fashion.

Insulin-like Growth Factors

Insulin-like growth factors (IGF) include IGF-I and IGF-II (see review by Goustin et al. 1986). Both these substances are members of the somatomedin family and are structurally related to insulin and produced by many fetal and adult tissues. IGF-I

Table 6.1. *Human Chorionic Gonadotropin in the Conditioned Media of Cultured Colon Cells*

Cell Line	Type	Beta hCG[a] (mIU/ml)
NCM 70	Normal epithelial cells	<1.0
LoVo	Adenocarcinoma	2.65
SW48	Adenocarcinoma	64.0
SW480	Adenocarcinoma	44.3
SW1116	Adenocarcinoma	24.5
SW403	Adenocarcinoma	100.5
SW620	Adenocarcinoma	26.0

Abbreviation: hCG, human chorionic gonadotropin.

[a] Determined by radioimmunoassay.

Data presented by B. Boman at the Molecular Biology of Large Bowel Cancer Workshop (Organ Systems Program of NCI), Houston, Texas, May 1985.

corresponds to somatomedin C and IGF-II corresponds to somatomedin A. It has been proposed that IGF-I is the adult somatomedin and IGF-II is the embryonic form. Because the IGFs stimulate cell growth in culture, it is hypothesized that they may function in an autocrine fashion in malignant cells.

A recent study by Tricoli et al. (1986) examined the expression of IGFs in colon tissues. The results showed that normal adult colonic mucosa had low levels of IGF-I and IGF-II expression but that expression of both was elevated in several colon tumors. Interestingly, IGF-II expression was more often enhanced in tumors from the rectosigmoid regions, particularly in Dukes stage C lesions in this location. Possibly a stage-specific mechanism is responsible for this enhanced expression.

GROWTH-INHIBITORY FACTORS

It has been postulated that the normal control of cell growth may involve both stimulatory growth factors and inhibitory growth factors so that the regulation of cell growth represents a balance between positive and negative cellular signaling (Goustin et al. 1986). Several growth-inhibitory factors have been identified that act on nontransformed and malignant cells in vitro. Levine et al. (1985) described a polypeptide synthesized by the Moser human colon cancer cell line that inhibits the growth of the better-differentiated colon cancer cell lines. Characterization of this substance is in progress, but the preliminary results indicate that it is different from TGF beta, another factor that has growth-inhibitory activity.

Transforming Growth Factor Beta

TGF beta is a relatively ubiquitous protein that is detected in most normal tissues (Goustin et al. 1986). It appears to be synthesized from an inactive precursor substance so that an activation mechanism may be an important regulatory step. TGF beta is structurally unrelated to EGF and does not compete with EGF for binding to specific cell-surface receptors. It has a mitogenic effect on a variety of cell types, including fibroblasts. This mitogenic activity in AKR-2B cells is believed to occur indirectly by inducing the synthesis of another growth substance, platelet-derived growth factor (PDGF) (Leof et al. 1986). The growth-stimulatory effect of TGF beta appears to be direct in cultured mesothelial cells (Gabrielson et al. 1986). TGF beta has also been shown to inhibit 3T3 T-mesenchymal stem-cell differentiation (Sparks and Scott 1986).

In a variety of other cell types, including several epithelial cell types, TGF beta is growth inhibitory. It inhibits the growth of cultured normal human prokeratinocytes but does not affect a squamous carcinoma cell line (Shipley et al. 1986). TGF beta also induces differentiation of cultured, normal, human bronchial epithelial cells but not of bronchogenic carcinoma cell lines (Masui et al. 1986). Therefore, researchers have proposed that the loss of the inhibitory response to TGF beta may, in some circumstances, give transformed cells a selective growth advantage (Goustin et al. 1986). The loss of the inhibitory response may result in part from the inability of a cell to activate the precursor TGF beta (Moses et al. 1985). Another possibility is that a cell may lose cell-surface receptors for TGF beta and therefore become unresponsive to this factor.

Coffey, Shipley, and Moses (1986) showed that colon cancer cell lines SW480, SW620, and WIDR secrete TGF beta into growth medium. In this study, SW620 and WIDR cells possess specific binding activity for TGF beta, but SW480 cells appear to lack these receptors. Exogenous beta TGF did not have any effect on the soft agar growth of these cell lines. Therefore, the colon cancer lines in these studies appear to have lost their response to TGF beta.

Another recent study by Brattain and coworkers (Hoosein et al. in press) showed that the growth of the Moser colon cancer line is inhibited by TGF beta in a nontoxic and dose-dependent manner. Binding studies revealed that these cells possess TGF beta-specific receptors. Treatment of Moser cells with exogenous TGF beta induced a differentiated cellular morphology and increased production of fibronectin. Further studies on several other colon cancer cell lines, using the previously described classification system (Brattain et al. 1984), showed that the aggressive undifferentiated colon cancer cell lines were resistant to the inhibitory effects of TGF beta (Levine et al. 1986). In contrast, the least aggressive, well-differentiated cell lines were sensitive to TGF beta–induced growth inhibition. These results, together with those cited for TGF alpha, show that the aggressive undifferentiated colon cancer lines are more growth factor-independent and also are resistant to growth-inhibitory factors in vitro.

HORMONE RECEPTORS

A third way that a tumor may gain a selective growth advantage is through the abnormal synthesis of receptors for peptide or steroid hormones. One possibility is the inappropriate expression of hormone receptors that do not occur in normal colonic epithelial cells. In this manner the colon carcinoma may respond to circulating hormones, resulting in abnormal cell proliferation. Also, it is possible that hormone receptors that are present in normal cells are abnormally regulated or structurally

Table 6.2. *Steroid Receptors in Colon Cancer (N = 40)*

Receptors	Carcinomas	Adjacent Normal Mucosa
ER$^+$ PGR$^+$	6	2
ER$^+$ PGR$^-$	3	1
ER$^-$ PGR$^+$	10	2
ER$^-$ PGR$^-$	21	35

Source: Lointier et al. 1985.
Abbreviations: ER, estrogen receptor; PGR, progesterone receptor.

modified in the colon cancer cell so that its response to circulating hormones is altered. Recent research on steroid and polypeptide hormones and colon cancer appears to support this mechanism.

Steroid Receptors

Several studies have shown that colon carcinomas often contain detectable estrogen, progesterone, and androgen receptors. In a recent study, Lointier et al. (1985) showed that estrogen, progesterone, and androgen receptors can be detected in primary colon carcinomas by a competitive binding assay (table 6.2). A smaller proportion of the adjacent mucosa samples were also positive for these receptors, whereas biopsy results from normal mucosa from 10 patients without cancer were negative. This indicates that colon carcinomas are able to produce steroid hormone receptors that are not expressed in the normal tissue of patients without cancer. The presence of steroid receptors in adjacent normal mucosa of patients with colon cancer indicates that the expression of steroid receptors may occur at an early or premalignant step in colon carcinogenesis.

To understand the role of steroid hormones in the growth of colon cancer, we have studied the LoVo colon carcinoma cell line. Scatchard analysis revealed the presence of relatively high quantitites of estrogen, androgen, progesterone, and glucocorticoid receptors with high specificity in LoVo cells (table 6.3). Yang (1987) has also detected estrogen receptors in several colon cancer cell lines, including LoVo.

To determine whether the expression of these receptors might be associated with a cellular response to steroids, we analyzed the growth effects of these steroid hor-

Table 6.3. *Steroid Receptors in LoVo Cells*

Receptor	Protein (FMOL/MG)	K$_D$ ($\times$ 10^{-9} M)
Estrogen	139	1.8
Progesterone	35	1.0
Androgen	14	0.5
Glucocorticoid	31	0.62

Note: Determined by Scatchard analysis.

mones on LoVo cells. The addition of a low concentration of estrogen analogues (10^{-11} M) stimulated slightly (10% to 15%) the LoVo cell growth (Lointier et al. 1986). A supraphysiologic concentration of estrogen analogues inhibited LoVo cell growth cultured in serum-free medium (Lointier et al. 1986). An independent study by Yang (1987) also showed a stimulation (25%) of LoVo cell growth at a slightly higher estrogen concentration (10^{-8} M) and a similar inhibition of LoVo cell growth at supraphysiologic estrogen concentrations. Androgen and progesterone did not affect the growth of LoVo cells, but glucocorticoid hormones (10^{-9} to 10^{-7} M) stimulated their growth (Lointier et al. 1986). These results show that a human colon cancer cell line has detectable steroid receptors and that these cells are responsive to estrogen analogues and glucocorticoid hormones. We hope that these in vitro studies will help to define the role of steroid hormones in colon cancer growth in vivo.

Polypeptide Hormone Receptors

Alterations in polypeptide hormone receptors, such as those for insulin and transferrin, may also be important in the growth of colon cancer. Wong and Holdaway (1985) studied normal and malignant colon tissues and reported a similar binding specificity for labeled insulin, indicating that the biochemical properties of the receptor are not altered during carcinogenesis. However, insulin receptors in malignant colon tissue showed less sensitivity to down-regulation by ambient insulin than did receptors in normal colon mucosal cells. This suggests that insulin-receptor regulation is altered in colon cancer cells.

Brattain's group (Brattain et al. 1984) studied the in vitro growth requirements of colon cancer lines for insulin and transferrin (Brattain, Matthews, and Brattain 1986; Boyd et al. in press). The least aggressive colon cancer cell lines were dependent upon insulin and transferrin for growth in vitro; however, the most aggressive colon cancer cell lines were able to grow in the absence of these substances. These results correlate with the EGF studies in that the most aggressive colon cancer cell lines possess mechanisms that override their requirement for exogenous growth factors and hormones.

The possible clinical relevance of transferrin- and insulin-receptor production in colon cancer is related to liver metastases. Transferrin is produced by hepatocytes (Struck et al. 1978), and the concentration of insulin in the liver is up to 10 times greater than in peripheral circulation because of the portal circulation from the pancreas (Felig, Havel, and Smith 1981). The fact that colon carcinomas show significant variability in their metastatic potential (Miller et al. 1985; Giavazzi et al. 1986) and in the growth rate of hepatic metastases (Wagner et al. 1984) may be a consequence of the presence of varying numbers of transferrin and insulin receptors on malignant colon cells.

Another example of a polypeptide hormone that may be important in colon cancer growth is gastrin. This hormone has trophic effects on normal colon epithelial cells in vivo and in vitro (Sirinek, Levine, and Moyer 1985; Johnson and Guthrie 1976) and also on colon cancer cells (Sirinek, Levine, and Moyer 1985). Gastrin stimulates the growth of the LoVo colon cancer cell line (Kusyk, McNiel, and Johnson 1986), and administration of gastrin to mice increased the growth of a transplantable colon cancer (Singh et al. 1986; Winsett et al. 1986). This growth was later inhibited by proglumide, a gastrin-receptor antagonist (Beauchamp et al. 1985). When hypergastrinemia was induced by antral exclusion in another animal model, the carcinogenic effect of 1,2 dimethylhydrazine (DMH) was augmented (McGregor et al. 1983; Karlin et al. 1985). The growth of colon cancer xenografts increased after the induction of hypergastrinemia, and secretin inhibited this increased growth response (Elwyn, Jones, and Romsdahl 1985). Another study showed that gastrin-induced colon carcinoma cells maintain high levels of gastrin receptors that were lacking in the absence of gastrin (Singh et al. 1985). These results support the possibility that abnormal gastrin-receptor expression affects the growth of colon carcinoma cells.

ONCOGENES

The cellular response to growth factors may also be altered by perturbing the growth factor–receptor intracellular signal pathway by activating or enhancing the expression of oncogenes. Oncogenes were initially described as the transforming genes of retroviruses. However, further studies have shown that cellular progenitors of these genes, termed proto-oncogenes, are also expressed in normal cells and play critical roles in cell division, growth control, and differentiation. Evidence now shows that proto-oncogene expression is important in the normal cellular response to growth factors as discussed below. The hypothesis that alterations in these genes (activation) could be important in malignant transformation was initially derived from studies of transfection of tumor cell DNA into NIH 3T3 cells. These cells can be altered from low to high tumorigenicity by a single activated proto-oncogene.

The association between oncogene expression and growth-control regulation has been studied using cultured cells characterized as having exogenous growth factor–controlled proliferation. Several investigators have reported that growth-stimulatory factors (EGF, PDGF, and serum) increase the transcription of the proto-oncogenes c-*myc* and c-*fos* (Greenberg and Ziff 1984; Kelly et al. 1983; Mueller et al. 1984; Armelin et al. 1984; Ran et al. 1986). Expression of c-*myc*, c-*fos*, and c-*ras* appears to be regulated in a cell cycle–dependent manner, increasing transiently during the G_1 phase (Campsi et al. 1984; Mulcahy, Smith, and Stacey 1985). Transfection of some cells with c-*ras* seems to bypass the requirement for exogenous EGF and is associated with enhanced production of TGF alpha in mouse mammary epithelial cells (Saloman et al. 1987). Sorrentino et al. (1986) revealed that c-*myc* transfection enhanced the response of cells to PDGF. Therefore, proto-oncogene expression seems to be important in the normal control of cellular growth, and oncogene activation or enhanced expression may mimic or enhance the response to growth factors, thus possibly significantly reducing the need for growth factors.

The cellular function of some of the oncogene products has been defined. The c-*sis* oncogene product is the beta chain of PDGF (Doolittle et al. 1983), which in some malignant cells probably acts in an autocrine manner. Elevated expression of c-*sis* has not been identified in colon carcinomas (Spandidos and Kerr 1984). Other oncogenes have sequence homology with genes that code for hormone receptors; these include c-*erb* B1 with the EGF receptor (Downward, Schlessinger, and Waterfield 1984), c-*erb* A with steroid and thyroid hormone receptors (Green et al. 1986; Weinberger et al. 1986; Sap et al. 1986), and the c-*src* oncogene family with the tyrosine kinase domain of the insulin receptor. The c-*erb* B1/EGF receptor has not been found to be overexpressed in human colon cancer lines (Wan, Brattain, and Yeoman 1986) or amplified in human colon carcinomas in vivo (Yokota et al. 1986). The enzymatic activity of the phosphoprotein product of the c-*src* oncogene is activated in the majority of colon carcinomas analyzed (Bolen et al. 1987). This activation is not the result of increased expression of c-*src* but rather is due to deregulation of this phosphoprotein's tyrosine kinase activity. The homology of these oncogene products with growth factor–receptor proteins supports the concept that their function is directly related to growth factor–signaling pathways. It seems likely that activation of these oncogenes in colon cancer cells may give them a selective growth advantage.

The cellular functions of many of the other oncogene products are not as well defined. The c-*ras* oncogene product is located in the cytoplasm and may affect a transmembrane signaling mechanism by activating phospholipase (Preiss et al. 1986). Activation of the c-*ras* oncogenes in some cells is associated with the acquisition of anchorage-independent growth (Land, Parada, and Weinberg 1983). The c-*myc* oncogene product is a nuclear protein, and its activation appears to be associated with cellular immortalization (Land, Parada, and Weinberg 1983). In most studies the activation of *ras* or *myc* alone was insufficient to achieve tumorigenic conversion when untransformed diploid recipient cells were employed for transfection. However, the *myc* gene was shown to complement the *ras* oncogene in producing a fully malignant phenotype in some normal cells (Land, Parada, and Weinberg 1983).

c-*ras* Oncogene

Oncogene activation in malignant cells may occur through gene mutation or enhanced expression. Mutation of the c-*ras* oncogene has been reported in several colon cancer cell lines (Der and Cooper 1983; Greenhalgh and Kinsella 1985; McCoy, Bargmann, and Weinberg 1984; Capon et al. 1983) and has been found in a significant proportion of primary colonic carcinoma tissue (Feinberg et al. 1983; McCoy et al. 1983; Pulciani et al. 1982; Forrester et al. 1987; Bos et al. 1987). Several investigators have also reported enhanced expression of *ras* oncogenes in primary colon carcinomas as compared to normal colon mucosa (Slamon et al. 1984; Kerr et al. 1985; Gallick et al. 1985; Thor et al. 1984; Spandidos and Kerr 1984; Hand et al. 1984). Feinberg and Vogelstein (1983) have shown that the *ras* oncogenes are hypomethylated in colon carcinomas, which may be related to enhanced *ras* expression. Normal colonic mucosa has low levels of *ras* expression, and its crypts stain uniformly for *ras* by immunohistochemistry techniques (Kerr et al. 1985). Some studies have reported increased *ras* expression in adenomas (Spandidos and Kerr 1984; Williams et al. 1985), but others have not confirmed this (Thor et al. 1984). A property unique to colon carcinomas (Gallick et al. 1985; 1986) is that their metastases appear to have lower levels of *ras* expression than do their early-stage carcinomas.

c-*myc* Oncogene

Enhanced expression of the c-*myc* oncogene has been found in several colon cancer cell lines (Schwab et al. 1986; Untawale, Blick, and Pathak 1986; Yoshimoto, Hirohashi, and Fekiya 1986). The enhanced expression of c-*myc* in some of these cell lines was associated with gene amplification (Lin et al. 1985; Alitalo et al. 1983; Untawale, Blick, and Pathak 1986), and the CoLo 320 cell line had a c-*myc* gene rearrangement (Schwab et al. 1986). The *myc* oncogene has also been found to have higher expression in colon cancers than in normal mucosa (Erisman et al. 1985; Calabretta et al. 1985; Yander et al. 1985; Untawale, Blick, and Pathak 1986). Two-fold to five-fold amplification of the *myc* locus was observed in two of nine primary human colon tumors relative to adjacent normal colon tissue controls (Alexander, Buxbaum, and Raicht 1986). The c-*myc* gene is believed to play a role in cell division and differentiation (Stewart 1986).

Normal colonic mucosa expresses the *myc* oncogene product with maximal immunohistochemical staining in the mid-zone of the crypts, implying involvement of this oncogene product in crypt maturation, a differentiation process (Stewart et al. 1986). Adenomatous polyps stain intensely for *myc* in areas of dysplasia correlating with increased cell proliferation (Stewart et al. 1986). The more differentiated colon carcinomas have been reported to stain more intensely for the *myc* oncogene product than anaplastic tumors (Stewart et al. 1986). Enhanced *myc* expression is more common in tumors located in the left colon (Rothberg et al. 1985). Possibly an anatomic site-specific mechanism is responsible for this enhanced expression.

Because the c-*ras* and c-*myc* oncogenes are expressed in normal colonic mucosa, they are probably involved in the regulation of normal colonic epithelial cell growth. Enhanced expression or activation of c-*ras* and c-*myc* oncogenes in premalignant or malignant colonic tumors suggests a role in colon carcinogenesis. This may result in perturbations of the growth factor–receptor intracellular signal pathway, thus giving a malignant colon cell a selective growth advantage. Further studies in this area should help to define whether these oncogenes play a primary role in malignant transformation, progression, and metastasis in colon tumorigenesis.

SUMMARY

Colon carcinoma cells may gain a selective growth advantage through alterations that occur in the cellular response to growth factors. This may occur at any or all of the four levels discussed in this chapter (see fig. 1): (1) autocrine production of growth-stimulatory factors, (2) resistance to growth-inhibitory factors, (3) abnormal synthesis or regulation of hormone/growth-factor receptors, and (4) oncogene activation that may mimic growth factor–signaling pathways.

Further investigation of these mechanisms should aid in our understanding of the steps involved in colon tumorigenesis, including malignant transformation, pro-

82 BRUCE M. BOMAN ET AL.

gression, and metastasis. Studies in this area may also be clinically useful in terms of identifying subtypes of colon cancer, predicting the biologic behavior of colon carcinomas, and pinpointing potential therapeutic targets.

REFERENCES

Alexander RJ, Buxbaum JN, Raicht RF. 1986. Oncogene alterations in primary human colon tumors. *Gastroenterology* 91:1503–1510.

Alitalo K, Schwab M, Lin C, et al. 1983. Homogeneously staining chromosomal regions contain amplified copies of an abundantly expressed cellular oncogene (c-*myc*) in malignant neuroendocrine cells from a human colon carcinoma. *Proc Natl Acad Sci USA* 80:1707–1711.

Anzano MA, Roberts AB, Smith JM, et al. 1983. Sarcoma growth factor from conditioned medium of transformed cells is composed of both type alpha and beta transforming growth factors. *Proc Natl Acad Sci USA* 80:6264–6268.

Armelin HA, Armelin MCS, Kelly K, et al. 1984. Functional role for c-*myc* in mitogenic response to platelet-derived growth factor. *Nature* 310:655–660.

Bartocci A, Welker RD, Schlick E, et al. 1983. Immunosuppressive activity of human chorionic gonadotropin preparations *in vivo:* Evidence for gonadal dependence. Cell Immunol 82:334–342.

Beauchamp RD, Townsend CM, Singh P, et al. 1985. Proglumide, a gastrin receptor antagonist, inhibits growth of colon cancer and enhances survival in mice. *Ann Surg* 202:303–308.

Bolen JB, Veillette A, Schwartz AM, et al. 1987. Activation of pp60[c-src] protein kinase activity in human colon carcinoma. *Proc Natl Acad Sci USA* 84:2251–2255.

Bos JL, Fearon ER, Hamilton SR, et al. 1987. Prevalence of *ras* gene mutations in human colorectal cancer. *Nature* 327:293–297.

Boyd D, Brattain DE, Matthews K, et al. In press. Two human intratumoral colon carcinoma cell lines have different growth requirements in monolayer and soft agarose. *Cancer Res.*

Brattain DE, Matthews MK, Brattain MG. 1986. Growth factor requirements of human colon carcinoma cells (abstract). *Proceedings of the American Association for Cancer Research* 27:42.

Brattain MG, Levine AE, Chakrabarty S, et al. 1984. Heterogeneity of human colon carcinoma. *Cancer Metastasis Rev* 3:177–191.

Buckley CH, Fox H. 1979. An immunohistochemical study of the significance of HCG secretion by large bowel adenocarcinomata. *J Clin Pathol* 32:368–372.

Calabretta B, Kaczmarek L, Ming PML, et al. 1985. Expression of c-*myc* and other cell cycle dependent genes in human colon neoplasia. *Cancer Res* 45:6000–6004.

Campo E, Palacin A, Benasco C, et al. 1987. Human chorionic gonadotropin in colorectal carcinoma. *Cancer* 59:1611–1616.

Campsi J, Gray HE, Pardee AB, et al. 1984. Cell-cycle control of c-*myc* but not c-*ras* expression is lost following chemical transformation. *Cell* 36:241–247.

Capon DJ, Seeburg PH, McGrath JP, et al. 1983. Activation of Ki-*ras*2 gene in human colon and lung carcinomas by two different point mutations. *Nature* 304:507–512.

Coffey RJ, Derynck R, Wilcox JN, et al. In press. Production and auto-induction of TGF alpha in human keratinocytes. *Nature.*

Coffey RJ, Shipley GD, Moses HL. 1986. Production of transforming growth factors by human colon cancer lines. *Cancer Res* 46:1164–1169.

Cohen S. 1962. Isolation of a mouse submaxillary gland protein accelerating incisor eruption and eyelid closing in the new-born animal. *J Biol Chem* 237:1555–1562.

DeLarco JE, Todaro GJ. 1978. Growth factors from murine sarcoma virus-transformed cells. *Proc Natl Acad Sci USA* 75:4001–4005.

Der CJ, Cooper GM. 1983. Altered gene products are associated with activation of cellular *ras*^k genes in human lung and colon carcinomas. *Cell* 32:201–208.

Derynck R, Bringman TS, Linquist PB, et al. 1987. Transforming growth factor alpha: Cellular expression and processing of the precursor and tissue specific distribution (abstract). *J Cell Biochem* 11A:4.

Doolittle RF, Hunkapiller MW, Hood LE, et al. 1983. Simian sarcoma virus onc gene v-*sis* is derived from the gene encoding a platelet-derived growth factor. *Science* 221:275–277.

Downward J, Schlessinger J, Waterfield MD. 1984. Close similarity of epidermal growth factor and v-*erb*B oncogene protein sequences. *Nature* 307:521–527.

Elwyn KE, Jones RD, Romsdahl MM. 1985. Inhibitory effects of secretin on gastrin-stimulated rat colon neoplasma. *Cancer* 55:1186–1189.

Erisman MD, Rothberg PG, Drehl RE, et al. 1985. Deregulation of c-*myc* is not accompanied by amplification or rearrangement of the gene. *Mol Cell Biol* 5:1969–1976.

Feinberg AP, Vogelstein B. 1983. Hypomethylation of *ras* oncogenes in primary human cancers. *Biochem Biophys Res Commun* 111:47–54.

Feinberg AP, Vogelstein B, Droller MJ, et al. 1983. Mutation affecting the 12th amino acid of the c-Ha-*ras* oncogene product occurs infrequently in human cancer. *Nature* 220:1175–1177.

Felig P, Havel RJ, Smith LH. 1981. Hormonal regulation. In *Pathophysiology: The Biologic Principles of Disease,* pp. 527–538. Philadelphia: W. B. Saunders.

Forrester K, Almoguerra C, Han K, et al. 1987. Detection of high incidence of K-*ras* oncogenes during human colon tumorigenesis. *Nature* 327:298–303.

Friedman EA, Higgins PJ, Lipkin M, et al. 1981. Tissue culture of human epithelial cells from benign colonic tumors. *In Vitro* 17:632–644.

Fukayama M, Hayashi Y, Koike M. 1987. Human chorionic gonadotropin in the rectosigmoid colon. *Am J Pathol* 127:83–89.

Gabrielson EW, Lechner JF, Gerwin BI, et al. 1986. Transforming growth factor type beta (TGF-beta), platelet-derived growth factor (PDGF), and epidermal growth factor (EGF) stimulate DNA synthesis in cultured human mesothelial cells (abstract). *Proceedings of the American Association for Cancer Research* 27:214.

Gallick GE, Kurzrock R, Gutterman JU. 1986. Expression of p21^ras gene products in fresh primary and metastatic human tumor tissue. In *Biochemistry and Molecular Biology of Cancer Metastasis,* K Lapis, LA Liotta, and AS Rabson, eds., pp. 65–72. Boston: Martinus Nijhoff.

Gallick GE, Kurzrock R, Kloetzer WS, et al. 1985. Expression of p21 *ras* in fresh primary and metastatic human colorectal tumors. *Proc Natl Acad Sci USA* 82:1795–1799.

Giavazzi R, Campbell DE, Jessup JM, et al. 1986. Metastatic behavior of tumor cells isolated from primary and metastatic human colorectal carcinomas implanted into different sites in nude mice. *Cancer Res* 46:1928–1933.

Goustin AS, Leof EB, Shipley GD, et al. 1986. Growth factors and cancer. *Cancer Res* 46:1015–1029.

Green S, Walter P, Kumar V, et al. 1986. Human estrogen receptor cDNA: Sequence, expression and homology of v-*erb*-A. *Nature* 320:134–139.

Greenberg ME, Ziff EB. 1984. Stimulation of 3T3 cells induces transcription of the c-*fos* proto-oncogenes. *Nature* 311:433–438.

Greenhalgh DA, Kinsella AR. 1985. C-Ha-*ras* not c-Ki-*ras* activation in three colon tumor cell lines. *Carcinogenesis* 6:1533–1535.

Gregory H. 1975. Isolation and structure of urogastrone and its relationship to epidermal growth factors. *Nature* 257:325–327.

Hand PH, Thor A, Wunderlich D, et al. 1984. Monoclonal antibodies of predefined specificity detect activated *ras* gene expression in human mammary and colon carcinomas. *Proc Natl Acad Sci USA* 81:5227–5231.

Heilig K, Goustin AS, Moses HL, et al. 1986. Transforming growth factor alpha expression by human colon cancer but not by normal colonic epithelium (abstract). *Gastroenterology* 90:1455.

Hoosein NM, Brattain DE, Matthews KM, et al. In press. Characterization of the inhibitory effects of transforming growth factor *beta* on a human colon carcinoma cell line. *Cancer Res.*

Hussa RO. 1981. Human chorionic gonadotropin, a clinical marker: Review of its biosynthesis. *Ligand Review* 3:5–44.

Johnson LR, Guthrie PD. 1976. Stimulation of DNA synthesis by big and little gastrin. *Gastroenterology* 71:599–602.

Karlin DA, McBath M, Jones RD, et al. 1985. Hypergastrinemia and colorectal carcinogenesis in the rat. *Cancer Lett* 29:73–78.

Kelly K, Cochran BH, Stiles CD, et al. 1983. Cell-specific regulation of the c-*myc* gene by lymphocyte mitogens and platelet-derived growth factor. *Cell* 35:603–610.

Kerr IB, Lee FD, Quintanella M, et al. 1985. Immunocytochemical demonstration of p21 *ras* family oncogene product in normal mucosa and in premalignant and malignant tumours of the colorectum. *Br J Cancer* 52:695–700.

Kusyk CJ, McNiel NO, Johnson LR. 1986. Stimulation of growth of a colon cancer cell line by gastrin. *Am J Physiol* 251:6597–6601.

Land H, Parada LF, Weinberg RA. 1983. Cellular oncogenes and multi-step carcinogenesis. *Science* 222:771–778.

Leof EB, Proper JA, Goustin AS, et al. 1986. Induction of c-*sis* mRNA and activity similar to platelet-derived growth factor by transforming growth factor B. A proposed model for indirect mitogenesis involving autocrine activity. *Proc Natl Acad Sci USA* 83:2453–2457.

Levine A, Brattain M, Crandall C, et al. 1986. Growth factors in human colon carcinoma (abstract). *Proceedings of the American Association for Cancer Research* 26:41.

Levine AE, McRae LJ, Hamilton DA, et al. 1985. Identification of endogenous growth factors from a human colon carcinoma cell line. *Cancer Res* 45:2248–2254.

Lin CCK, Alitab M, Schwab D, et al. 1985. Evolution of karyotypic abnormalities and c-*myc* amplification in human colonic carcinoma cell lines. *Chromosoma* 92:11–15.

Lointier P, Chipponi J, Robial PG, et al. 1985. Recepteurs des steroids sexuels dans les adenocarcinomes digestifs (abstract). *Gastroenterol Clin Biol* 9:78A.

Lointier P, Raynaud JP, Levin B, et al. 1986. The effects of steroid hormones on human colon carcinoma cells in vitro (abstract). *Proceedings of the American Association for Cancer Research* 27:227.

McCoy MS, Bargmann CI, Weinberg RA. 1984. Human colon carcinoma Ki-*ras*2 oncogene and its corresponding proto-oncogene. *Mol Cell Biol* 4:1577–1582.

McCoy MS, Toole JJ, Cunningham JM, et al. 1983. Characterization of a human colon/lung carcinoma oncogene. *Nature* 302:79–81.

McGregor DB, Jones RD, Karlin DA, et al. 1983. Comparison of effects of pentagastrin and gastrin on rat colon mucosa. *J Surg Res* 34:325–331.

Marquardt H, Hunkapiller MW, Hood LE, et al. 1984. Rat transforming growth factor type 1: Structure and relation to epidermal growth factor. *Science* 223:1079–1082.

Masui T, Wakefield LM, Lechner JF, et al. 1986. Type *beta* transforming growth factor is the primary differentiation-inducing serum factor for normal human bronchial epithelial cells. *Proc Natl Acad Sci USA* 83:2438–2442.

Melmed S, Braunstein GD. 1983. Human chorionic gonadotropin stimulates proliferation of Nb 2 rat lymphoma cells. *J Clin Endocrinol Metab* 56:1068–1070.

Miller W, Ota D, Giacco G, et al. 1985. Absence of a relationship of size of primary colon carcinoma with metastasis and survival. *Clin Exp Metastasis* 3:189–196.

Moses HL, Tucker RF, Leof EB, et al. 1985. Type beta transforming growth factor is a growth stimulator and a growth inhibitor. *Cancer Cells* 3:65–71.

Mueller R, Bravo R, Burckhardt J, et al. 1984. Induction of c-*fos* gene and protein by growth factor precedes activation of c-*myc*. *Nature* 312:716–720.

Mukherjee K, Das S. 1984. A placental glycoprotein, human chorionic gonadotropin, as a growth stimulant of murine tumor cells. *IRCS Journal of Medical Science* 12:1101–1102.

Mulcahy LS, Smith MR, Stacey DW. 1985. Requirement for *ras* proto-oncogene function during serum-stimulated growth of NIH 3T3 cells. *Nature* 313:241–243.

Preiss L, Loomis CR, Bishop WR, et al. 1986. Quantitative measurement of 1,2 diacylglycerol present in platelets, hepatocytes and *ras*- and *sis*-transformed normal rat kidney cells. *J Biol Chem* 261:8597–8600.

Pulciani S, Santos E, Lauver AV, et al. 1982. Oncogenes in solid human tumours. *Nature* 300:539–542.

Ran W, Dean M, Levine RA, et al. 1986. Induction of c-*fos* and c-*myc* mRNA by epidermal growth factor or calcium ionophore is cAMP dependent. *Proc Natl Acad Sci USA* 83:8216–8220.

Rose SP, Pruss RM, Herschmann HR. 1975. Initiation of 3T3 fibroblast cell division by epidermal growth factor. *J Cell Physiol* 86:593–598.

Rosen SW. 1975. Placental proteins and their subunits as tumor markers. *Ann Intern Med* 82:71–82.

Rothberg PG, Spandorfer JM, Erisman MD, et al. 1985. Evidence that c-*myc* expression defines two genetically distinct forms of colorectal adenocarcinoma. *Br J Cancer* 52:629–632.

Saloman DS, Perroteau I, Kidwell WR, et al. 1987. Loss of growth responsiveness to epidermal growth factor and enhanced production of alpha-transforming growth factors in *vos*-transformed mouse mammary epithelial cells. *J Cell Physiol* 130:397–409.

Sap J, Munoz A, Damm K, et al. 1986. The c-*erb*-A protein is a high-affinity receptor for thyroid hormone. *Nature* 324:635–640.

Schwab M, Klempnauer KH, Alitalo K, et al. 1986. Rearrangement at the 5[1] end of amplified c-*myc* in human CoLo 320 cells is associated with abnormal transcription. *Mol Cell Biol* 6:2752–2755.

Sherwin SA, Twardzik DR, Bohn WH, et al. 1983. High-molecular-weight transforming growth factor activity in the urine of patients with disseminated cancer. *Cancer Res* 43:403–407.

Shipley GD, Childs CB, Volkenant ME, et al. 1984. Differential effects of epidermal growth factor, transforming growth factor and insulin on DNA and protein synthesis and morphology in serum-free culture of AKR-2B cells. *Cancer Res* 44:710–716.

Shipley GD, Pittelkow MR, Wille JJ, et al. 1986. Reversible inhibition of normal human prokeratinocyte proliferation by type *beta* transforming growth factor-growth inhibitor in serum-free medium. *Cancer Res* 46:2068–2071.

Shousha S, Chappell R, Mathews J, et al. 1986. Human chorionic gonadotropin expression in colorectal adenocarcinoma. *Dis Colon Rectum* 29:558–560.

Singh P, Rae-Venter B, Townsend CM, et al. 1985. Gastrin receptors in normal and malignant gastrointestinal mucosa: Age-associated changes. *Am J Physiol* 249:G761–G769.

Singh P, Walker JP, Townsend CM, et al. 1986. Role of gastrin and gastrin receptors on the growth of a transplantable mouse colon carcinoma (MC-26) in BALB/c mice. *Cancer Res* 46:1612–1616.

Singletary SE, Baler FL, Spitzer G, et al. 1987. Biological effect of epidermal growth factor on the in vitro growth of human tumors. *Cancer Res* 47:403–406.

Sirinek KR, Levine BA, Moyer MP. 1985. Pentagastrin stimulates in vitro growth of normal and malignant human colon epithelial cells. *Am J Surg* 149:35–39.

Slamon DJ, deKernion JB, Verma IM, et al. 1984. Expression of cellular oncogenes in human malignancies. *Science* 224:256–262.

Sorrentino V, Drozooff V, McKinney MD, et al. 1986. Potentiation of growth factor activity by exogenous c-*myc* expression. *Proc Natl Acad Sci USA* 83:8167–8171.

Spandidos DA, Kerr IB. 1984. Elevated expression of the human *ras* oncogene family in premalignant and maligant tumours of the colorectum. *Br J Cancer* 49:681–688.

Sparks RL, Scott RE. 1986. Transforming growth factor type beta is a specific inhibitor of 3T3 T mesenchymal stem cell differentiation. *Exp Cell Res* 165:345–352.

Stewart J, Evan G, Watson J, et al. 1986. Detection of the c-*myc* oncogene product in colonic polyps and carcinomas. *Br J Cancer* 53:1–6.

Stromberg K, Pigott DA, Ranchalis JE, et al. 1982. Human term placenta contains transforming growth factors. *Biochem Biophys Res Commun* 106:354–361.

Struck DK, Suita PB, Lane MD, et al. 1978. Effect of tunicamycin on the secretion of serum proteins by primary cultures of rat and chick hepatocytes. *J Biol Chem* 253:5332–5337.

Tam JP. 1985. Physiological effects of transforming growth factor in the newborn mouse. *Science* 229:673–675.

Thor A, Horan Hand PH, Wunderlich D, et al. 1984. Monoclonal antibodies define differential *ras* gene expression in malignant and benign colonic diseases. *Nature* 311:562–565.

Todaro GJ, DeLarco JE, Cohen S. 1976. Transformation by murine and feline sarcoma viruses specifically blocks binding of epidermal growth factors to cells. *Nature* 264:26–31.

Tricoli JV, Rall LB, Karakoousis CP, et al. 1986. Enhanced levels of insulin-like growth factor messenger RNA in human colon carcinomas and liposarcomas. *Cancer Res* 46:6169–6173.

Untawale S, Blick M, Pathak S. 1986. Cytogenetic and molecular analysis of colon cancer (abstract). *Am J Hum Genet* 39:A45.

Wagner JS, Adson MA, VanHeerden JA, et al. 1984. The natural history of hepatic metastases from colorectal cancer. *Ann Surg* 199:502–508.

Wan CW, Brattain MG, Yeoman LC. 1986. Epidermal growth factor receptor levels vary among human colon tumor cell lines with differing rates of growth (abstract). *J Cell Biol* 103:155a.

Weinberger C, Thompson CC, Ong ES, et al. 1986. The c-*erb*-A gene encodes a thyroid hormone receptor. *Nature* 324:641–646.

Williams ARW, Piris J, Spandidos DA, et al. 1985. Immunohistochemical detection of the *ras* oncogene p21 product in an experimental tumour and in human colorectal neoplasms. *Br J Cancer* 52:687–693.

Willson JKV, Bittner G, Oberly T, et al. 1987. Human colon neoplastic cells in culture. *Cancer Res* 47:2704–2713.

Winsett OE, Townsend CM, Glass EJ, et al. 1986. Gastrin stimulates growth of colon cancer. *Surgery* 99:302–307.

Wong M, Holdaway IM. 1985. Insulin binding by normal and neoplastic colon tissue. *Int J Cancer* 35:335–341.

Yander G, Halsey H, Kenna M, et al. 1985. Amplification and elevated expression of c-*myc* in a chemically induced mouse colon tumor. *Cancer Res* 45:4433–4438.

Yang KP. 1987. Estrogen receptors in human colon cancer cell lines (abstract). *Proceedings of the American Association for Cancer Research* 28:245.

Yokota J, Toyoshima K, Sugimura T, et al. 1986. Amplification of c-*erb*B-2 oncogene in human adenocarcinomas in vivo. *Lancet* 1:765–767.

Yoshimoto K, Hirohashi J, Fekiya T. 1986. Increased expression of the c-*myc* gene without gene amplification in human lung cancer and colon cancer cell lines. *Jpn J Cancer Res* 77:540–545.

Annual Clinical Conference on Cancer, Vol. 30
Gastrointestinal Cancer: Current Approaches to Diagnosis and Treatment
© 1988 by The University of Texas System Cancer Center

7. Development of an In Vivo Model to Study the Biology of Human Colorectal Carcinoma Metastasis

Isaiah J. Fidler, Kiyoshi Morikawa, Sen Pathak,
Raffaella Giavazzi, and J. Milburn Jessup

The spread of human colorectal carcinoma (HCC) cells from a primary site to distant organs and the production of metastases is the most devastating aspect of this cancer. Metastasis involves the release of cells from the primary tumor followed by their dissemination to distant sites, arrest in the microcirculation of organs, extravasation and infiltration into the stroma of those organs, and survival and growth into new tumor foci (fig. 7.1). The outcome of the process has been shown to depend on both host factors and tumor cell properties, and the balance of these interactions varies among different tumor systems (Poste and Fidler 1980; Fidler and Poste 1985).

Although our understanding of the process of metastasis has increased considerably, comparable improvement in the treatment of metastatic disease produced by colorectal carcinoma has been unsatisfactory. Despite major advances in general patient care, in surgical techniques, and in adjuvant therapies, most deaths from colorectal carcinoma are caused by the growth of metastases resistant to therapy. The biggest obstacle to the effective treatment of metastases is the nonuniformity of the cells that populate both primary and secondary neoplasms. By the time of diagnosis, and certainly in clinically advanced lesions, primary colorectal cancers are likely to contain multiple cell populations exhibiting a wide range of biologic characteristics; the populations differ, for example, in their cell surface properties, antigenicity, immunogenicity, growth rate, karyotype, sensitivity to various cytotoxic drugs, and ability to invade and metastasize (Fidler 1984). Biologic heterogeneity is equally prominent between the cell populations in metastases (Fidler and Hart 1982; Heppner 1984). Indeed, in a given patient, metastases in different organs or even multiple metastases within the same organ can exhibit diversity in hormone receptors, antigenicity, immunogenicity, and sensitivity to various chemotherapeutic drugs, for example (Fidler and Poste 1985).

In colorectal carcinoma, the major goal of surgical and medical oncologists is the prevention or eradication of metastases. In fact, metastasis is likely to have occurred by the time of diagnosis in many patients (August, Ottow, and Sugarbaker 1984). New therapeutic approaches are needed, and thus models that allow study of the biology and therapy of this disease must be developed. Adequate animal models for

THE PATHOGENESIS OF
COLORECTAL CARCINOMA METASTASIS

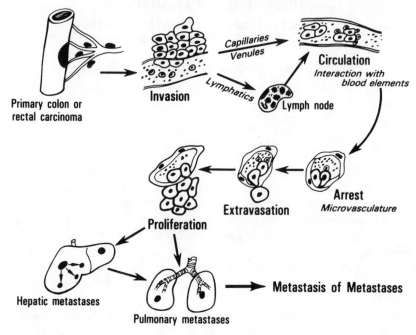

Fig. 7.1. The pathogenesis of colorectal cancer metastasis.

in vivo studies of human neoplasia in general, and of metastasis in particular, have been lacking. However, the discovery of the athymic T-cell deficient nude mouse and its use in studies of tissue transplantation have proved most valuable for examining several aspects of metastatic human tumors in vivo (Fidler 1986).

The nude mouse displays congenital thymic aplasia and, accordingly, T lymphocyte-related deficiencies (Flanagan 1966; Hansen 1978; Pantelouris and Hair 1970). Indeed, over the past two decades the nude mouse has been used in the study of various neoplasms and experimental cancer therapies (Bogden et al. 1982; Fidler 1986; Giovanella and Fogh 1978, 1985; Sharkey and Fogh 1984; Povlsen and Rygaard 1976; Rygaard and Povlsen 1982; Sordat, Ueyama, and Fogh 1982).

The usefulness of nude mice in the study of colorectal cancers has been limited. Like other human tumor cell lines, HCC cells transplanted into nude mice rarely metastasize, regardless of their degree of malignancy in the patient. In most such studies, however, tumor cells were implanted into the subcutis of nude mice. Recent reports have shown that the growth rate and incidence of metastasis produced by human tumors transplanted into nude mice can be manipulated by the route of implantation and that different organ environments contribute to the growth and expression of metastatic phenotypes of implanted tumor cells (Kozlowski et al. 1984; Giavazzi et al. 1986a; Naito et al. 1986; Fidler 1986).

The most common site of HCC metastasis is the liver. For this reason, there has been an urgent need to develop an experimental model to study HCC hepatic metastases. In the nude mouse model, the injection of human and murine tumor cell lines into the spleen has been shown to produce grossly evident tumor foci in the liver (Kozlowski et al. 1984; Kopper, Van Hanh, and Lapis 1982; Giavazzi et al. 1986a). The ideal in vivo model for studying human HCC metastasis should allow the interaction of relevant HCC cells with a relevant organ environment, namely, the liver. In this chapter, we review data from our laboratories that deal with human colorectal tumors xenografted into nude mice, and we discuss our efforts to determine the suitability of the nude mouse for use as an in vivo model in studies on the biology and treatment of HCC metastasis.

HUMAN COLORECTAL CARCINOMAS TRANSPLANTED INTO NUDE MICE

The first success in the transplantation of a human tumor into nude mice was reported in 1969 (Rygaard and Povlsen 1969). Since then, successful transplantation of colorectal tumors into these animals has been reported by many investigators (Povlsen and Rygaard 1971; Povlsen et al. 1975; Giovanella et al. 1978; Sharkey and Fogh 1984; McBain et al. 1984; Giovanella and Fogh 1985). In fact, only human melanomas have shown better takes in nude mice (Sharkey and Fogh 1984). Xenografts of colon tumors in nude mice have been produced either directly from surgical specimens (Povlsen and Rygaard 1971; Giovanella, Stehlin, and Williams 1974; Carrel, Sordat, and Merenola 1976; Fogh et al. 1979; Bhargava and Lipkin 1981; Spremulli and Dexter 1983; Spremulli et al. 1983; Neulat-Duga et al. 1984; Whitehead et al. 1985; Giavazzi et al. 1986a, 1986b) or from cell lines established in culture (Zalcberg et al. 1983; Carrel, Sordat, and Merenola 1976; Leibovitz et al. 1976; Tom et al. 1976; Fogh, Fogh, and Orfeo 1977; Kimball and Brattain 1980; Kyriazis et al. 1978, 1981; Namba et al. 1983; Brattain et al. 1983, 1984; Klug et al. 1984; Kozlowski et al. 1984; Kirkland 1985; Pimm et al. 1985; Drewinko et al. 1986). Whether fresh specimens or cell lines provide the better model for HCC in nude mice is still debated. Tumor growth in nude mice has been commonly accepted as verification of the tumorigenicity of cell lines that have been established in vitro (Giovanella, Stehlin, and Williams 1974; Fogh, Fogh, and Orfeo 1977; Freedman and Shin 1978). However, not all cultured colorectal cancer lines are tumorigenic in nude mice (Rutzky et al. 1983; Brattain et al. 1984). Cultured cell lines have, by necessity, undergone adaptation to the culture environment, changes that may or may not correlate with growth in vivo. Nevertheless, morphologically, some human colon tumors taken from culture and grown in nude mice do not differ from those tumors initiated in nude mice by the direct inoculation of cells from surgical specimens (Carrel, Sordat, and Merenola 1976; Leibovitz et al. 1976; Fogh et al. 1979; Kirkland 1985; Giavazzi et al. 1986b).

Growth of human colorectal carcinomas in nude mice occurs more frequently if the cells are derived from metastases or from sites of tumor recurrence rather than from primary neoplasms. Colon tumors derived either from primary or metastatic lesions have been established as continuous lines in vivo in nude mice (Povlsen and Rygaard 1971; Giovanella, Stehlin, and Williams 1974; Fogh et al. 1979; Spremulli et al. 1983; Neulat-Duga et al. 1984; Giavazzi et al. 1986a). Fogh and coworkers studied 10 primary tumors and 12 metastases of HCC and reported only a slightly higher rate of takes for metastases (58%) than for primary tumors (50%). However, from these growing tumors, tumors derived from metastases both were established as continuous lines at a higher rate (100%) and grew faster than tumors derived from primary colon cancers (with only a 40% establishment of continuous lines) (Fogh et al. 1979).

Tumorigenicity of Freshly Isolated Cells

In our initial study (Giavazzi et al. 1986a), we transplanted 15 primary cancers and 11 metastases into nude mice. In eight (53%) of the mice that received primary-derived tumor and in eight (72%) of the mice that received metastasis-derived tumor, continuously growing tumor developed. We did not find significant correlations between the Dukes stage classification of the original neoplasms and tumorigenicity in nude mice. Even from the first passage, tumor lines derived from metastases grew faster than those derived from primary tumors. In the second serial passage, an increased rate of tumor take and a decrease in latency time were observed, changes that have been described before (Fogh et al. 1979; Neulat-Duga et al. 1984) and that could well have been due to host selection pressures (Fidler 1986). Nonetheless, the differences in doubling time observed between primary tumors (median doubling time, 7.5 days; range, 5.0–8.0 days) and metastases (median doubling time, 4.0 days; range, 3.5–5.0 days) were maintained even on further passages.

The synthesis of carcinoembryonic antigen (CEA) and its release by human colon cell lines established in vitro or in vivo have often been reported. CEA production was found in cultured cells of HCC, and it was maintained in xenografted colon tumors (Mach et al. 1974; Carrel, Sordat, and Merenola 1976; Spremulli et al. 1983; Pimm et al. 1985). Moreover, the synthesis of CEA was shown to be stable in HCCs serially transplanted into nude mice (Egan and Todd 1972; Tomkins et al. 1974; Carrel, Sordat, and Merenola 1976; Leibovitz et al. 1976; Spremulli and Dexter 1983; Spremulli et al. 1983; Namba et al. 1983; Brattain et al. 1984; Pimm et al. 1985; Drewinko et al. 1986).

Serum levels of CEA that exceed 5 ng/ml are associated with a poor prognosis in patients with adenocarcinoma of the colon or rectum. An elevated concentration of CEA in serum often indicates the presence of visceral metastases (Sugarbaker, Gunderson, and Wittes 1985). Moreover, Wanebo et al. (1978) have found, in patients with disease limited to the bowel wall or regional lymph nodes, that the prognosis is worse when there is an elevated CEA level than when the CEA value is normal. These authors speculate that the poorer outlook may be due either to the presence of occult metastases or to a greater biologic aggressiveness of the primary tumor. In our laboratory, we examined whether colorectal adenocarcinomas from patients with a preoperative serum CEA level that exceeded 5 ng/ml would be more tumorigenic in nude mice than cells isolated from tumors of patients who had normal concentrations of serum CEA. A carcinoma was considered biologically aggressive if injection of 2×10^6 of its viable cells into the flank of a nude mouse produced a progressively growing tumor nodule within six months. This method of analysis can be applied equally to primary tumors and to metastases because it does not require consideration of the various steps of metastasis formation.

Our study utilized tumors from 25 patients, whose clinical characteristics are presented in table 7.1. In 14 patients, cells were harvested only from the primary; in 8, only from a metastasis; and in 3, from both the primary and a simultaneously excised metastasis. The 17 primary tumors sampled were 1 Dukes A, 1 Dukes B1, 5 Dukes B2, 2 Dukes B3, 4 Dukes C2, and 4 Dukes D, and all but 2 of the 11 metastases were taken from the liver. The tumorigenicity of cells from metastases was not significantly greater than that of cells from primary neoplasms (82% and 59%, respectively, demonstrated biologic aggressiveness). When primary colorectal carcinomas and metastases were considered together, tumors from patients whose preoperative serum CEA exceeded 5 ng/ml were significantly more tumorigenic in nude mice than tumors isolated from patients with normal levels of CEA (15 of 17 biologically aggressive in the former case, 4 of 11 in the latter; $p < .005$, 8.24 by the chi-square test). The association of serum CEA concentration with the tumorigenicity of metastases could not be evaluated, since 8 of 11 metastases were harvested from patients with an elevated CEA value. However, evaluation was possible with the primary tumors: eight of nine primary neoplasms from patients with an elevated CEA level were biologically aggressive in the nude mice, compared with only two of eight tumors from patients with a normal CEA value ($p < .01$, 7.14 by the chi-square test). Tumorigenicity did not correlate with standard prognostic factors such as histological parameters or stage of disease, nor did serum concentration of CEA correlate with the size of the primary tumor (Jessup et al., unpublished data).

These data suggest that CEA might be associated with growth regulation of HCC. Although we did not measure serum CEA in the recipient mice, CEA has been identified in the serum of nude mice bearing HCC xenografts (Martin and Halpern 1984). Since CEA concentration did not correlate with tumor size in our patients, the CEA level may either reflect a stage of evolution in the neoplastic progression of colorectal cancer or actually be a substance that can regulate neoplastic growth of HCC.

Characterization of Cells Growing in the Mice

Before the nude mouse can be used as a relevant model for studies of the biology and therapy of human tumors, it is necessary to ascertain that the tumors maintain their characteristics after passage in nude mice (Povlsen, Rygaard, and Fogh 1982; Fogh et al. 1979; Giovanella and Fogh 1985; Sharkey and Fogh 1984). The histological parameters of HCCs propagated in nude mice have been reported to resemble those of the tumors of origin (Povlsen and Rygaard 1971; Giovanella,

Table 7.1. Clinical Characteristics of Patients with Colorectal Carcinoma

Patient No.	Age (yr)	Dukes Stage	Site	No. of Nodes	Sex	Race	Size of Primary (cm)	CEA (ng/ml)	Biologically Aggressive
Primary tumor sampled									
1	73	B1	S	0	F	W	3.0	1.4	No
2	61	B2	R	0	F	W	2.0	1.5	No
3	71	C2	S	2	M	W	7.0	1.5	No
4	71	A	R	0	M	W	1.0	1.7	No
5	58	C2	R	7	M	W	4.0	2.2	No
6	69	C2	R	1	F	W	6.5	3.6	No
7	53	D	R	6	F	H	2.5	172.4	No
8	42	B2	RC	0	M	B	5.0	1.9	Yes
9	51	B2	R	0	F	W	3.5	3.5	Yes
10	56	B2	RC	0	M	W	9.0	6.7	Yes
11	70	B3	R	0	M	W	7.0	8.2	Yes
12	41	B3	R	0	F	W	6.5	9.6	Yes
13	67	C2	S	10	M	O	3.0	21.3	Yes
14	74	B2	R	0	M	W	7.5	30.4	Yes
15	45	D	S	2	M	W	6.0	31.6	Yes
16	69	D	RC	0	F	W	5.0	37.7	Yes
17	67	D	LC	7	F	H	3.0	1906.0	Yes
Metastasis sampled									
18	58	D	L		M	W		2.2	No
19	57	D	L		M	W		84.8	No
20	68	D	L		F	W		1.5	Yes
21	53	D	L		M	B		2.4	Yes
22	65	D	L		M	W		8.6	Yes
23	50	D	L		F	W		9.1	Yes
15	45	D	L		M	W		31.6	Yes
24	49	D	L		F	W		48.6	Yes
7	53	D	P		F	H		172.4	Yes
25	45	D	L		M	W		173.9	Yes
14	67	D	MS		F	H		1906.0	Yes

Abbreviations: CEA, carcinoembryonic antigen; S, sigmoid colon; R, rectum; RC, right colon; LC, left colon; L, liver; P, perineum; MS, mesentery; W, white; H, Hispanic; B, black; O, Oriental.

Stehlin, and Williams 1974; Carrel, Sordat, and Merenola 1976; Leibovitz et al. 1976; Sharkey and Fogh 1979; Povlsen, Rygaard, and Fogh 1982). In general, the cytological appearance by light and ultrastructural microscopy is also maintained (Fogh et al. 1978; Povlsen, Rygaard, and Fogh 1982; Spremulli et al. 1983). Moreover, the synthesis of specialized products has been shown to be stable after transplantation of tumor into nude mice (Povlsen, Rygaard, and Fogh 1982; Spremulli and Dexter 1983; Sharkey and Fogh 1984; Giovanella and Fogh 1985). Differences in the degree of morphological differentiation between the original human tumor and the tumor growing in a nude mouse have also been reported (Hajdu and Fogh 1978; Horten, Basler, and Shapiro 1981; Spremulli et al. 1983; Sharkey and Fogh 1984). Changes most often occurred early in the first transplant generation, after which the histological differentiation was quite stable. In general, the morphological differentiation of the HCC does not correlate with transplantability (Povlsen and Rygaard 1971), but, for some HCC cells, the lack of differentiation has been associated with successful transplantation into immunodeficient animals (Houghton and Taylor 1978; Drewinko et al. 1986).

We histologically analyzed 30 HCCs that had been successfully transplanted into nude mice. The evaluation revealed a high degree of identity with the human tumor of origin, although occasionally a higher or lower degree of differentiation was found. Morphological characteristics were maintained after several passages in the nude mouse at different sites of tumor growth and in the metastatic lesions (Giavazzi et al. 1986a, 1986b). Moreover, the degree of tumor necrosis and the capacity to produce such cell products as mucin were maintained in the transplanted tumors.

Recently, a method has been described that allows, by the use of polymorphic enzymes, the determination of the human origin of tumors proliferating in nude mice (Wright, Daniels, and Fogh 1981). Isoenzyme mobility patterns, which have been considered the most reliable identification of individual tumors, have been shown to be stable even after several passages of tumors in nude mice (Povlsen, Rygaard, and Fogh 1982; Fogh et al. 1979). For instance, tissue-specific isoenzymes maintained stable expression within an individual colorectal cell line, although their pattern of expression in some cases varied between lines of different origin (Rutzky and Siciliano 1982). We analyzed 6 polymorphic enzymes in HCC cells recovered from a total of 30 primary tumors and metastases growing in nude mice; without exception, all the tumors proved to be of human origin.

Metastatic Behavior in the Mice

For many years it had been reported that malignant human tumors did not metastasize in the nude mouse, thus casting doubt on the validity of this model in tumor biology. Since the initial report that human tumor cell lines would produce metastases in nude mice (Giovanella and coworkers' 1973 findings of melanoma spread to lungs and lymph nodes) there has been an increasing number of reports of such metastasis with a variety of tumors (Kyriazis et al. 1978; Sordat, Merenola, and Carrel 1977; Sharkey and Fogh 1979; Kozlowski et al. 1984; Fidler, Pollack, and Hanna 1984; Giovanella and Fogh 1985; Lockshin et al. 1985; Fidler 1986). And, indeed colon cancer lines can produce spontaneous or experimental metastasis in nude mice

(Kyriazis et al. 1978; Kimball and Brattain 1980; Sordat, Ueyama, and Fogh 1982; Sordat and Wang 1984; Wang et al. 1984; Spremulli and Dexter 1983; Kozlowski et al. 1984; Fermor et al. 1986; Giavazzi et al. 1986a, 1986b).

The production of metastasis depends both on the intrinsic tumor cell properties and on the host response, the experimental technique, and the origin, health, and maintenance of the nude mice (Giovanella, Stehlin, and Williams 1974; Kyriazis et al. 1981; Hanna 1982; Hanna, Davis, and Fidler 1982; Sordat, Ueyama, and Fogh 1982; Sharkey and Fogh 1984; Sordat and Wang 1984; Kerbel, Man, and Dexter 1984; Fidler 1986). The importance of the health of the recipient mouse for the success of such studies cannot be overemphasized. Nude mice infected by a pathogenic virus (e.g., hepatitis virus) can resist xenografted tumors and, hence, metastasis formation (Hanna, Davis, and Fidler 1982; Sharkey and Fogh 1984). Thus, nude mice must be housed under specific pathogen–free conditions and the injected tumor cells free of pathogenic murine viruses and *Mycoplasma* infections (Fidler 1986).

As mentioned above, the first steps in metastasis involve the detachment of tumor cells from the primary tumor and the invasion of host stroma and entrance into the circulation. For this reason, the implantation site of tumor cells in nude mice influences not only the growth of the local tumor but also the production of metastases (Giavazzi et al. 1986a, 1986b). Most solid tumors grafted into nude mice grow locally but show limited invasiveness (Naito et al. 1986). This lack of invasion, as well as the consequent lack of metastases, has been often associated with the development of a dense, fibrous capsule around the tumor (DeVore et al. 1980).

Indeed, the metastatic capacity of human tumor cells implanted subcutaneously into the nude mouse has been found to correlate with invasion of the body wall (Kyriazis et al. 1978; Sharkey and Fogh 1979; Neulat-Duga et al. 1984). Moreover, tumor cells implanted subcutaneously into the cranial aspect of the nude mouse grow faster and produce more metastases than tumor cells implanted subcutaneously into the posterior body aspect (Kyriazis et al. 1981). The intraperitoneal injection of human solid tumor cells can produce ascitic growth with local infiltration followed by production of distant metastases (Takahashi et al. 1978; Sordat, Ueyama, and Fogh 1982; Lockshin et al. 1985); these very same tumor cells, however, were not invasive when implanted subcutaneously. Similarly, Kyriazis et al. (1978) described a human colon tumor line that upon subcutaneous injection evoked a host response manifested by formation of a dense capsule composed of connective tissue. Metastases were observed only after there had been extensive invasion of the capsule, although they were limited to regional lymph nodes. Following intraperitoneal injection, 60% of the mice developed metastases in the mediastinal lymph nodes and the lungs (Kyriazis et al. 1978). Successful production of lung tumor colonies after intravenous injection of human tumor cells into nude mice has not been accomplished. These findings agree with earlier studies that demonstrated that fewer pulmonary tumor colonies would develop in homozygous mice than in heterozygous littermates or syngeneic mice (Fidler, Caines, and Dolan 1976; Richie, McDonald, and Gittes 1981). Variability in results has been attributed to variations in experimental techniques and in host immune response (mainly natural killer–cell activity) (Hanna 1982).

Most HCCs studied in nude mice have been implanted into the subcutis, a site that is readily accessible to experimental manipulation but that in most cases does not correspond with the anatomic origin of the tumor. Several published studies of transplanted human tumors document the importance of the correct implantation site for growth and eventual metastasis. A human pancreatic tumor cell line injected into the duodenal lobe of the pancreas of nude mice produced local and distant metastases, but no metastases were observed after subcutaneous transplantation (Mong and Chu 1985). Injection of a hormone-responsive human mammary carcinoma into the mammary fat pad of nude mice resulted in 100% tumor growth, with metastases to lung, liver, and spleen (Shafie and Liotta 1980). The same human mammary carcinoma cells injected into the uterus or intracerebrally proliferated rapidly and were highly invasive, but at a subcutaneous injection site the cells grew locally and there was no evidence of invasion into adjacent tissue (Levy, White, and McGrath 1982).

The orthotopic transplantation of colon tumor has been described for a chemically induced murine adenocarcinoma (Tom et al. 1976; Goldrosen 1980; Thombre and Deodhar 1984). The colon tumor cells were injected into different sites along the small and large intestines of syngeneic mice. The highest rate of tumor take occurred in the cecum, and about 50% of positive mice with a local tumor developed liver metastases. The same tumor implanted subcutaneously grew locally and produced pulmonary but not hepatic metastases. In this tumor system, the direct intraportal injection of tumor cells did not produce hepatic metastases, suggesting that the primary tumor promoted the formation of hepatic metastases (Wang et al. 1984; Sordat and Wang 1984).

Hepatic metastases account for many of the deaths from colorectal carcinoma. To develop a reproducible model of hepatic metastasis, tumor cells have been implanted into the spleens of nude mice. From this site of injection, tumor cells gain access to the bloodstream and thence reach the liver to proliferate into secondary tumor colonies. Formation of hepatic metastases subsequent to intrasplenic injection of tumor cells was first described by Leduc in 1959. More recently, a variety of murine tumors implanted into the spleens of syngeneic mice were also shown to produce liver tumor growths (Kopper, Van Hanh, and Lapis 1982; LaFreniere and Rosenberg 1986). In our laboratory, Kozlowski and coworkers (1984) investigated the metastatic behavior of 11 human cell lines of different histological origin and the production of lung and liver metastases in the nude mouse. The extent of metastasis depended on the nature of the tumor cells, with the most dramatic expression of malignancy found for two variants of the HT-29 HCC cell line subsequent to intrasplenic injection. Merely implanting human tumor cells into the spleens of nude mice does not guarantee that metastasis to the liver will occur. A more recent study from our laboratory demonstrated that variant lines established from a surgical specimen of a human renal cell carcinoma produced extensive metastasis if the cells were implanted into the kidneys of nude mice. In contrast, intrasplenic implantation of these cells produced only tumors in the spleen, but not metastasis (Naito et al. 1986).

Correlation of Experimental Metastatic Behavior with Clinical Staging

During the last three years, we have investigated the biologic behavior of cells isolated from surgical specimens of HCC by implantation into nude mice. The major goal of the study has been to examine the malignant behavior of colorectal carcinoma cells, whether isolated from primary neoplasms or metastases of patients. For these experiments, four tumor lines were derived from primary colorectal carcinomas, three from hepatic metastases, and one from a mesenteric lymph node metastasis. Tumor cells of each line were injected into multiple sites in nude mice: the spleen, the subcutis, muscle, and the venous system (Giavazzi et al. 1986a, 1986b). All the inoculi consisted of single-cell suspensions obtained by enzymatic dissociation of solid tumors. In the course of these experiments, we have examined by autopsy approximately 500 mice that had a growing HCC.

Implantation of HCC into the spleen resulted in macroscopic tumor in the spleen and then in the liver. In contrast, subcutaneous injection, although successful in initiating local tumor growth, in only one case yielded visceral metastasis, in lung (table 7.2). In 10 of the 53 mice in the subcutaneous group, histological examination revealed invasion of lymph nodes draining the injection site.

Metastases of colorectal cancer may occur late in the disease, and this occurrence is often after surgical excision of the primary tumor. In some reports of experimental tumor systems in rodents, multiple metastases developed subsequent to surgical removal of a local tumor. Similarly, the incidence of lung metastases was shown to increase with the prolonged survival of nude mice that had locally recurrent HCC at the site of injection-resection (Sordat, Ueyama, and Fogh 1982). In our experiments with nude mice, we injected HCC into a hind thigh and amputated the

Table 7.2. *Metastatic Behavior of Human Colorectal Carcinoma Cells Injected Subcutaneously into Nude Mice*

Tumor Origin[a]	Dukes Stage	Median Survival of Mice in Days (Range)	Mice with Macroscopic Metastasis/ Total Mice
Primary			
Rectum	B1	64 (46–90)	0/7
Rectum	B2	77 (43–77)	0/6
Rectum	B3	58 (—)	0/6
Rectum	B3	55 (55–63)	1/6[b]
Metastasis			
Lymph node	C2	30 (30–57)	0/6
Liver	D	82 (74–83)	0/6
Liver	D	49 (49–61)	0/6
Liver	D	50 (47–72)	0/10

[a] Each tumor represents disease from a different patient.
[b] The metastasis was to lung and consisted of multiple lesions.

Table 7.3. *Metastatic Behavior of Human Colorectal Carcinoma Cells Injected Intravenously into Nude Mice*

Tumor Origin[a]	Dukes Stage	Mice with Lung Colonies/ Total Mice	Median Lung Tumor Foci (Range)
Primary			
Rectum	B1	9/9	3 (1−26)
Rectum	B2	6/6	15 (5−29)
Rectum	B3	3/10	0 (0−8)
Rectum	B3	8/8	48 (7−150)
Metastasis			
Lymph node	C2	7/10	1 (0−12)
Liver	D	0/6	0
Liver	D	6/10	2 (0−21)
Liver	D	8/9	51 (0−161)

[a]The tumor cell lines are the same as those in table 7.2.

leg when the tumors reached 1.5−2 cm in size. Although most of the mice developed recurrent tumor at the incision site, metastases were found in lung in only two mice, even though all mice survived six months after the initial tumor cell injection. Neither cells from primary colon cancers nor cells from metastases produced metastasis in nude mice subsequent to subcutaneous or intramuscular implantation. When the HCC cells were administered intravenously, no correlation was found between the experimental lung metastases and the clinical stage of the original neoplasms (table 7.3).

The intrasplenic injection of HCC cells followed by the formation of tumor lesions in the liver allowed us to distinguish human carcinomas with different malignant potentials. Thirty days after the injection of tumor cells derived from two human liver metastases, the mice became moribund. At autopsy, their livers were completely replaced by tumor (fig. 7.2). Mice injected with cells from primary colorectal carcinomas developed few visible tumor foci in the liver by 90 days after intrasplenic injection (table 7.4). Cells of one primary tumor produced visible liver tumor in all the injected mice, but this required 90 days. The cells recovered from the liver lesions were of human origin (karyotype and isoenzyme analyses).

In Vivo Model for Liver Metastasis

The previous studies demonstrated that the intrasplenic injection of HCC cells can lead to the production of discrete tumor nodules in the liver. To further delineate the malignancy of tumors of different origin, we compared the behavior of HCC cells enzymatically dissociated from surgical specimens of one primary colorectal carcinoma (Dukes stage B2), one hepatic metastasis, and one mesenteric lymph node metastasis.

In this experiment (table 7.5), intrasplenically injected cells isolated from a patient's liver metastasis produced a rapid growth of tumor cells in the liver of all the injected mice, whereas those derived from a primary colorectal carcinoma produced but a few liver tumor foci and these after a longer period of time. The cells from a

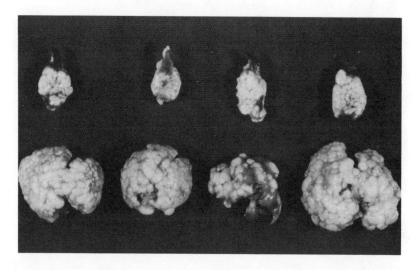

Fig. 7.2. Growth of human colorectal carcinoma cells in the spleens and livers of nude mice subsequent to intrasplenic injection. The cells were derived from metastases in human liver.

patient's lymph node metastasis failed to colonize the liver. All cells produced spleen tumors. All three cell lines were serially passaged in nude mice, and we repeated the experiment at different passages. The three lines maintained their characteristic malignant behavior.

That not all the mice in this experiment developed tumor growths in the liver could not be merely attributed to the absence of tumor cells reaching the liver after

Table 7.4. *Metastatic Behavior of Human Colorectal Carcinoma Cells Injected Intrasplenically into Nude Mice*

Tumor Origin[a]	Dukes Stage	Autopsy Day	Mice with Spleen Tumors/ Total Mice	Mice with Liver Tumors/ Total Mice	Liver Tumor Foci
Primary					
Rectum	B1	90	8/9	4/9	<10
Rectum	B2	90	9/10	0/10	<10
Rectum	B3	90	8/10	7/10	<10
Rectum	B3	90	5/5	5/5	<10
Metastasis					
Lymph node	C2	90	6/6	1/6	<10
Liver	D	90	6/6	2/6	<10
Liver	D	40	6/6	6/6	>200
Liver	D	30	9/9	9/9	>10, <200

[a] The tumor cell lines are the same as those in table 7.2.

Table 7.5. *Production of Liver Tumor Foci by Human Colorectal Carcinoma Cells Injected Intrasplenically into Nude Mice*

Tumor Origin	Autopsy Day	Mice with Liver Tumor/ Total Mice	Median Liver Tumor Foci (Range)
Primary	50	4/5	9 (0–11)
(Dukes B1)	90	5/6	11 (10–100)
Lymph node metastasis	50	2/5	0 (0–4)
(Dukes C)	90	1/5	0 (0–2)
Hepatic metastasis	30	8/8	all > 300
(Dukes D)	30	5/5	300 (10–>300)

intrasplenic injection. We base this conclusion on the data from two studies. First, studies on the fate and distribution of [^{125}I] IdUrd–labeled HT-29 cells showed that 61% of the cells reached the liver by five minutes after intrasplenic injection (table 7.6) and grossly evident spleen, pancreas, and liver tumors grew by day 42 after intrasplenic injection. Second, splenectomy carried out 24 hours after intrasplenic injection of cells neither impaired cell growth in the liver nor enhanced the expression of malignancy of HCC-M-14328 cells (table 7.7). These two experiments suggest that in this system HCC cells can reach the liver subsequent to intra-

Table 7.6. *Distribution, Arrest, and Survival of [^{125}I] IUDR-labeled HT-29 Tumor Cells Subsequent to Intrasplenic Injection*

Time after Injection	Radioactivity Retained (Percentage of Injected Cells)		
	Spleen	Liver	Lung
5 min	21	61	0.05
1 hr	12	53	0.06
4 hr	5	26	0.05
24 hr	0.8	7.1	
72 hr	0.09	0.1	

Table 7.7. *Production of Liver Tumors in Nude Mice Intrasplenically Injected with Human Colorectal Carcinoma Cells and Then Splenectomized*

Tumor Line	Splenectomy	Autopsy Day	Mice with Liver Tumor/ Total Mice	Median Liver Tumor Foci (Range)
HCC-M14328	−	60	1/5	0 (0–2)
(lymph node)	+	90	3/5	0 (0–3)
HCC-M1410	−	28	6/6	62 (0–>300)
(liver)	+	28	6/6	15 (1–>300)

splenic injection. Thus, highly malignant HCC cells are distinguished by their ability to rapidly proliferate in the liver (fig. 7.1).

The histological parameters of the original tumors were maintained in the livers of the nude mice; human origin was ascertained by karyotype and isoenzyme analyses. The method of karyotype analysis of the original tumor cells directly established in culture and of the same tumor first grown in the nude mouse and then established in culture is discussed in detail below.

Collectively, these data suggest that the intrasplenic injection of HCC and liver tumor formation could provide an experimental model to study the biology and therapy of hepatic metastasis.

Karyotype Analysis

Some human colon tumor cells xenografted into nude mice manifest increased tumorigenicity upon repeated passages. The acquisition of xenotropic murine C-type viruses by human tumors may account for this phenomenon (Tompkins, Rao, and Tompkins 1979). The induction of murine stromal neoplasms in the presence of transplanted human tumors has also been reported (Bowen et al. 1983). This process has been designated *horizontal oncogenesis* and is thought to represent a form of genetic transfer from human to murine cells (Goldenberg and Pavia 1981, 1982). Although this type of oncogenesis is apparently a rare event, the implications of the finding warrant the intensive investigation currently under way in many laboratories.

Karyotype analysis of two cells has been routinely used by us to confirm the human origin of the tumors. Two primary HCCs and two metastases of HCC were analyzed cytogenetically before and after implantation into different organs of nude mice. After dissociation, tumor cells were grown in Eagle's minimal essential medium and harvested for chromosome preparations according to the standard air-drying technique. Eight- to ten-day-old slide preparations were subjected to Q- and G-banding techniques according to routine procedures developed in our laboratory (Pathak 1976).

The purpose of this analysis was to identify the marker chromosomes and determine the stemline chromosome numbers, and thus to assure the human origin of the tumors growing in the nude mice. All four HCCs exhibited altered karyotypes, including numerical and structural rearrangements. The modal chromosome numbers in these carcinomas ranged from 43 to 75. The most consistent similarity, seen in three of four HCCs, was the presence of an altered chromosome 12. In the two metastases of HCC, the short arm of one of the homologues of chromosome 12 was replaced by large and small segments, respectively, with homogeneously staining regions. This marker chromosome was present in more than 98% of the cells analyzed.

Other chromosomes involved in structural rearrangements were chromosomes 1, 3, 4, and 17. Monosomy of chromosome 22 was one of the frequent numerical anomalies observed. Rearrangement of the long arm of chromosome 17 in the form of an isochromosome deserves special mention. This chromosomal rearrangement is one reported in a number of leukemias, lymphomas, and solid tumors at late stages of development, notably in the blastic phase of chronic myelogenous leukemia and in breast carcinoma (Pathak and Goodacre 1986). In the HCCs we assessed, three copies of normal chromosome 17 or two normal copies and long-arm isochromosome were sometimes present. Since the growth-hormone gene is mapped on the long arm of chromosome 17, it is possible that an increase in the copy number provides selective growth advantage to these tumors.

All the colorectal carcinomas we studied consisted of cells with human karyotypes, including those cells that had grown in nude mice. Some metaphase spreads exhibited a higher number of chromosomes as compared with that of the original tumor cells. This last observation indicates that the evolution of karyotype continues with tumor growth either in nude mice or in vitro.

CONCLUSIONS

The metastatic behavior of human colorectal neoplasms can be studied in athymic mice. The neoplasms must be free of mouse pathogens and the mice must be kept in specific pathogen-free conditions. Careful consideration must be given to the anatomic particulars of implantation, because the metastatic potential of HCC is dependent on both intrinsic properties of the tumor cells and host factors.

The intrasplenic implantation of HCC cells that leads to the production of liver metastases distinguishes those cells with a high malignant potential from those with a low potential. The human origin of all tumors growing in the spleens and livers of mice must be determined by both isoenzyme and karyotype analysis. Studies with radiolabeled HCC cells demonstrate that tumor cells can reach the mouse liver within minutes of intrasplenic administration. Thus, the production of HCC lesions in the livers of nude mice is determined by the tumor cells' ability to proliferate in the liver parenchyma rather than by their ability to reach the liver.

Clinically, the liver is the organ most often involved by HCC metastasis. Taken together, our results show that HCC can produce liver metastases in nude mice; in particular, HCC cells obtained from a liver metastasis and implanted intrasplenically are aggressive in that production. The animal model we describe can be used to study some aspects of liver metastasis such as the tumor cells' invasion of and growth in the liver environment and the interaction of the cells with the host organ environment, including with local defense cells. Finally, this nude mouse model could prove valuable for therapy studies because of HCC cells' proliferation in the relevant metastatic site of the liver.

ACKNOWLEDGMENTS

This research was supported by grants from SmithKline Beckman Corporation, the AMOCO Foundation Inc., and by funds from the National Cancer Institute Cancer Center Support Grant (CA-16672)-Centralized Histopathology Laboratory.

We thank Debra Campbell, Lisa Daniels, and Shirley Walker for expert technical assistance, and Emily Rondon for help in the preparation of this manuscript.

REFERENCES

August DA, Ottow RT, Sugarbaker PH. 1984. Clinical perspective of human colorectal cancer metastases. *Cancer Metastasis Rev* 3:303–324.

Bhargava DK, Lipkin M. 1981. Transplantation of adenomatous polyps, normal colonic mucosa and adenocarcinoma of colon into athymic mice. *Digestion* 21:225–231.

Bogden AE, Houchens DP, Ovejera AA, et al. 1982. Advances in chemotherapy studies with the nude mouse. In *The Nude Mouse in Experimental and Clinical Research*, vol. 2, J Fogh, BC Giovanella, eds., pp. 367–400. New York: Academic Press.

Bowen JM, Cailleau R, Giovanella B, et al. 1983. A retrovirus-producing transformed mouse cell line derived from a human breast adenocarcinoma transplanted in nude mice. *In Vitro* 19:635–641.

Brattain MG, Levine AE, Chakrabarty S, et al. 1984. Heterogeneity of human carcinoma. *Cancer Metastasis Rev* 3:177–191.

Brattain MG, Marks ME, McCombs J, et al. 1983. Characterization of human colon carcinoma cell lines isolated from a single primary tumour. *Br J Cancer* 47:373–381.

Carrel S, Sordat B, Merenola C. 1976. Establishment of a cell line (CO-115) from a human colon carcinoma transplanted into nude mice. *Cancer Res* 36:3978–3984.

DeVore DP, Houchens DP, Ovejera AA, et al. 1980. Collagenase inhibitors retarding invasion of a human tumor in nude mice. *Exp Cell Biol* 48:367–373.

Drewinko B, Moskwa P, Lotzova E, et al. 1986. Successful heterotransplantation of human colon cancer cells to athymic animals is related to tumor cell differentiation and growth kinetics and to host natural killer cell activity. *Invasion Metastasis* 6:69–82.

Egan ML, Todd CW. 1972. Carcinoembryonic antigen: Synthesis by a continuous line of adenocarcinoma cells. *JNCI* 49:887–889.

Fermor B, Umpleby HC, Lever JV, et al. 1986. Proliferative and metastatic potential of exfoliated colorectal cancer cells. *JNCI* 76:347–439.

Fidler IJ. 1984. The evolution of biological heterogeneity in metastatic neoplasms. In *Cancer Invasion and Metastasis: Biologic and Therapeutic Aspects*, GL Nicolson, L Milas, eds., pp. 5–17. New York: Raven Press.

Fidler IJ. 1986. Rationale and methods for the use of nude mice to study the biology and therapy of human cancer metastasis. *Cancer Metastasis Rev* 5:29–49.

Fidler IJ, Caines S, Dolan Z. 1976. Survival of hematogenously disseminated allogeneic tumor cells in athymic nude mice. *Transplantation* 22:208–212.

Fidler IJ, Hart IR. 1982. Biologic diversity in metastatic neoplasms: Origins and implications. *Science* 217:998–1003.

Fidler IJ, Pollack VA, Hanna N. 1984. The use of nude mice for studies of cancer metastasis. In *Immune Deficient Animals*, B Sordat, ed., pp. 328–338. Basel: Karger A. G.

Fidler IJ, Poste G. 1985. The cellular heterogeneity of malignant neoplasms: Implications for adjuvant chemotherapy. *Semin Oncol* 12:207–222.

Flanagan SP. 1966. Nude, a new hairless gene with pleiotropic effects in the mouse. *Genet Res* 8:295–299.

Fogh J, Fogh JM, Orfeo T. 1977. One hundred and twenty-seven cultured human tumor cell lines producing tumors in nude mice. *JNCI* 59:221–226.

Fogh J, Orfeo T, Tiso J, et al. 1979. Establishment of human colon carcinoma lines in nude mice. *Exp Cell Biol* 47:136–144.

Freedman VH, Shin S. 1978. Use of nude mice for studies on the tumorigenicity of animal cells. In *The Nude Mouse in Experimental and Clinical Research*, vol. 1, J Fogh, BC Giovanella, eds., pp. 353–384. New York: Academic Press.

Giavazzi R, Campbell DE, Jessup JM, et al. 1986a. Metastatic behavior of tumor cells isolated from primary and metastatic human colorectal carcinomas implanted into different sites in nude mice. *Cancer Res* 46:1928–1933.

Giavazzi R, Jessup JM, Campbell DE, et al. 1986b. Experimental nude mouse model in human colorectal cancer liver metastases. *JNCI* 77:1303–1308.

Giovanella BC, Fogh J. 1978. Present and future trends in investigations with nude mouse as a recipient of human tumor transplants. In *The Nude Mouse in Experimental and Clinical Research* vol. 1, J Fogh, BC Giovanella, eds., pp. 282–312. New York: Academic Press.

Giovanella BC, Fogh J. 1985. The nude mouse in cancer research. *Adv Cancer Res* 44: 70–120.

Giovanella BC, Stehlin JS, Williams LJ Jr. 1974. Hetero-transplantation of human malignant tumors in "nude" thymusless mice. II. Malignant tumors induced by injection of cell cultures derived from human solid tumors. *JNCI* 52:921–930.

Giovanella BC, Stehlin JS Jr, Williams LJ Jr, et al. 1978. Heterotransplantation of human cancers into nude mice. *Cancer* 42:2269–2281.

Giovanella BC, Yim SO, Morgan AC, et al. 1973. Mctastases of human melanomas transplanted in "nude" mice. *JNCI* 50:1051–1053.

Goldenberg D, Pavia R. 1981. Malignant potential of murine stromal cells after transplantation of human tumors into nude mice. *Science* 212:65–67.

Goldenberg D, Pavia R. 1982. In vivo horizontal oncogenesis by a human tumor in nude mice. *Proc Natl Acad Sci USA* 79:2389–2394.

Goldrosen MH. 1980. Murine colon adenocarcinoma immunobiology of metastases. *Cancer* 45:1223–1228.

Hajdu SI, Fogh J. 1978. The nude mouse as a diagnostic tool in human tumor cell research. In *The Nude Mouse in Experimental and Clinical Research*, vol. 1, J Fogh, BC Giovanella, eds., pp. 235–266. New York: Academic Press.

Hanna N. 1982. Role of natural killer cells in control of cancer metastasis. *Cancer Metastasis Rev* 1:45–64.

Hanna N, Davis TW, Fidler IJ. 1982. Environmental and genetic factors determine the level of NK activity of nude mice and affect their suitability as models for experimental metastasis. *Int J Cancer* 30:371–376.

Hansen CT. 1978. The nude gene and its effects. In *The Nude Mouse in Experimental and Clinical Research*, vol. 1, J Fogh, BC Giovanella, eds., pp. 1–13. New York: Academic Press.

Heppner GH. 1984. Tumor heterogeneity. *Cancer Res* 44:2259–2265.

Horten BC, Basler GA, Shapiro WR. 1981. Xenograft of human malignant glial tumors into brains of nude mice: A histological study. *J Neuropathol Exp Neurol* 40:493–511.

Houghton JA, Taylor DM. 1978. Maintenance of biological and biochemical characteristics of human colorectal tumours during serial passage in immune-deprived mice. *Br J Cancer* 37:199–206.

Kerbel RS, Man MS, Dexter D. 1984. A model of human cancer metastasis: Extensive spontaneous and artificial metastasis of a human pigmented melanoma and derived variant sublines in nude mice. *JNCI* 72:93–108.

Kimball PM, Brattain MG. 1980. Isolation of a cellular subpopulation from a human colonic carcinoma cell line. *Cancer Res* 40:1574–1579.

Kirkland SC. 1985. Dome formation by a human colonic adenocarcinoma cell line (HCA-7). *Cancer Res* 45:3790–3795.

Klug TL, Salzmans S, Quinn A, et al. 1984. Tumorigenicity in athymic mice of the human colon carcinoma cell line SW 1116 expressing the tumor-associated antigenic determinant CA 19-9. *Cancer Res* 44:5212–5218.

Kopper L, Van Hanh T, Lapis K. 1982. Experimental model for liver metastasis formation using Lewis lung tumor. *J Cancer Res Clin Oncol* 103:31–38.

Kozlowski JM, Fidler IJ, Campbell D, et al. 1984. Metastatic behavior of human tumor cell lines grown in the nude mouse. *Cancer Res* 44:3522–3529.

Kyriazis AP, DiPersio L, Michael GJ, et al. 1978. Growth patterns and metastatic behavior of human tumors growing in athymic mice. *Cancer Res* 38:3186–3190.

Kyriazis AP, Kyriazis AA, McCombs WB III, et al. 1981. Biological behavior of human malignant tumors grown in the nude mouse. *Cancer Res* 41:3995–4000.

Lafreniere R, Rosenberg SA. 1986. A novel approach to the generation and identification of experimental hepatic metastases in a murine model. *JNCI* 76:309–315.

Leduc EH. 1959. Metastasis of transplantable hepatomas from the spleen to the liver in mice. *Cancer Res* 19:1091–1095.

Leibovitz A, Stinson SC, McCombs WB III, et al. 1976. Classification of human colorectal adenocarcinoma cell lines. *Cancer Res* 36:4562–4569.

Levy JA, White AC, McGrath CM. 1982. Growth and histology of a human mammary-carcinoma cell line at different sites in the athymic mouse. *Br J Cancer* 45:375–383.

Lockshin A, Giovanella BC, De Ipolyi PD, et al. 1985. Exceptional lethality for nude mice of cells derived from a primary human melanoma. *Cancer Res* 45:345–350.

Mach JP, Carrel B, Merenda C, et al. 1974. In vivo localization of radiolabelled antibodies to carcinoembryonic antigen in human colon carcinoma grafted into nude mice. *Nature* 248:704–706.

Martin KW, Halpern SE. 1984. Carcinoembryonic antigen production, secretion, and kinetics in BALB/c mice and a nude mouse-human tumor model. *Cancer Res* 44:5475–5481.

McBain JA, Weese JL, Meisner LF, et al. 1984. Establishment and characterization of human colorectal cancer cell lines. *Cancer Res* 44:5813–5821.

Mong HT, Chu TM. 1985. Characterization of the tumorigenic and metastatic properties of a human pancreatic tumor cell line (ASPC-1) implanted orthotopically into nude mice. *Tumour Biol* 6:89–98.

Naito S, von Eschenbach AC, Giavazzi R, et al. 1986. Growth and metastasis of tumor cells isolated from a human renal cell carcinoma implanted into different organs of nude mice. *Cancer Res* 46:4109–4115.

Namba M, Miyamoto K, Hyodoh F, et al. 1983. Establishment and characterization of a human colon carcinoma cell line (KmS-4) from a patient with hereditary adenomatosis of the colon and rectum. *Int J Cancer* 32:697–702.

Naulat-Duga I, Sheppel A, Marty C, et al. 1984. Metastases of human tumor xenografts in nude mice. *Invasion Metastasis* 4:209–224.

Pantelouris EM, Hair J. 1970. Thymus dysgenesis in nude (nu/nu) mice. *J Embryol Exp Morphol* 24:615–621.

Pathak S. 1976. Chromosome banding techniques. *J Reprod Med* 17:25–28.

Pathak S, Goodacre A. 1986. Specific chromosome anomalies and predisposition to human breast, renal cell and colorectal carcinoma. *Cancer Genet Cytogenet* 19:29–36.

Pimm MV, Armitage NC, Perkins AC, et al. 1985. Localization of an anti-CEA monoclonal antibody in colo-rectal carcinoma xenografts. *Cancer Immunol Immunother* 91:8–17.

Poste G, Fidler IJ. 1980. The pathogenesis of cancer metastasis. *Nature* 283:139–146.

Povlsen CO, Rygaard J. 1971. Heterotransplantation of human adenocarcinomas of the colon and rectum to the mouse mutant nude. A study of nine consecutive transplantations. *Acta Pathologica et Microbiologica Scandinavica. Section A, Pathology* 79:159–169.

Povlsen CO, Rygaard J. 1976. Growth of tumors in the nude mouse. In *In Vitro Methods of Cell-Mediated and Tumor Immunity*, BB Bloom, JR David, eds., pp. 701–711. New York: Academic Press.

Povlsen C, Rygaard J, Fogh J. 1982. Long-term growth of human tumors in nude mice: Evaluation of stability. In *The Nude Mouse in Experimental and Clinical Research*, vol. 2, J Fogh, BC Giovanella, eds., pp. 79–93. New York: Academic Press.

Povlsen CO, Visfeldt J, Rygaard J, et al. 1975. Growth patterns and chromosome constitutions of human malignant tumours after long-term serial transplantation in nude mice. *Acta Pathologica et Microbiologica Scandinavica. Section A, Pathology* 83:709–716.

Richie JP, McDonald J, Gittes RF. 1981. Resistance to intravenous tumor metastases in the athymic mouse: A paradoxic response. *Surgery* 90:214–220.

Rutzky LP, Giovanella BC, Tom BH, et al. 1983. Characterization of a human colonic adenocarcinoma cell line, LS123. *In Vitro* 19:99–107.

Rutzky LP, Siciliano MJ. 1982. Various isozyme gene expression patterns among human colorectal adenocarcinoma cell lines and tissues. *JNCI* 68:81–90.

Rygaard J, Povlsen CO. 1969. Heterotransplantation of a human malignant tumour in "nude" mice. *Acta Pathologica et Microbiologica Scandinavica. Section A* 77:758–760.

Rygaard J, Povlsen CO. 1982. Athymic (nude) mice. In *The Mouse in Biomedical Research,* vol. 4, *Experimental Biology and Oncology,* HL Foster, ed., pp. 51–67. New York: Academic Press.

Shafie SM, Liotta LA. 1980. Formation of metastasis by human breast carcinoma cells (MCF-7) in nude mice. *Cancer Lett* 11:81–87.

Sharkey FE, Fogh J. 1979. Metastasis of human tumors in athymic nude mice. *Int J Cancer* 24:733–738.

Sharkey FE, Fogh J. 1984. Considerations in the use of nude mice for cancer research. *Cancer Metastasis Rev* 3:341–360.

Sordat B, Merenola C, Carrel S. 1977. Invasive growth and dissemination of human solid tumors and malignant cell lines grafted subcutaneously to newborn nude mice. In *Proceedings of the Second International Workshop on Nude Mice,* T Nomura, N Ohsawa, N Tamaoki, R Fujiwara, eds., pp. 311–316. Tokyo: University of Tokyo Press.

Sordat BCM, Ueyama Y, Fogh J. 1982. Metastasis of tumor xenografts in the nude mouse. In *The Nude Mouse in Experimental and Clinical Research,* vol. 2, J Fogh, BC Giovanella, eds., pp. 95–147. New York: Academic Press.

Sordat B, Wang WR. 1984. Human colorectal tumor xenografts in nude mice: Expression of malignancy. *Behring Inst Mitt* 74:291–300.

Spremulli EN, Dexter DL. 1983. Human tumor cell metastasis. *J Clin Oncol* 1:496–509.

Spremulli EN, Scott C, Campbell DE, et al. 1983. Characterization of two metastatic sub-populations originating from a single human colon carcinoma. *Cancer Res* 43:3828–3835.

Sugarbaker PH, Gunderson LL, Wittes RE. 1985. Colorectal cancer. In *Cancer Principles and Practice of Oncology,* VT deVita Jr, S Hellman, SA Rosenberg, eds., pp. 795–884. Philadelphia: J. B. Lippincott.

Takahashi S, Konishi Y, Nakatani K, et al. 1978. Brief communication: Conversion of a poorly differentiated human adenocarcinoma to ascites form with invasion and metastasis in nude mice. *JNCI* 60:925–927.

Thombre PS, Doedhar SD. 1984. Inhibition of liver metastases in murine colon adenocarcinoma by liposomes containing human C-reactive protein or crude lymphokines. *Cancer Immunol Immunother* 16:145–150.

Tom BH, Rutzky LP, Jakstys MM, et al. 1976. Human colonic adenocarcinoma cells. I. Establishment and description of a new line. *In Vitro* 12:180–191.

Tompkins MB, Rao GV, Tompkins WAE. 1979. Increased tumorigenicity and resistance to antibody lysis of human colon tumor cells xenografted in congenitally athymic mice. *Cancer Res* 39:2160–2166.

Tompkins WAE, Watrach AM, Schmale JD, et al. 1974. Cultural and antigenic properties of newly established cell strains derived from adenocarcinomas of the human colon and rectum. *JCNI* 52:1101–1110.

Wanebo HJ, Rao B, Pinsky CM, et al. 1978. Preoperative carcinoembryonic antigen level as a prognostic indicator in colorectal cancer. *N Engl J Med* 299:448–451.

Wang WR, Sordat B, Piquet D, et al. 1984. Human colon tumors in nude mice: Implantation site and expression of the invasive phenotype. In *Immune-Deficient Animals,* 4th International Workshop on Immune-Deficient Animals in Experimental Research, Chexbres, October 31–November 3, 1982, ed. B Sordat, pp. 239–245. Basel, New York: S Karger.

Whitehead RH, Macrae FA, St John DJB, et al. 1985. Colon cancer cell line (LIM 1215) derived from a patient with inherited nonpolyposis colorectal cancer. *JNCI* 74:759–765.

Wright WC, Daniels WP, Fogh J. 1981. Distinction of seventy-one cultured human tumor cell lines by polymorphic enzyme analysis. *JNCI* 66:239–247.

Zalcberg JR, Thompson CH, Lichtenstein M, et al. 1983. Localization of human colorectal tumor xenografts in the nude mouse with the use of radiolabeled monoclonal antibody. *JNCI* 71:801–808.

Annual Clinical Conference on Cancer, Vol. 30
Gastrointestinal Cancer: Current Approaches to Diagnosis and Treatment
© 1988 by The University of Texas System Cancer Center

8. In Vitro Study of Adenomas: Effect of Fat Derivatives in Colon Cancer Development

Eileen A. Friedman

There is substantial clinical and experimental evidence that colon adenomas contain premalignant cells that are the direct precursors of colon carcinoma in man. Those adenomas classified as villous by histopathology have a much greater probability of giving rise to a carcinoma than the generally smaller tubular adenomas that appear less aberrant (Muto, Bussey, and Morson 1975). Detailed study of the cells within sectioned adenomas led to the conclusion that the dysplastic cells within adenomas were of the type that directly precede carcinoma (Konishi and Morson 1982).

We were able to study the relationships among adenomas of different histological classes, normal cells, and carcinomas by developing tissue culture techniques that allowed us to place into primary culture these epithelial cells (Friedman et al. 1981; Friedman, Gillin, and Lipkin 1984). About 90% of all normal and adenoma tissues and 50% of carcinomas were cultureable, so the results were representative. The epithelial cells migrated within 24 hours as a continuous sheet from partially digested explants to form round "patch" colonies (fig. 8.1). The cells were identified as epithelial by general morphology and the presence of characteristic epithelial subcellular structures including junctional complexes (tight junctions, gap junctions, and desmosomes), interlocking adjacent cells, a brush border on the apical side facing the medium, mucous secretion, and goblet cells interspersed between the transporting cells within the epithelial sheets cultured from cells of normal patients. The cells were also functionally epithelial. They transported water through their apical surfaces and discharged it through their basal surfaces. The accumulated fluid caused a bulging of the epithelial sheet into readily apparent fluid-filled domes.

The cells were studied without passage, so the only selection was for viable cells able to migrate onto the surface of the dish. Migration is a normal characteristic of colon epithelial cells, which move up the colonic crypt as they differentiate and divide. The lymphocytes, which make up the lamina propria, were lost upon digestion of the colon tissue, and the few fibroblasts that line the crypts did not migrate from the explants unless the epithelial cells that migrated first had died. The cellular sheets were monolayers of pure epithelial cells.

The normal, adenoma, and carcinoma cells looked grossly similar by phase microscopy; however, close examination showed they differed in several respects. Under the same culture conditions normal cells remained viable for only a few days, but adenoma and carcinoma cells could be maintained for over a month. The cells also differed structurally. The cytoskeleton in each cell was visualized by per-

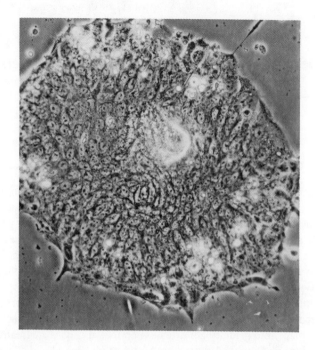

Fig. 8.1. Phase micrograph of living adenoma patch colony showing intact curved colony boundary (×200).

meabilizing the cell with the detergent NP40 and then staining with rhodamine-conjugated phalloidin. This toxic drug binds very tightly to actin molecules polymerized into filaments that are then stacked into bundles. These actin "cables" are then visualized using fluorescence microscopy. Nonpolymerized actin molecules were unstained. Carcinomas had the lowest number of cables, adenomas the most, and normal cells an intermediate number. The presence of actin cables within adenoma cells was more readily seen than the tiny actin filaments underneath the cell membrane of carcinoma cells (fig. 8.2). We quantified the method by photographing random fields of each cell type and scored the photographs blindly using a score of 0 (no cables) to 5 (extensive cable network). Normal cells cultured from five subjects had an actin score of $2.66+/-0.42$; cells of 15 adenomas had a score of $4.41+/-0.11$; cells of seven carcinomas had a score of $0.90+/-0.80$. Adenomas of the tubular class (4.1) could not be distinguished from adenomas of the villous (4.5) or villotubular classes (4.3) (Friedman et al. 1984, 1985).

Certain adenoma cells could be induced to have an actin phenotype like carcinoma cells if they were treated with the promoting agent 12-O-tetradecanoylphorbol-13-acetate (TPA), or phorbol. The adenomas that responded to TPA exhibited either moderate or severe dysplasia, or infiltrating or in situ carcinoma. The TPA-responsive adenoma cells became rounded or detached from the plate and lost their actin cables.

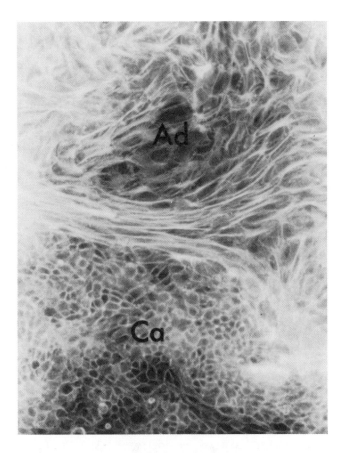

Fig. 8.2. Cocultivation of HT29 carcinoma cells (*Ca*) with adenoma cells (*Ad*). The cells were permeabilized with NP40, and then the actin cables were stained with rhodamine-conjugated phalloidin. The cells are readily distinguished (×815).

A similar phenotypic change induced by TPA had been seen earlier (Friedman 1981; Friedman, Urmacher, and Winawer 1984) and had been correlated to the induction of secretion of the protease plasminogen activator. Twenty-nine of 30 adenomas (16 villotubular, 8 villous, and 6 tubular) that contained moderate-to-severe dysplasia or carcinoma responded like carcinoma cells (each of 12 tested) to TPA (tables 8.1 and 8.2). The cultured adenoma cells released plasminogen activator, rounded up, and lost some attachment to the petri dish. Some even detached. We hypothesize that the secreted protease from the dysplastic or carcinoma cells within the adenoma selectively clips adenoma cell membrane proteins. The adenoma cells would then be partially or completely released from the dish. Presumably, the transmembrane actin-anchoring proteins would also be partly digested, and the actin cable network would rapidly unravel. We hypothesize that the responses to TPA are physiologically relevant responses to a nonphysiological agent (TPA) that mimics an

Table 8.1. *Summary of Plasminogen Activator Secretion and Morphological Changes Induced by TPA in Primary Cultures of Adenomas and Carcinomas*

Pathology	No. of Specimens	Percent Specimens Secreting Plasminogen Activator	TPA Effects on Morphology
Adenocarcinomas	13	100	Some cell detachment
Villous adenomas with in situ or infiltrating carcinoma or severe to moderate dysplasia	8	100	Many monolayer cells detached
Villotubular adenomas with in situ or infiltrating carcinoma or moderate to severe dysplasia	16	94	Many monolayer cells detached
Tubular adenomas with in situ or infiltrating carcinoma or moderate to severe dysplasia	6	100	Many monolayer cells detached
Tubular adenomas with only mild dysplasia	21	5	No cells detached

Abbreviation: TPA, 12-*O*-tetradecanoylphorbol-13-acetate.

endogenous compound. We further propose that the physiological agents are products of a partial breakdown of triglycerides found within the colon.

Consider the background for the use of synthetic tumor-promoting agents like TPA. Investigation of carcinogenesis originally began with an experimental animal and a putative carcinogen, and two questions were asked: Would the compound cause a tumor, and if so, where? This very necessary work simplified tumorigenesis into a one-step phenomenon. The introduction of promoting agents, which were initially observed to be cellular irritants, allowed tumor development to be broken up into stages so that it more closely approximated the multistage development of human cancer. A dose of a carcinogen too low to cause a tumor was selected. When this carcinogen was followed by repeated applications of a promoting agent, a tumor appeared. Either protocol alone did not produce a tumor, and reversing the order of

Table 8.2. *Effect of TPA on Established Human Colon Carcinoma Cell Line HT29*

TPA Concentration	Plasminogen Activator Secreted per 10^6 Cells (mU)	Morphological Changes
0	6.5	None
25 ng/ml	12.0	Cells rounded but attached
50 ng/ml	15.0	Cells rounded but attached
100 ng/ml	23.0	Cells rounded but attached

Abbreviation: TPA, 12-*O*-tetradecanoylphorbol-13-acetate.

application was ineffective. Effective carcinogens were mutagens, so an interpretation of the results was that a mutated cell was further modified by the promoting agent to become tumorigenic. A further improvement of the system using mouse skin in in vivo experiments has been described (Hennings et al. 1983). A low dose of a mutagen followed by repeated applications of a promoter led to papillomas. A second mutagen then converted the papillomas to carcinomas. Experimental carcinogenesis was now divided into three stages.

Additional evidence suggests that tumor promotion has relevance to human cancer development. It is not limited to skin carcinogenesis. TPA-mediated tumor promotion also occurs in the gastrointestinal tract (Goerttler et al. 1979) and other organs (Blumberg et al. 1984). This is not surprising because tumor promoters bind to a cellular receptor found on all nucleated vertebrate cells, including human cells (Blumberg et al. 1984). This receptor has been identified as the enzyme protein kinase C (Niskizuka 1984), which is important in cellular regulation. Tumor promoters like TPA somehow adventitiously bind to and activate a normal cellular regulator and subvert its activity. However, the relevance of this finding to colon carcinoma is that the endogenous activators of protein kinase C are a class of compounds called *diacylglycerols* that are derived intracellularly from membrane phospholipids.

Diacylglycerols, or diglycerides, have another source in the colon. They are partially digested triglycerides and come from dietary fat. Diglycerides are also derived from the degradation of the cellular membranes of desquamated colon epithelial cells. The diglycerides in the colon must include arachidonic and stearic residues from membrane digestion. Fat breakdown would yield diglycerides with stearic, oleic, palmitic, myristic, and lauric fatty acid moieties. Chain lengths shorter than 12 would be very rare. We found that the synthetic diglyceride dimyristin induced plasminogen activator secretion from carcinoma cells in an effect parallel to that of TPA, which itself has a myristic acid residue.

What does this mean in biologic terms for tumor development? The careful histopathology studies cited above from Morson's group (Konishi and Morson 1982; Muto, Bussey, and Morson 1975) have shown that colon carcinoma in man begins within a focus of moderate to severely dysplastic cells. Dysplastic cells in the majority of instances, except in some cases of ulcerative colitis (Riddell et al. 1983), lie within an adenoma, most often a villous adenoma. These are the classes of adenoma cells that secrete plasminogen activator when promoted. Also, all carcinomas tested also secreted this protease, functionally linking the premalignant dysplastic cells with malignant cells. When the carcinoma cell arises, probably by mutation of a preexisting adenoma cell, it is surrounded by adenoma cells that form a tightly interwoven cell network. The carcinoma cell would be, we hypothesize, prevented from dividing by the contact inhibition of the surrounding adenoma cells if it and the surrounding cells did not secrete plasminogen activator when promoted. The protease secretion probably is not a one-step procedure, but a continuous process that slowly allows the carcinoma focus to grow within the adenoma. Diacylglycerols from desquamated cell membranes and dietary fat would, of course, be repeatedly present in the fecal matter.

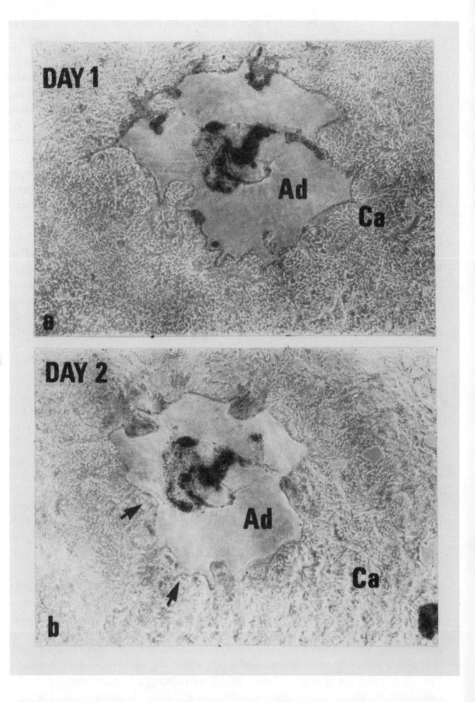

Fig. 8.3. Phase photomicrographs of adenoma cells cocultivated with invading HT29 colon carcinoma cells. *a,* The rounded adenoma colony has been photographed slightly out of phase so that the entire colony appears as one sheet and its outline is clear. The carcinoma cells have slightly deformed the adenoma colony. *b,* This is the same cocultivation 24 hours later. Note how the carcinoma (*Ca*) cell invasion has produced a depression in the adenoma (*Ad*) colony (*arrows*) (×304).

The carcinoma cells must penetrate the adenoma to become invasive. The effect of the protease on adenoma cells is quite dramatic, and in our study few adenoma cells after protease release remained viable for an extended period. In contrast, carcinoma cells from an established line (HT29) continued to proliferate after repeated treatments with TPA. Our cocultivation of HT29 carcinoma cells with adenoma cells has shown that the adenoma cells are invaded and destroyed by proteolysis (fig. 8.3) while the carcinoma cells flourish. Addition of the tumor promoter TPA enhanced the rate of adenoma destruction. These experiments, we believe, demonstrate that carcinoma cells can overgrow and destroy the adenoma within which they arise. This theory may also explain why most carcinomas exhibit little if any adenomatous regions by the time they are resected. Therefore, absence of adenoma tissue from a carcinoma would in no way disprove the adenoma-carcinoma sequence. Our data predict the destruction of most, if not all, of the host adenoma by the emerging carcinoma.

REFERENCES

Blumberg PM, Dunn JA, Jaken S, et al. 1984. Specific receptors for phorbol ester tumor promoters and their involvement in biological responses. In *Mechanisms of Tumor Promotion*, vol. 3, TJ Slaga, ed., pp. 1–91. Boca Raton, Fla.: CRC Press.

Friedman EA. 1981. Differential response of premalignant epithelial cell classes to phorbol ester tumor promoters. *Cancer Res* 41:4588–4599.

Friedman EA, Gillin S, Lipkin M. 1984. 12-*O*-Tetradecanoylphorbol-13-acetate stimulation of DNA synthesis in cultured preneoplastic familial polyposis colonic epithelial cells but not in normal colonic epithelial cells. *Cancer Res* 44:4078–4086.

Friedman EA, Higgins PJ, Lipkin M, et al. 1981. Tissue culture of human epithelial cells from benign colonic tumors. *In Vitro Cell Dev Biol* 17:632–644.

Friedman E, Urmacher C, Winawer S. 1984. A model for human colon carcinoma evolution based on the differential response of cultured preneoplastic, premalignant, and malignant cells to 12-*O*-tetradecanoylphorbol-13-acetate. *Cancer Res* 44:1568–1578.

Friedman E, Verderame M, Lipkin M, et al. 1985. Altered actin cytoskeletal patterns in two premalignant stages in human colon carcinoma development. *Cancer Res* 45:3236–3242.

Friedman E, Verderame M, Winawer S, et al. 1984. Actin cytoskeletal organization loss in the benign-to-malignant tumor transition in cultured human colonic epithelial cells. *Cancer Res* 44:3040–3050.

Goerttler K, Loehrke H, Schweizer J, et al. 1979. Systemic two-stage carcinogenesis in the epithelium of the forestomach of mice using 7,12-dimethylbenz[*a*]anthracene as initiator and the phorbol ester 12-*O*-tetradecanoylphorbol-13-acetate as promoter. *Cancer Res* 39:1293–1295.

Hennings H, Shores R, Wemk ML, et al. 1983. Malignant conversion of mouse skin tumors is increased by tumor initiators and unaffected by tumor promoters. *Nature* 304:67–71.

Konishi F, Morson BC. 1982. Pathology of colorectal adenomas: A colonoscopic survey. *J Clin Pathol* 35:830–841.

Muto T, Bussey HJR, Morson BC. 1975. The evolution of cancer of the colon and rectum. *Cancer* 36:2251–2270.

Nishizuka Y. 1984. The role of protein kinase C in cell surface signal transduction and tumour promotion. *Nature* 308:693–698.

Riddell RH, Goldman H, Ransohoff DF, et al. 1983. Dysplasia in inflammatory bowel disease. *Hum Pathol* 14:931–968.

Annual Clinical Conference on Cancer, Vol. 30
Gastrointestinal Cancer: Current Approaches to Diagnosis and Treatment
© 1988 by The University of Texas System Cancer Center

9. Familial Colon Cancer: Delineation of Clinical Subsets with Etiologic and Treatment Considerations

Henry T. Lynch, Patrice Watson, Stephen J. Lanspa,
Joseph N. Marcus, Tom E. Smyrk, Robert J. Fitzgibbons, Jr.,
Mary Kriegler, Jane F. Lynch, Churnfang A. Chen,
and Patrick M. Lynch

The etiology of colon cancer remains enigmatic. Its incidence is second only to lung cancer in Western industrialized nations (Silverberg 1984). It has shown a steady increase since the turn of the century (Byers and Graham 1984). Most epidemiologists agree that dietary factors (Lynch and Lynch 1985), including such trace metals as selenium, play an important etiologic role in accounting for broad ethnic and international differences in its incidence. However, a significant subset of the colon cancer burden is clearly the result of primary genetic factors (Correa and Haenszel 1978). Furthermore, when one considers the fact that only a fraction of patients exposed to specific environmental influences develop colon cancer, to conclude that some individuals are more susceptible to this disease than others seems logical. This reasoning implies that environmental and genetic factors are not mutually exclusive as causes of colon cancer, a concept that has been voluminously documented at the infrahuman level in experimental carcinogenesis (Autrup and Williams 1983) and has been inferential for humans (Harris 1980).

Unfortunately, with the exception of familial multiple adenomatous polyposis coli (FPC), the role of genetics in the etiology of colorectal cancer has been severely neglected (Lynch et al. 1984; Lynch and Lynch 1985; Lynch, Rosen, and Schuelke 1985).

Survival from colon cancer has not improved in the last two decades (Moore and Lamont 1984). A major problem is its early detection. Surveillance programs that focus on high-risk groups would logically show a higher cancer yield and thereby become more cost-effective. Identification of high-risk groups, inclusive of research on biomarkers that correlate with cancer susceptibility, should therefore become a high priority in our national cancer effort (Lynch 1976; Lynch and Lynch 1985).

Our purpose here is to focus attention on that fraction of patients with colon cancer who, by virtue of the characteristics of their family history, are at increased risk of colorectal cancer (and, occasionally, cancer of other anatomic sites). Special attention will be given to hereditary *non*polyposis colorectal cancer.

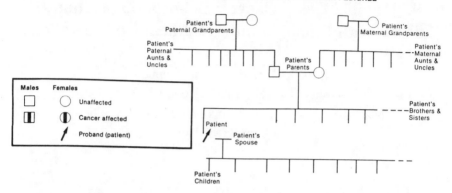

Fig. 9.1. Diagram representing a simple, modified nuclear pedigree for clinical use. Reprinted, by permission, from S. Karger, AG; Basel, Switzerland, from Lynch HT, Rozen P, Schuelke GS, et al., Hereditary colorectal cancer review: Colonic polyposis and nonpolyposis colonic cancer (Lynch syndromes I and II). *Survey of Digestive Diseases* 1984; 2:244–260.

STRATEGIES FOR FAMILY HISTORY COLLECTION

During the past two decades, we have had an opportunity to study thousands of families with virtually all forms of hereditary cancer and precancer syndromes (Lynch 1976, 1981; Lynch and Fusaro 1982). We concluded from this experience that investigations of cancer-prone families should include as an absolute minimum the collection of genealogic, general medical, and cancer history, with maximal attention to cancer verification (at all anatomic sites) in the proband, his or her siblings, progeny, parents, both paternal and maternal grandparents, aunts, and uncles (fig. 9.1). When considering the later age of cancer onset in the general population, older relatives (grandparents, aunts, and uncles) will logically be more informative than younger kin (siblings, progeny, and cousins) who have not reached the cancer-risk age. To recognize hereditary cancer syndromes, the investigator may, in certain situations, have to extend this basic, minimal pedigree much farther, particularly when physical signs or biomarkers for a particular syndrome are wholly lacking. Furthermore, because cancer is common in the general population, certain familial cancer clusters, characterized by two or more first-degree relatives affected by the same form of cancer but lacking Mendelian-inherited segregation patterns in the kindred, might result from chance alone.

CLASSIFICATION OF HEREDITARY COLORECTAL CANCER

We have operationally classified hereditary colon cancer into two major categories: those *with* multiple polyps of the colon (familial polyposis coli, FPC); and those *without* multiple colon polyps, referred to as hereditary nonpolyposis colorectal cancer syndromes (HNPCC), with subclassifications into Lynch syndromes I and II, to be discussed.

We recently reviewed the subject of hereditary cancers of the entire gastrointestinal tract (Lynch et al. in press). In this paper, we shall focus attention on hereditary cancers of the colorectum and tumors integral to these syndromes.

FAMILIAL POLYPOSIS COLI

Cancer genetics research has advanced at an almost explosive pace during the past two decades (Lynch 1976, 1981; Lynch and Fusaro 1982; Lynch and Lynch 1985). There has been particular progress in the realm of gastrointestinal cancer (Lynch and Lynch 1985). Herein, probably no precancerous disease has received greater attention than familial multiple adenomatous polyposis coli (FPC), a disease or group of diseases that is exceedingly heterogeneous. Several putatively distinct diagnostic categories of FPC exist, based in part on differences in polyp histological expression (adenomatous, hamartomatous, mixed adenomatous-hamartomatous) and extracancer manifestations (cutaneous and osseous signs in so-called Gardner's syndrome). Although colon cancer is the predominant neoplastic lesion in FPC, patients with these disorders exhibit a variable tumor spectrum involving gastrointestinal as well as other organs (for example, intracranial neoplasms in Turcot's syndrome). The full complement of tumors integral to the FPC genotypes remains undefined (Lynch 1976; Lynch 1981; Lynch and Fusaro 1982; Lynch and Lynch 1985; Lynch et al. in press).

The gastrointestinal polyposis phenotype in FPC is extremely variable, ranging from isolated polyps in obligate gene carrier adults to the more florid polyposis expression characterized by carpeting of the entire mucosal surface—the so-called "textbook" picture. Disturbingly, however, patients who have only isolated or several adenomatous polyps but are obligate gene carriers of one of the FPC syndromes remain at an inordinately high risk of colon cancer as well as other phenotypic facets of the syndrome. The vexing problem is that physicians may not consider them to be genotypically affected and, hence, destined to manifest colon cancer since their colon polyp phenotype is incomplete. These individuals will therefore not be engaged in intensive surveillance/management programs of the type mandated for their brethren who show florid FPC manifestations. An example of the variable tumor spectrum and colon polyp variation in this syndrome is shown in the pedigree in figure 9.2. The important point is that a detailed family study with particular attention to a full examination of the entire colon mucosa as well as a search for cancer of differing anatomic sites is mandatory when managing patients and families at risk of FPC. The old clinical saw that FPC requires 100, 200, or more polyps for its diagnosis must be abandoned, given the fact of variable expressivity of the polyposis colon mucosal phenotype (Lynch, Lynch, and Harris 1977; Lynch and Lynch 1985). Rather, greater attention must be given to all facets of the phenotypic findings in individual patients within the context of the pedigree, with the full realization that autosomal dominantly inherited disorders are noteworthy for extreme variability in phenotypic expression.

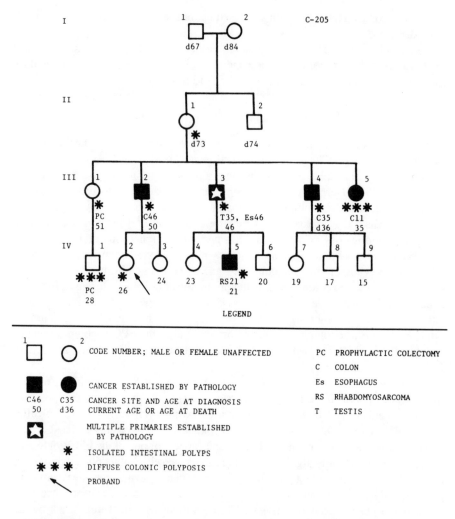

Fig. 9.2. Pedigree of a familial polyposis coli family showing variable colonic polyp expression. Reprinted, by permission, from Lynch HT, Rozen P, Schuelke GS, Hereditary colon cancer: Polyposis and nonpolyposis variants. *CA* 1985; 35:95–115.

An excellent example of such variable expressivity of phenotype was clearly depicted in a recent study of 18 patients who showed unusual and recurring features of FPC and so-called Gardner's syndrome. These patients revealed manifestations that included upper gastrointestinal polyposis, small bowel obstruction secondary to desmoid tumors or adhesions, recurring pancreatitis, and adenomas of the ampulla of Vater (Stevenson and Reid 1986). In twins, one had features of Gardner's syndrome while the other had FPC and no extracolonic manifestations of Gardner's syndrome. A woman with an ileorectal anastomosis developed multiple rectal adenomas during each of three pregnancies, and these adenomas regressed after each delivery. In addition, her daughter had multiple rectal adenomas that occurred on two occasions while she was taking birth control pills. These are some examples of the variable clinical nuances of FPC.

PHENOTYPIC OVERLAP IN VARIABLE HEREDITARY COLON CANCER DISORDERS

Many of the phenotypic features of FPC *overlap* among allegedly discrete precancer FPC syndromes, making their classification onerous. Thus, the nosology of what heretofore were considered clearly discrete syndromes now seem to be blurred and less clearly defined. Indeed, their ultimate classification often relates to the energy and ingenuity of the investigator and the time he or she is able to devote to ferreting out tumor patterns and clinical signs in families prone to polyps of the gastrointestinal tract. This phenomenon is seen in high relief in context with a newly disclosed phenotypic finding in Gardner's syndrome. A brief background sketch is in order.

The historical evolution of phenotypic findings emanating from the original 1951 description by Eldon Gardner of a large colon cancer–prone family, subsequently designated *Gardner's syndrome,* has been remarkable (Gardner 1951). Continuous investigation of this and similar kindreds has revealed, in addition to colon cancer and multiple colon polyps, a variety of other features, including benign epidermoid cysts of the skin, desmoid tumors, osteomas, abnormalities of the teeth (delayed eruption of teeth, extra teeth, and abnormally shaped teeth), tumors of the gums and palate, and a broad spectrum of cancers (cancer of the small bowel, stomach, pancreas, and cancer of extragastrointestinal sites as in brain tumors, carcinoma of the thyroid and adrenal glands, and sarcomas) (Lynch and Lynch 1985). As clinicians continued to intensively evaluate at-risk and affected patients with suspected or proven Gardner's syndrome, they added in a mushrooming fashion to its phenotypic complement. For example, in 1980, Blair and Trempe described intraocular findings during a routine examination of a patient affected by Gardner's syndrome, in whom they observed a number of "freckles" located behind the retina. These were described as *congenital hypertrophy of the retinal pigment epithelium* (CHRPE) as shown in figure 9.3. These pigmentations may occur in between one in 200 and one in 500 individuals in the general population in whom they will be restricted to one eye only; very rarely a normal, healthy person may have two or more patches of CHRPE. These pigmentary lesions vary in color from gray to jet black, and their

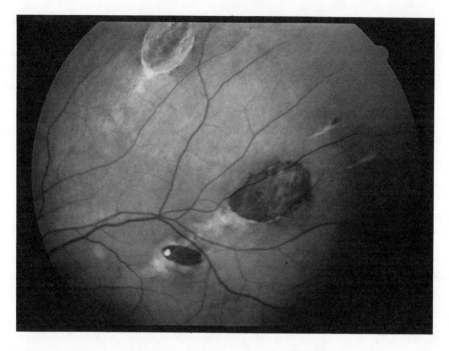

Fig. 9.3. An example of congenital hypertrophy of the retinal pigment epithelium. Courtesy of Richard A. Lewis, M.D., Baylor College of Medicine, Houston, Texas.

size ranges from less than 1 mm to 5 or 6 mm in diameter. They do not impair vision and have no known malignant predisposition.

Lewis et al. (1984) studied three families in which all patients who showed the phenotypic features consistent with Gardner's syndrome also had multiple and bilateral patches of CHRPE. Among these three kindreds, 11 adults with Gardner's syndrome and CHRPE had children available for examination. Among the 28 living offspring of these patients, 15 (54%) showed CHRPE and 13 (46%) showed an absence of CHRPE, a finding consonant with the anticipated bimodal expression of this trait in a dominantly inherited disease such as Gardner's syndrome. Interestingly, all children of CHRPE-unaffected Gardner's patients had no CHRPE. The youngest recognized individual with CHRPE in the three kindreds was two years old, a finding the authors used to emphasize the probable congenital aspect of CHRPE. In addition to their findings in the three Gardner's syndrome kindreds, Lewis et al. (1984) found, among eight Gardner's-affected individuals from four other kindreds, that all of these patients showed an *absence* of CHRPE. This is consonant with genetic heterogeneity and suggests at least two distinctive entities—Gardner's syndrome kindreds with CHRPE and, contrariwise, Gardner's syndrome kindreds showing an absence of CHRPE. These authors called attention to the value of CHRPE in linkage studies and suggested the possibility that Gardner's syndrome is caused by at least two different alleles with pleiotropic expression at a single locus.

Lewis et al. (1984) emphasized the need to reassess affected and at-risk individuals in Gardner's syndrome kindreds with attention to complete ophthalmic examination, including indirect stereo-ophthalmoscopy. Further investigation should be conducted of CHRPE in other Gardner's syndrome kindreds, including families with FPC who lack phenotypic aspects of Gardner's syndrome as well as patients with Lynch syndromes I and II.

Overlap of phenotype in colon cancer per se, as well as in hereditary colon cancer–predisposing syndromes, has been particularly noteworthy in the case of *mandibular osteomas*. Specifically, an excessive number of mandibular osteomas have been observed in consecutively examined patients with so-called sporadic colon cancer (Søndergaard et al. 1985) compared with controls, in patients with Gardner's syndrome (Bulow et al. 1984), in individuals with FPC in the absence of extracolonic signs suggestive of Gardner's syndrome (Søndergaard et al. 1985), and finally, in patients with HNPCC (Søndergaard et al. 1986). These observations are intriguing in that they suggest an etiologic connection between genotypes that predispose to colon cancer in the context of colon polyps or extracolonic signs or both, as well as to colon cancer *without* colon polyps, all occurring in concert with cancer of variable anatomic sites in a variety of putatively distinct genotypic cancer-prone settings. One might therefore raise the question as to what other physical markers may appear in common with an individual's proneness to colon cancer. For example, skin tags have been suggested to correlate with susceptibility to colon cancer (Chobanian et al. 1985; Luk and Colon Neoplasia Work Group 1986). These types of clinical and pathologic correlations are extremely perplexing for the so-called "lumpers" versus the "splitters" when the classification of hereditary colon cancer syndromes is attempted. Biomarker research, particularly the study of restriction fragment length polymorphisms (RFLP), may one day resolve these problems in hereditary cancer syndrome classification.

HEREDITARY NONPOLYPOSIS COLORECTAL CANCER
(LYNCH SYNDROMES I AND II)

The HNPCC syndromes may be divided into two subcategories: (a) Lynch syndrome I—hereditary site–specific colon cancer (HSSCC) (fig. 9.4), and (b) Lynch syndrome II—colon cancer in association with *other* forms of cancer, particularly endometrial and ovarian carcinoma (Boland and Troncale 1984; Lynch and Lynch 1985). This was originally termed the Cancer Family Syndrome (CFS) (fig. 9.5). In both hereditary nonpolyposis colorectal cancer syndromes, there is *proximal* predominance of colon cancer (making sigmoidoscopy an ineffective screening tool), vertical transmission, early age at cancer onset, an excess of multiple primary cancer, and significantly improved survival when compared stage for stage with the American College of Surgeons Audit Series (Albano et al. 1982; Russell et al. 1984). In Lynch syndrome I, the multiple primary cancers are restricted to the colon/rectum (about one third will involve the distal colon inclusive of the rectum). In Lynch syndrome II, in addition to colorectal cancer as in the former category, *other* anatomic sites may also be involved, including the endometrium and ovaries

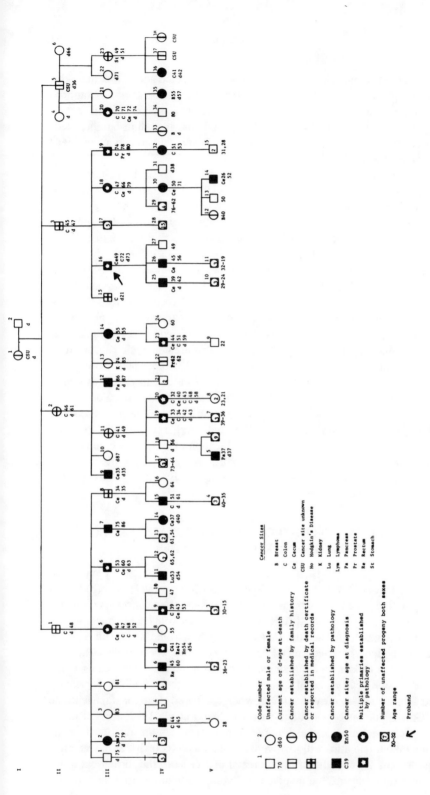

Fig. 9.4. Pedigree of a Lynch syndrome I family. This family history has been updated since it was originally reported. Reprinted, by permission, from Lynch HT, Harris RE, Bardawil WA, et al., Management of hereditary site–specific colon cancer. *Arch Surg* 1977; 112:170–174, Copyright 1977, American Medical Association.

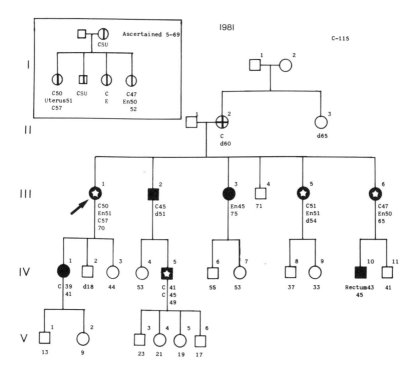

Fig. 9.5. Pedigree of a family showing the classic features found in a Lynch syndrome II family. See figure 9.4 for explanation of symbols. Reprinted, by permission, from Lynch PM, Lynch HT, eds., *Colon Cancer Genetics.* New York: V. N. Reinhold.

(Lynch et al. 1981), and organs such as pancreas (Lynch et al. 1985a). As in FPC, the full tumor spectrum in Lynch syndrome II remains elusive, suggesting the likelihood of heterogeneity.

Diagnostic Criteria for HNPCC Syndromes

The diagnosis of Lynch syndrome I or II is necessarily predicated on a full understanding of the natural history in context with the patient's position in the pedigree, since premorbid physical signs and biomarkers of clinically acceptable sensitivity and specificity are lacking. When the pedigree is extended, one is then able to make certain predictions about the likelihood of cancer occurrences by age at onset, anatomic site, and patterns of tumor combinations, all in concert with knowledge of these statistical expectations in the general population. When seen in the context of the developing pedigree, particularly as multiple first- or second-degree relatives become affected in accord with a known hereditary cancer syndrome phenotype, one is then able to identify hereditary cancer syndrome affecteds. Given the autosomal dominant mode of genetic transmission of Lynch syndromes I and II, one can

then predict risk (50%) to parents, siblings, and progeny of the putative genotypically affected individuals.

As a practical matter, the clinician is vitally concerned with this question: What
is the minimal amount of information that will be required to diagnose Lynch syndrome I or II with a reasonable degree of confidence? We have provided actual
clinical examples that illustrate the manner in which cumulative knowledge of the
evolution of cancer, with attention to age at onset, site, and multiple primary cancer
patterns within the context of the pedigree, can lead to confidence in hereditary
cancer syndrome diagnosis.

A family consistent with Lynch syndrome I was initially referred to us in 1975 by
the proband's physician when his patient at age 72 developed a second primary
colon cancer, an adenocarcinoma of the sigmoid. At age 49, he had undergone a
hemicolectomy for carcinoma of the cecum. His son at age 45 had recently also
undergone an operation for "adenocarcinoma of the cecum" (fig. 9.6A).

The cancer history provided by the proband on his first-degree relatives (fig.
9.6B) was sufficient to lead us to suspect that we were dealing with a colon
cancer–prone family. When the pedigree was extended to include second-degree
relatives (fig. 9.6C), there was little doubt that this family represented a hereditary
colon cancer syndrome. The full pedigree is seen in figure 9.4. The fact that multiple polyps of the colon were not present in any of the patients excluded the FPC
syndromes. Finally, there was a paucity of cancer of extracolonic sites, including an
absence of carcinoma of the endometrium and ovary, tumors that are integral to
Lynch syndrome II. Therefore, this is an example of an HNPCC kindred that shows
a predominance of early-onset carcinoma of the colon with predilection for the

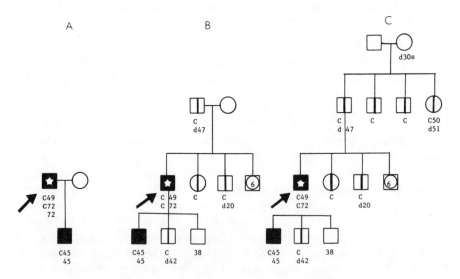

Fig. 9.6. Schematic diagram of the development of the family history leading to recognition of a
family with Lynch syndrome I seen in figure 9.4.

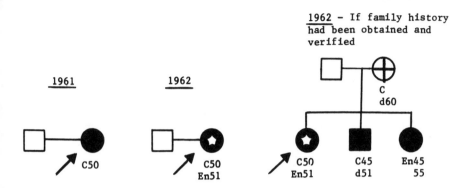

Fig. 9.7. Schematic diagram of clues leading to confirmation of the family representing Lynch syndrome II seen in figure 9.5. See figure 9.4 for explanation of symbols.

proximal colon and multiple primary colonic cancers, thereby fulfilling the criteria for Lynch syndrome I.

Findings clearly depicting medical genetic features consistent with Lynch syndrome II are seen in figure 9.5. The developing family history is seen in figure 9.7. Note that the proband had colon cancer at age 50 and developed a primary carcinoma of the endometrium (En) at age 51. If the cancer family history had been obtained and verified at the time of her second cancer diagnosis (1962), it would have revealed that her mother had had colon cancer and died from the disease at age 60. A brother had had a hemicolectomy for carcinoma of the cecum at age 45 and died from metastatic disease at age 51. In addition, a sister had undergone a panhysterectomy for adenocarcinoma of the endometrium at age 45 and was alive and well at age 55. This amount of information would have made us suspect a hereditary colon cancer syndrome. The family, however, was not referred to us by the proband's physician until 1969 when she developed a second carcinoma of the colon at age 57 and two sisters had developed multiple primary cancers of the colon and endometrium. The history the physician gave us is shown in the inset in figure 9.5. The extended, verified pedigree (1981) shows incidences of colorectal carcinoma that had been diagnosed since 1969 (fig. 9.5). Current (1986) updated information, not shown in figure 9.5, revealed that patient III-6 developed a second primary colon cancer that was diagnosed at age 67. Her sister (III-3), who had stomach cancer diagnosed at age 78, died of metastatic disease.

Segregation Analysis of HNPCC

Segregation analysis was performed on a set of 11 extended families with HNPCC (9 of these families were sampled for biomarkers discussed below) to elucidate the role of a major gene in colorectal cancer susceptibility (Bailey-Wilson et al. 1986). Segregation analysis is performed on a trait that is expressed as a dichotomy, namely, affected versus normal. In the matter of concern here, it pertains to cancer consistent with HNPCC. Allowance is made for variable age at onset, and an attempt is then made to determine whether Mendelian segregation of a single gene can account for the presence of multiple cases of HNPCC in the respective families. There was no significant departure at the 0.05 significance level from Mendelian autosomal dominant transmission ($\chi^2 = 2.62$, 2–3 df, $p > 0.20$), but there was significant departure from the hypothesis of Mendelian autosomal recessive transmission ($\chi^2 = 32.88$, 2 df, $p < 0.0005$) and from the hypothesis of no intergenerational transmission ($\chi^2 = 60.27$, 1–2 df, $p < 0.0005$). The estimate of gene frequency of the putative susceptibility allele was 0.0155. We signify "A" as the autosomal dominant cancer–predisposing allele and "a" as the recessive normal allele. The estimates of the mean of the age-of-onset distribution were 46.82 for individuals of genotype AA and Aa and 100.78 for individuals of genotype aa. The common variance for these age-of-onset distributions is 101.385. Most patients will not survive to age 100, which implies that only the lower tail of the distribution with a mean of 100.78 and variance of 101.385 is relevant to human data. The findings show, therefore, that sporadic cases of HNPCC may exist under this mode, but the age of onset for such sporadic cases is substantially greater than that of the genetic cases. The estimate of the susceptibility was 0.785.

Biomarkers and HNPCC

We initiated comprehensive studies dealing specifically with the genetic features and biomarker associations in HNPCC (Lynch et al. 1985b) and obtained the following biomarker results: (A) Putative linkage of Lynch syndrome II with Jk (Kidd) blood group with a lod score of 3.0. A lod score is used to express results of linkage analysis. It is the logarithm (to base 10) of the odds for linkage of a genetic polymorphism to the gene of concern; in this case, the gene for the Lynch syndrome II. A lod score of 1 indicates that linkage is 10 times as likely as free recombination, a lod score of 2 indicates linkage is 100 times as likely, and finally, a lod score of 3 indicates that linkage is 1000 times as likely. Most geneticists require a lod score of 3 or more to indicate significance of linkage. If our findings are correct, this would place the Lynch syndrome II gene on chromosome 2. (B) Increased in vitro tetraploidy of cultured skin fibroblasts (lod score 3.5) for Lynch syndromes I and II. (C) Positive association of tritiated thymidine labeling uptake pattern of the distal colonic mucosal crypt compartments with cancer risk status in Lynch syndrome I and II kindreds. (D) A high incidence of polymorphisms of centromeric heterochromatin, including complete inversion in cytogenetic studies of peripheral blood leukocytes in HNPCC. "Genetic polymorphism" pertains to genetically determined traits that show frequent qualitative differences such as the ABO and Rh blood groups. The term polymorphism may also apply to chromosomal differences, many of which have been revealed by recent advances in chromosomal banding techniques. The degree of polymorphism may be quantified by the heterozygosity of the system (the portion of the population heterozygous for the genetic locus in question). In the case of polymorphism of centromeric heterochromatin, we are referring to individual differences in the amount of heterochromatin in that area of the centromere revealed by C-banding techniques. Little is known about this heterochromatic region's function in the host. (E) Methionine dependence observed in dermal fibroblasts in tissue culture in HNPCC.

Pathology and HNPCC

The pathology of colorectal carcinoma in HNPCC differs in several respects from that of sporadic cases. The first difference in HNPCC is a predilection for the proximal colon. Recently updated data from 10 HNPCC families revealed 116 patients with colon or rectal carcinoma. In the 159 separate primary carcinomas found in these patients for which a subsite was identified, 79 (67%) were at or proximal to the splenic flexure (the generally accepted dividing point between right and left colon). The cecum alone accounted for 53 of the 159 (33%). Among the general population, adenocarcinoma of the cecum is said to make up between 4.5% and 20% of colorectal carcinomas (Gennaro 1977; Beart et al. 1983). Although there has been a recent, well-documented shift from distal to proximal carcinoma in the general population (Beart et al. 1983; Mamazza and Gordon 1982), there is evidence that this shift is age-related. For example, Eide and Stalsberg (1978) demonstrated that adenomatous polyps were more common in the distal colon in patients younger than age 65 and more common in the proximal colon in older patients. Snyder et al. (1977) found the greatest increase in right-sided colon cancers in people older than 65 years. Investigators at the University of Kansas (Butcher et al. 1985) found a similar relationship between age and colorectal cancer, although the data were significant only for female patients. Because the mean age at initial colorectal cancer diagnosis for our patients was 45.6 years and because many of the cases were diagnosed before 1960 (when distal carcinoma was clearly predominant in the general population), the predominance of right-sided tumors is even more striking.

Why should the cecum, which accounts for between 5% and 10% of the colon surface area, be the site of so many tumors? There are, of course, embryological and physiological differences between the right and left colons. The left colon is a derivative of the hindgut; the right colon, along with most of the small bowel, is derived from the midgut. Small bowel adenocarcinoma, a very rare lesion, has been reported in CFS kindreds (Love, Gilchrist, and Morrissey 1985). The population study of HNPCC at our institution includes patients with adenocarcinoma of the ileum.

Physiologically, the left colon simply transports fecal material to the rectum, while the right colon has mixing and absorbing functions. In fact, the cecum is probably the major storage and absorptive site in the large bowel (Magee and Dalley 1986). Fecal passage through the right colon may take days; passage through the left colon is more rapid.

There are also subtle histological differences between right and left colon, as reported by Shamsuddin, Phelps, and Trump (1982). They showed that goblet-type mucous cells are more numerous in the left colon and that the apical vesicles of these cells are electron-dense in the ascending colon and electron-lucent in the sigmoid and rectum. The histochemical properties of colonic mucin also differ according to site, with neutral mucin predominating in the ascending colon and acidic mucin predominating in the rectum. Endocrine cells are also more numerous in the rectum. Paneth cells, a normal inhabitant of the small bowel, may be seen in tissue from the proximal colon (Whitehead 1985). Interestingly, we recently reviewed a villous adenoma from the cecum of one of our patients, which was composed, in large part, of Paneth cells. Paneth cell metaplasia is also mentioned occasionally in the pathology reports for other patients in our kindreds; we have not had the chance to review those cases. Paneth cell numbers are known to be increased in goblet-cell carcinoids of the appendix, but the significance of Paneth cells in other neoplastic proliferations of the large intestine is unknown. Bansal et al. (1984) recently concluded that the Paneth cell may be a reserve cell from which goblet cells can develop. At this time, no etiologic connection can be drawn between the right-sided colon cancer predominance in HNPCC and embryological, physiological, and morphological differences between right and left colon.

In view of the right-sided colon cancer predominance in HNPCC, it is instructive to look at other conditions or biomarkers that exhibit right- or left-side polarity in the colon and to address the issue of any possible pathogenetic relation to HNPCC. Of special interest is the report that, in patients developing asynchronous multiple primary colon tumors, the first tumor is frequently in the right colon (Thomas, Dockerty, and Waugh 1948). These patients also develop cancers at an earlier age than does the general population. Among the tumor biomarkers, squamous cell carcinoma is decidedly right-sided (Lundquest et al. unpublished data), but its incidence is extremely rare (about 0.05% of adenocarcinoma). Particularly interesting is the propensity for c-*myc* oncogene mRNA expression to be higher in left-sided tumors and the suggestion that HNPCC neoplasms, regardless of their site, might have consistently low c-*myc* expression (Rothberg et al. 1985). The presence of marker chromosomes is a mainly left-sided phenomenon (Reichmann, Levin, and Martin 1982). The authors of this study also reported that 10 of 12 familial non-polyposis colon cancers showed a near diploid karyotype. Although the relationship of tumor ploidy, as assessed by flow cytometry, to clinical behavior is not yet crystallized, at least one report (Kokal et al. 1986) shows aneuploidy to be an unfavorable prognostic variable, more strongly so than tumor stage. HNPCC has a less aggressive clinical course than sporadic colon cancer. One must wonder whether HNPCC will be characterized by low c-*myc* oncogene expression and near diploid karyotypes, but so far, this has not been directly demonstrated. Clearly, much work needs to be done.

In addition to preference for the right colon, colorectal carcinoma in HNPCC shows an apparently increased frequency of mucinous histology in selected families. This distinctive subtype, characterized by abundant pools of extracellular mucin that usually far exceed the epithelial component, comprises about 15% of all colorectal cancer (Symonds and Vickery 1976; Sundblad and Paz 1982). It is numerically more common in the left colon, but tends to make up a higher percentage of those cancers found in the right colon. Its prevalence in familial cancer was highlighted in a recent report (Budd and Fink 1982) describing a family in which 14 individuals developed colon cancer; 7 of these tumors were mucinous adenocarcinomas. The mucinous subtype is also encountered quite frequently in our own work, making up more than 30% of colon cancers in some kindreds, a phenomenon consonant with heterogeneity. In one kindred, 10 of 15 mucinous adenocarcinomas were located in the right colon.

These two features, right-sided predominance and mucinous histology, are strikingly reminiscent of the situation seen in the colon carcinomas of children and adolescents. In a recent review of 30 patients aged 8 to 25 years, 15 had tumors in the right colon, and 25 were mucinous (Rao et al. 1985). Previous reports on the topic have given similar results (Enker, Paloyan, and Kirsner 1977; Kottmeier and Clatworthy 1975). One might speculate that these patients suffer from a spontaneous occurrence of the same defect that affects HNPCC patients.

In the general population, one feature of mucinous adenocarcinoma that deserves mention here is an association with adenomas. Although it is generally accepted that adenomatous polyps are precursor lesions to adenocarcinoma, the actual identification of a residual polyp in a resected colon cancer is a comparatively rare event. Sundblad and Paz (1982), for example, reported such a finding in 14 of 223 cases. A startling 11 of those 14 tumors were mucinous adenocarcinomas. Moreover, the authors were able to identify mucous hyperplasia in all 11 adenomas that contained mucinous adenocarcinoma. Similarly, Symonds and Vickery (1976) found an intimately associated villous adenoma in 31% of their 132 cases of mucinous adenocarcinoma.

This information may be useful in the continuing search for a marker to identify which members of an HNPCC kindred do, in fact, carry the cancer susceptibility genotype. Currently, it is possible by family history to identify those at 50% risk. An ideal marker would separate that group into those at nearly 100% risk and those at nearly 0% risk. In the absence of that, a marker for identifying incipient neoplasia in the 50% risk patient is desirable. Candidate markers are described elsewhere in this paper; relevant to this section is a report from the University of Wisconsin concerning a screening program with colonoscopy in CFS kindreds (Love and Morrissey 1984). Of 42 asymptomatic individuals who underwent colonoscopy, 7 (17%) were found to have adenomatous or villous polyps. Two of these polyps contained carcinoma. Recall that CFS was dubbed "hereditary *non*polyposis colon cancer" to separate it from familial conditions characterized by numerous polyps and an increased cancer risk, for example, familial polyposis coli. In truth, however, it is not known whether the cancers in HNPCC arise in flat mucosa or in polyps. HNPCC kindreds have been suggested to have actually fewer polyps than do patients in the general population (Mecklin, Järvinen, and Peltokallio 1986b). Indeed, some might use the Wisconsin data to argue in favor of that opinion by comparing it to such studies as the large autopsy study by Rickert et al. (1979), which showed a 46.9% incidence of adenomatous polyps in 518 autopsied colons. The prevalance of adenomatous polyps increases with age, however. The Rickert study included a preponderance of patients over age 50, whereas the 42 patients mentioned above had a median age of 29.5 years.

Although a dysplasia-carcinoma sequence in flat mucosa is presumed to occur in ulcerative colitis and sporadic reports of small, nonpolypoid colon cancers (Crawford and Stromeyer 1983) continue to appear, it may well be that HNPCC patients are polyp formers. The high frequency of mucinous adenocarcinomas in patients from certain HNPCC families, coupled with the strong association between mucinous adenocarcinoma and adenomatous polyps, suggests that regular colonoscopy with biopsy of all polypoid lesions may be the best screening method currently available.

One patient recently evaluated by us may be illustrative. A 39-year-old woman known to be at 50% risk of colorectal carcinoma was found to have a mucosal irregularity in the rectosigmoid. Biopsy showed a 2-cm sessile, tubulovillous adenoma with foci of high-grade dysplasia and large numbers of cells with prominent apical mucous vacuoles. Biopsy from the same area three months later again showed similar adenomatous change. There was high-grade dysplasia, and mucous hyperplasia was greater than the first biopsy examination had shown. The area containing the mucosal irregularity was fulgurated at the time of the second biopsy. Three months later, the patient was found to have a pedunculated, 1-cm polyp at the same site. Histological assay showed an adenomatous polyp with high-grade dysplasia but no mucous hyperplasia.

Surveillance in Concert with Clinical Aspects (Natural History) of HNPCC

The issues involved in justification of screening for colon cancer were summarized by Winawer, Schottenfeld, and Sherlock (1985). This depends heavily on incidence of disease in the population to be screened, the sensitivity and specificity of the tests used, and whether effective treatment is available. Ideally, screening tests should have high patient and physician acceptance and should be cost effective.

The potential benefits of colon cancer surveillance programs are difficult to evaluate. It is logical to conclude, however, that their yield will be greater when they involve high-risk target populations such as families affected by Lynch syndromes I and II. Because of ethical concerns, controlled trials of surveillance benefits cannot be done with high-risk populations. However, prospective evaluations of screening techniques for colon tumors in the general population should elicit results that will influence strategies for screening high-risk groups.

In the general population older than 40, the incidence of colon cancer is one to two cases per 1000 population. Incidence of adenomas is 50 to 100 patients per 1000 population, and in the subset with positive fecal occult blood tests, 25% to 30% have significant colon lesions (Schottenfeld and Winawer 1982). One study from Norway involving sigmoidoscopic screening of 400 patients between the ages of 50 and 59 yielded an 81% rate of compliance and showed that 35% of this population had rectosigmoid polyps (Hoff et al. 1985). To be able to identify subsets of the general population with even higher risks would be beneficial.

A detailed family history can increase the rate of positive findings in a screening program. Rozen et al. (1981) showed that, in asymptomatic young adults with a positive family history of colorectal cancer, the yield of tumors discovered in a screening program doubled compared with those without positive family history. In addition, Burt et al. (1985) found a 21% incidence of polyps in patients from colon cancer families as compared with 9% in controls using flexible sigmoidoscopy. The occurrence of the polyps in the study group followed an autosomal dominant inheritance pattern. In spite of the benefit of a detailed family history in detecting high-risk individuals, a paradoxical delay in diagnosis and treatment of such patients may occur because of fear, repression, and denial (Lynch and Krush 1968). Other limitations of the family history were shown by Mecklin, Järvinen, and Peltokallio (1986a) in a large Finnish population with Lynch syndrome II. Only 40% of these Lynch syndrome II patients had a positive family history demonstrable at the time of cancer diagnosis.

The frequency of the CFS (Lynch syndrome II) in this Finnish population was estimated as 1:20,000 and was believed to account for 0.4% of all colon cancers (Mecklin, Järvinen, and Peltokallio 1986a). In an accompanying editorial, Lynch (1986) proposed that the incidence of the CFS may have been greatly underestimated and might have been higher if modified diagnostic criteria or biomarkers had been used rather than the end point of colon cancer. Indeed, in a subset of this population, Mecklin, Järvinen, and Peltokallio (1986b) found an incidence 10 to 20 times that of their initial report.

In the Mecklin group's studies (1986b, 1986c), the greatest incidence of CFS was in the 30- to 50-year-old group, the youngest patient with colorectal cancer being 19 years old. Their recommendation was that in such families screening should begin at age 20 and continue until age 60. They emphasized the use of colonoscopy or air contrast barium enema over flexible sigmoidoscopy because of the demonstrated increased incidence of right colonic lesions.

In our population (Bailey-Wilson et al. 1986), the onset and distribution of colon cancers in Lynch syndromes I and II was similar to that of the Finnish group. Mean age at onset of the cancers was 47 years (SD ± 10 years). Lynch syndromes I and II did not differ in age at onset and in distribution. These data are similar to those of a population with HNPCC followed at Memorial Sloan-Kettering (Sherlock, Lipkin, and Winawer 1980). Therefore, if screening is to be undertaken of this high-risk population, it should begin during these individuals' twenties.

Few surveillance programs have been reported for Lynch syndrome populations. Love, Gilchrist, and Morrissey (1985) studied 34 at-risk patients (two had previous colon cancer) and found that two patients had colon cancers arising in polyps (youngest age, 20) and two had adenomas (youngest age, 28). Love and Morrissey (1984) evaluated the results of colonoscopies in 42 asymptomatic patients and found a 17% incidence of adenovillous polyps. Most were beyond the reach of a 25-cm sigmoidoscope. In a current surveillance study, we performed colonoscopies in 33 patients. Of eight obligate gene carriers, evidenced by previous colon cancer, four were found by surveillance colonoscopy to have adenomatous polyps. Of 25 asymptomatic patients, all at 50% risk for HNPCC by virtue of their position in the pedigree but without a history of colon cancer, five had adenomatous polyps and one had a hyperplastic polyp. The high incidence of tumors in relatively young patients argues for continuance of surveillance programs.

In a large screening program of Lynch syndrome patients in Brindisi, Italy (under the direction of Giuseppe Cristofaro, M.D., Associazione Provinciale Brindisina per la latta contro il Cancro, personal communication, 1986), a similar villous adenomatous lesion was found in a 25-year-old asymptomatic male. This was a 2-cm sessile lesion histologically described as "a severe dysplasia over flat mucosa."

A second patient in our series had many small, adenomatous polyps throughout the right colon and proximal/transverse colon and a 3-cm villous adenoma near the cecum. Although we do not consider the finding of single adenomatous polyps to connote the phenotypic expression of the syndrome (and to require subtotal colectomy), such patients warrant special consideration. Once colon cancer has been identified in these at-risk patients, however, a subtotal colectomy or total colectomy with ileoanal anastomosis is warranted.

SCREENING STRATEGIES

The effectiveness of diagnostic tools in colon cancer is difficult to evaluate. Simon (1985) recently reviewed fecal occult blood testing. The positive aspects of the Hemoccult test were that a sufficiently high prevalence of disease did exist, and longer patient survival and earlier disease staging were obtained in some studies. Furthermore, cancer could be aborted by the removal of polyps found during screening. The test is simple, safe, and cheap (about $3) and can definitely uncover asymptomatic cancer. Use of the fecal occult blood test can detect 3 to 20 cancers per 10,000 population. Only 5% to 10% of positive test results are, however, caused by cancer, and technical problems may interfere with the chemical reaction (Simon 1985). Another criterion at issue is improved patient survival, which may be related to lead time and length biases so that earlier detection may not necessarily reflect true, improved survival. Not all physicians accept the validity of occult blood testing (Kolata 1985). Nevertheless, Allison and Feldman (1985) showed it to be cost effective. In a Kaiser-Permanente health system, more than 14,000 patients older than 45 years of age were screened—representing 70% compliance—and 1.1% (112 patients) of the tests turned out positive. All of these patients were evaluated with colonoscopy. Twelve patients had colon cancers (50% Dukes A), 13 patients had polyps, and 45 had other gastrointestinal sources of blood loss. Adding four years for possible lead time bias, Allison and Feldman estimated an increased survival of 22 person-years and estimated savings at more than $14,000 each in the 12 people with cancer. Similar or even better results are likely to be obtained when the test is used in a higher-risk population, such as patients with Lynch syndromes. An improved fecal occult blood test (HemoQuant) was developed by Ahlquist et al.

(1985). The test is more sensitive and specific than the Hemoccult, and it has fewer technical problems. Although no data have been reported yet on use of the Hemo-Quant by Lynch syndrome populations, its use seems warranted.

Barium enema (BE) has been used to follow up patients who had positive fecal occult blood test results. Costs at Creighton University are $153 per test. With the single-contrast BE used at most institutions, however, half of all colon cancers and most adenomas are missed (Tedesco et al. 1978). Double-contrast BE improves the yield significantly (Miller 1974). Furthermore, any lesions seen with X ray must be evaluated with colonoscopy.

Colonoscopy ($550 at Creighton University) in the presence of a positive fecal occult blood test gives a higher yield than BE (Love and Morrissey 1984). Further-more, the ability to make a definitive tissue diagnosis of polyps and the proven benefit of polypectomy during colonoscopy argue for colonoscopy as the best ex-amination for patients with suspected disease. However, false-negatives do exist. Although the cecum can be reached in 95% of patients, this may be a blind spot as are the hepatic and splenic flexures. The rate of false-negative exams is difficult to determine, but in one study adenomas larger than 1 cm were reported to be missed 6% to 8% of the time (Leinicke et al. 1977). Colonoscopy and BE are complemen-tary tests, but the time and discomfort of two separate bowel preps limit compliance among patients. The complication rate of colonoscopy is 3% to 6% and consists of perforation, hemorrhage (rare), and drug reactions (Schrock 1983). Mortality is 0.02%. Because of the high incidence of right-sided colon lesions in the Lynch syn-dromes, we believe that colonoscopy or BE is required in a surveillance program because flexible sigmoidoscopy is insufficient. The choice of double-air contrast BE compared with colonoscopy depends on the relative quality of x-ray services in a particular area as well as the availability of colonoscopy. In our practice we rely on colonoscopy in managing the Lynch-syndrome kindreds.

SURGICAL IMPLICATIONS

Genetic knowledge can be used to make accurate predictions concerning the like-lihood of cancer developing in the colon remaining after partial colectomy and in selected extracolonic organs that are at risk. This information can be of value in deciding proper surgical management, that is, partial versus subtotal or total colec-tomy, or the addition of an oophorectomy or hysterectomy. Unfortunately, many clinicians are content with lumping all colon cancers together with the more com-mon sporadic form of the disease, making decisions without regard to the specific needs of the hereditary subset. Although the percentage of patients with hereditary colon cancer may be relatively small (about 7% of the total colon cancer burden), the absolute number is significant because of the high incidence of the disease (Lynch and Lynch 1985).

Surgical management of hereditary colon cancer syndromes requires a distinction to be made between syndromes in which the cancer is preceded by multiple neo-plastic polyps, of which familial polyposis (FPC) is best known, and those not asso-ciated with multiple colon polyps (HNPCC). Most surgeons are familiar with the polyposis syndromes because of their distinctive clinical features. However, the more subtle *non*polyposis varieties are about five times more common (Lynch et al. 1985c). Unfortunately, in many patients in the latter group, the nonpolyposis syndromes are not recognized and are treated subsequently as sporadic colon cancers, with partial colectomies and no consideration of extracolonic organs; in certain situations in which the family history is striking, the nonpolyposis syndromes are lumped together with the polyposis syndromes and treated by proctocolectomy. Either form of management may be inappropriate for patients afflicted with hereditary nonpolyposis colon cancer.

FPC and HNPCC must be distinguished, primarily because the polyposis syndromes place the entire colon from cecum to anus at risk of colon cancer, whereas the nonpolyposis syndromes have a predilection for proximal involvement of the colon, making a less morbid, rectum-sparing operation the procedure of choice.

Polyposis Syndromes

The most important of the polyposis syndromes is the autosomal dominantly inherited FPC and its so-called variant, Gardner's syndrome. Others include Turcot's syndrome, lymphosarcomatous polyposis, and leukemia polyposis (Bulow 1984). All are characterized by multiple, neoplastic colon polyps that precede the development of colon cancer. Associated extracolonic adenocarcinomas at such sites as the ampulla of Vater, small bowel, stomach, and other anatomic sites (full tumor spectrum, as mentioned, is unknown) require an effective surveillance program for early detection but do not mandate prophylactic surgery (Lynch et al. in press). The overriding consideration in treatment of the colon is that the entire organ is at risk. Thus, it is important that all of the colon, or as much as is practically possible, be removed. The commonly employed procedures used to achieve this aim are discussed below. There is little difference in the management of patients who present with a colon cancer, and the syndrome is recognized because of multiple associated polyps and the patient whose syndrome is recognized in the precancerous, polyp-only stage. Perhaps a more thorough lymphadenectomy is indicated in the former situation, however.

Proctocolectomy with Brooke Ileostomy

This is the most common procedure performed today. The entire colon, rectum, and anus are removed and the patient is left with a permanent stoma that is somewhat more difficult to manage than a colostomy because of the liquid nature of the effluent. The advantages are that all tissue at risk for cancer is removed and the operation has a relatively low morbidity. The major disadvantages are the practical inconvenience of caring for the stoma and the loss of self-image. The latter is an especially important consideration since many of the patients are young, that is, premarital. Sexual and urinary dysfunction may be minimized, if the rectum is not already involved with cancer, by employing an intrasphincteric technique for dissection of the rectum as has been described for inflammatory bowel disease (Bauer et al. 1983). The operation is safe and effective and must be considered the standard by which all other procedures are judged.

Proctocolectomy with Endorectal Pull Through

This procedure is similar to the standard proctocolectomy except that care is taken to preserve the rectal sphincteric musculature either by an intrasphincteric dissection or a mucosal stripping procedure. The end of the distal ileum is then sewn directly to the anus. Although effective in some surgeons' hands, most believe that the rate of rectal incontinence is too high, sometimes resulting in little better than a perineal ileostomy. This procedure is not widely used (Coran, Jordan, and Wesley 1986).

Proctocolectomy with Kock Pouch

This ingenious operation was developed by Professor Kock of Göteborg, Sweden, in 1969. It consists of a reservoir fashioned out of distal ileum with a nipple-valve arrangement proximal to an abdominal stoma at skin level. The reservoir is periodically emptied by intubating the pouch with a catheter. Its advantage over the Brooke ileostomy is that it alleviates the need for an external appliance. The disadvantages are the need for a permanent stoma and the frequently encountered failure of the nipple valve, which results in incontinence and requires corrective surgery. Its popularity has lessened with development of the ileoanal pouch procedures discussed below (Goligher 1984).

Colectomy with Mucosal Proctectomy and Ileo Pouch–Anal Anastomosis

This procedure involves removing all of the colon to the rectum and then stripping out the rectal mucosa. A pouch is fashioned using loops of ileum, and an anastomosis is accomplished between the pouch and the anus. This procedure is clearly growing in use, primarily because it is the most effective procedure for completely eliminating all colon tissue at risk of cancer and still allowing the normal route of defecation. The procedure is often chosen for and by patients who want to be spared any danger of cancer but consider an abdominal stoma a serious threat to their self-image (Buls and Goldberg 1983; Williams and Johnston 1985). These patients must be prepared to accept a significantly higher degree of morbidity compared with that of proctocolectomy and Brooke ileostomy. A recent report from the Mayo Clinic (Dozois 1986) noted that 49% of patients experienced some type of complication, which required a second procedure for 20% of these patients. This is in addition to the second operation needed routinely to close the temporary diverting ileostomy. Long-term follow-up revealed that patients had an average of 6 stools during the day and 1.2 stools at night. Twenty percent were occasionally incontinent of stool or gas or both, and 5% eventually required conversion to a Brooke ileostomy. In addition, bowel obstruction or infections of the pouch seem to plague some of the patients in long-term follow-up. Of concern is the potential complication rate of this procedure in the hands of surgeons who do not have the considerable experience of surgeons at the Mayo Clinic. Nevertheless, the majority of patients treated with this operation are satisfied with the results.

Subtotal Abdominal Colectomy with Ileorectal Anastomosis

In 1970, Moertel, Hill, and Adson reported their experience with ileorectal anastomosis for FPC, demonstrating a 59% incidence of cancer in the retained colon in 17 patients followed for 23 years. This widely quoted paper led to the general impression that this operation is inadequate for treating patients who have FPC. Other centers have not had such dismal results, however, and there have been some recent reports of no or very few rectal recurrences even with long-term follow-up (Bussey et al. 1985; Gingold and Jagelman 1981; Järvinen 1985). Although Moertel and colleagues (1970) do not say so specifically, it is assumed that a relatively long segment of colon was spared as was the custom at that time, that is, 25 cm, the length of a rigid proctoscope. Thus, the discrepancy may be explained in part by the very short rectal stumps that can be achieved with modern anastomotic stapling devices. Indeed, the anastomosis may be placed on the levator ani muscles, with the entire remaining rectum in reach of the examining finger. The operation is becoming more common again. Even Dr. Robert Beart, who heads the division of colorectal surgery at the Mayo Clinic, agrees it is the preferred procedure in patients who have relatively few rectal polyps (Beart 1985). Without question, when one considers rectal continence, stool frequency, sexual and urinary function, and the desire for a normal route of defecation, this operation yields the best results. Given the well-recognized phenomena of patients and their potentially affected relatives refusing even diagnostic workup, let alone definitive therapy, for fear of a mutilating operation, this procedure should at least be discussed (Albano et al. 1982; Boland and Troncale 1984; Lynch et al. in press). Of course, the surgeon must have a reasonable degree of confidence that the patient will comply with frequent rectal examinations with polypectomies.

Hereditary Nonpolyposis Colon Cancer Syndromes

Both Lynch I and Lynch II syndromes have several cardinal features that were mentioned previously but are important for emphasis because of their surgical implications: (1) proximal colonic involvement, (2) increased incidence of synchronous or metachronous lesions, (3) early age of onset, (4) autosomal dominant genetic transmission, and (5) a better prognosis when compared with the sporadic counterpart (Lynch et al. 1984). Surgical management decisions are based on these features. Thus, in either syndrome, a subtotal colectomy as opposed to a conventional right, left, or sigmoid resection is recommended. In Lynch syndrome II, prophylactic treatment must be considered for extracolonic organs, especially of the female genital tract. The real problem is not the treatment of these patients but rather the recognition of a genetically affected individual. It is tragic how often we see patients at the Creighton University Hereditary Cancer Institute with advanced female genital cancer, a readily obtainable personal history of a previous colon resection, and a family history of multiple genital and colon cancers consonant with Lynch syndrome II. It seems that, all too often when a diagnosis of colon cancer is made, thinking immediately shifts to such things as operative risk assessment, bowel preparation, blood component needs, and other preoperative necessities. In reality, these should be considered second. The first question should be, What type of colon cancer am I dealing with? Is it: (1) sporadic (2) associated with a polyposis syndrome, or (3) associated with a hereditary *non*polyposis syndrome? This is especially important in patients who are seen at an unusually young age with colon cancer or, for that matter, any adenocarcinoma associated with a hereditary cancer syndrome because, in certain at-risk patients, extracolonic cancers may be expressed first (Lynch et al. 1984).

What should one do when facing a patient who has a newly diagnosed malignancy and a significant Lynch syndrome I or II cancer family history? How does one decide which patient is truly part of a hereditary cancer syndrome family? Although intense investigation is under way, as yet no specific biomarkers are available that would allow one to diagnose the HNPCC syndromes with a simple blood test. Obviously, it is not possible for each of these patients to be seen by a geneticist. And certainly, one would not want to recommend a subtotal colectomy for a patient who, by chance, happens to have several relatives with colon cancer. Data are now being analyzed at the Hereditary Cancer Institute from more than 10,000 individual members of various hereditary cancer syndrome kindreds in an attempt to address these issues more fully. The hope is that precise criteria will eventually be developed for these disorders to allow the primary care physician to diagnose a hereditary cancer syndrome accurately and confidently, and with the least possible amount of information.

Once the diagnosis of HNPCC has been made, how should the patient be managed? This is determined entirely by which of the two HNPCC syndromes the patient has and at what point the patient is being seen. We shall discuss hypothetical cases to illustrate the proper management.

1. *A patient from a Lynch syndrome I family with a newly diagnosed colon cancer.* A subtotal colectomy with ileorectal anastomosis is the procedure of choice because of the high incidence of synchronous and metachronous colon cancer lesions. Because of the propensity of these cancers to involve the proximal colon, sacrifice of the rectum would not be routinely justified. Of some concern is the concept that by transferring the effluent of the distal ileum from the right colon to the rectum, one might be establishing the same environment in the genetically susceptible mucosa of the rectum that had previously existed in the right colon. This could result in a high incidence of cancer in the retained rectum (Albano and Lynch 1985). Unfortunately, no data exist to support this theory, and long-term follow-up information is only now maturing.

    Extracolonic cancers are not part of Lynch syndrome I, so no specific treatment other than management of the colon cancer is needed. Some researchers believe that bilateral oophorectomy is indicated for staging purposes in all postmenopausal patients with colon cancer. Any consideration of this would not be directly related to the hereditary component of the disease but would be similar to the management recommended for the sporadic counterpart (Herrera et al. 1982).

2. *A patient from a Lynch syndrome II kindred with a newly diagnosed colon cancer.* Treatment of the colon would be as outlined for patient 1. If the patient is a woman, however, attention must also be directed to the genital tract. Certainly, if the patient is perimenopausal or postmenopausal, hysterectomy and bilateral oophorectomy should be performed. More difficult is the situation of the younger patient, who is perhaps in her early thirties. Factors such as childbearing desires,

osteoporosis, carcinogenic effects of prolonged estrogen replacement therapy, and others complicate the management recommendations. The decision concerning removal of these organs must be made to suit each patient. If hysterectomy and oophorectomy are not done, a screening program consisting of biannual pelvic examinations with attention to the ovaries and yearly endometrial aspiration currettage, an office procedure, should be initiated. Finally, some families with Lynch syndrome II have shown increased incidence of stomach, pancreas, breast, and other adenocarcinomas. An appropriate screening program for these organs should be outlined as dictated by the patient's own pedigree.

3. *A patient from a Lynch syndrome II family with a newly diagnosed endometrial cancer.* Not infrequently, patients with this syndrome develop genital tract cancer before colon cancer. A total abdominal hysterectomy and bilateral salpingo-oophorectomy, with or without lymphadenectomy and/or irradiation depending on the stage, should be performed (Gusberg 1986). Assuming that treatment of the genital cancer is curative, a prophylactic subtotal colectomy at the same setting would be considered. The added morbidity is not great enough to outweigh the benefits of this potentially cancer-preventing procedure.

4. *A patient from either a Lynch syndrome I or II family who was treated for colon cancer before being recognized as having the syndrome.* It is not unusual to see a patient who has had a conventional partial resection for colon cancer in whose case the significance of the family history was not appreciated. At the very least, an aggressive screening program of the female genital tract and the remaining colon are recommended. Frequently, the individual family's pedigree is so dramatic that the remaining colon is at 100% risk for a metachronous cancer. Conversion to subtotal colectomy is mandatory.

SUMMARY OF MANAGEMENT STRATEGIES FOR THE LYNCH SYNDROMES

The following is a summary of our management procedures in caring for patients from a Lynch syndrome kindred. Genetic counseling is undertaken in the mid-teens. At this age, patients are able to understand the implications of their family history and are encouraged to follow habits that promote health. This also allows them to become accustomed to the idea of health maintenance and attention to a surveillance program we believe should begin at age 25. Ideally, we recommend that intensive screening begin at age 25 and continue on to age 60. This consists of a yearly Hemo-Quant examination. In our practice, colonoscopy is conducted every two years and whenever the HemoQuant test is positive. Double air-contrast barium enema is an alternative. If polyps are found, they are removed endoscopically and surveillance is increased to yearly colonoscopy (Love 1986). If cancer is detected, a subtotal colectomy is recommended or, in patients under age 50, consideration is given to total colectomy and ileoanal anastomosis (see previous section for detailed surgical recommendations). If the patient has had no phenotypic expression of the syndrome by age 60, he or she is followed according to the recommendations of the American Cancer Society for managing risk in the general population. Because of the risk of ovarian and endometrial cancer, we perform annual pelvic examinations. There is no effective screening program for ovarian cancer, although we have experimented with ultrasonographic examination of the ovaries. For endometrial cancer screening, we recommend annual endometrial vacuum aspiration beginning after age 30, but with careful exclusion of pregnant women. At present, we do not screen for the myriad extraintestinal cancers that are part of the syndrome (Lynch et al. in press) except by thorough yearly history-taking and physical examination.

Compliance with cancer screening programs ranges from 15% to 75%. The problems involved with compliance have been detailed by Sherlock, Lipkin, and Winawer (1980) and include general health motivation as well as problems with perceived susceptibility and perceived benefit of screening procedures. Further public education is warranted to identify patients at risk and to let them know that colon cancer is a disease that can be cured. A further problem we have seen in our practice is that for financial concerns and because of worries over ability to get insurance, patients do not want to be identified as high-risk subjects.

As discussed earlier, identification of reliable biomarkers to identify patients that are obligate cancer gene carriers would allow our surveillance program to be even more highly targeted and would reduce the cost, time, and patient discomfort by half.

ACKNOWLEDGMENTS

The authors gratefully acknowledge support from the National Cancer Institute, Grant No. 1 RO1 CA41371; the Council for Tobacco Research, Grant No. 1297BR1; and the Health Futures Foundation, Inc.

REFERENCES

Ahlquist DA, McGill DB, Schwartz S, et al. 1985. Fecal blood levels in health and disease: A study using HemoQuant. *N Engl J Med* 312:1412–1428.

Albano WA, Lynch HT. 1985. Clinical management of hereditary colon cancer. In *Colon Cancer Genetics,* PM Lynch, HT Lynch, eds., pp. 99–110. New York: V. N. Reinhold.

Albano WA, Recabaren JA, Lynch HT, et al. 1982. Natural history of hereditary cancer of the breast and colon. *Cancer* 50:360–363.

Allison JE, Feldman R. 1985. Cost benefits of Hemoccult screening for colorectal cancer. *Dig Dis Sci* 30:860–865.

Autrup H, Williams GM. 1983. *Experimental Colon Carcinogenesis.* Boca Raton: CRC Press.

Bailey-Wilson JE, Elston RC, Schuelke GS, et al. 1986. Segregation analysis of hereditary nonpolyposis colorectal cancer. *Genet Epidemiol* 2:27–38.

Bansal M, Fenoglio CM, Robboy SJ, et al. 1984. Are metaplasias in colorectal adenomas truly metaplasias? *Am J Pathol* 115:253–265.

Bauer JJ, Gelernt IM, Salky B, et al. 1983. Sexual dysfunction following proctocolectomy for benign disease of the colon and rectum. *Ann Surg* 197:363–367.

Beart RW Jr. 1985. Familial polyposis. *Br J Surg* 72 (Suppl):S31–S32.

Beart RW, Melton LJ, Maruta M, et al. 1983. Trends in right and left-sided colon cancer. *Dis Colon Rectum* 26:393–398.

Blair NP, Trempe CL. 1980. Hypertrophy of the retinal pigment epithelium associated with Gardner's syndrome. *Am J Ophthalmol* 90:661–667.

Boland CR, Troncale FJ. 1984. Familial colonic cancer in the absence of antecedent polyposis. *Ann Intern Med* 100:700–701.

Budd DC, Fink DL. 1982. Autosomal dominant mucoid colon carcinoma: A study of a case and a kindred. *Am Surg* 48:180–183.

Bulow S. 1984. Colorectal polyposis syndromes. *Scand J Gastroenterol* 19:289–293.

Bulow S, Søndergaard JO, Witt I, et al. 1984. Mandibular osteomas in familial polyposis coli. *Dis Colon Rectum* 27:105–108.

Buls JG, Goldberg SM. 1983. Surgical options in ulcerative colitis. *Postgrad Med* 74:175–189.

Burt RW, Bishop T, Cannon L, et al. 1985. Dominant inheritance of adenomatous colonic polyps and colorectal cancer. *N Engl J Med* 312:1540–1544.

Bussey HJR, Eyers AA, Ritchie SM, et al. 1985. The rectum in adenomatous polyposis: The St. Mark's policy. *Br J Surg* 72:(suppl):S29–S35.

Butcher D, Hassanein K, Dudgeon M, et al. 1985. Female gender is a major determinant of changing subsite distribution of colorectal cancer with age. *Cancer* 56:714–716.

Byers T, Graham S. 1984. The epidemiology of diet and cancer. *Adv Cancer Res* 41:1–69.

Chobanian SJ, Van Ness MM, Winters C, et al. 1985. Skin tags as a marker for adenomatous polyps of the colon. *Ann Intern Med* 103:892–893.

Coran AG, Jordan FT, Wesley JR. 1986. The endorectal pull-through for the management of familial polyposis. *Int Rev Exp Pathol* 28:217–248.

Correa P, Haenszel W. 1978. The epidemiology of large bowel cancer. *Adv Cancer Res* 26:1–141.

Crawford BE, Stromeyer FW. 1983. Small nonpolypoid carcinomas of large intestine. *Cancer* 51:1760–1763.

Dozois RR. 1986. Restorative proctocolectomy and ileal reservoir. *Mayo Clin Proc* 61:283–286.

Eide TJ, Stalsberg H. 1978. Polyps of the large intestine in northern Norway. *Cancer* 42:2839–2848.

Enker WE, Paloyan E, Kirsner JB. 1977. Carcinoma of the colon in adolescents: A report and an analysis of the literature. *Am J Surg* 133:737–741.

Gardner EJ. 1951. A genetic and clinical study of intestinal polyposis, a predisposing factor for carcinoma of the colon and rectum. *Am J Hum Genet* 3:167–176.

Gennaro AR. 1977. Carcinoma of the cecum. *Surg Gynecol Obstet* 144:504–506.

Gingold BS, Jagelman DG. 1981. Sparing the rectum in familial polyposis: Causes for failure. *Surgery* 89:314–318.

Goligher JC. 1984. The changing face of colitis surgery. In *Advances in Gastrointestinal Surgery,* JS Najarian, JP Delaney, eds. Chicago: Year Book Medical.

Gusberg SB. 1986. Current concepts in the control of carcinoma of the endometrium. *CA* 36:245–253.

Harris CC. 1980. Individual differences in cancer susceptibilities. *Ann Intern Med* 92:809–825.

Herrera LO, Ledesma EJ, Nataraja N, et al. 1982. Metachronous ovarian metastases from adenocarcinoma of the colon and rectum. *Surg Gynecol Obstet* 154:531–534.

Hoff G, Vatn M, Gjone E, et al. 1985. Epidemiology of polyps in the rectum and sigmoid colon: Design of a population screening study. *Scand J Gastroenterol* 20:351–355.

Järvinen HJ. 1985. Time and type of prophylactic surgery for familial adenomatosis coli. *Ann Surg* 202:93–97.

Kokal W, Sheibani K, Terz S, et al. 1986. Tumor DNA content in the prognosis of colorectal carcinoma. *JAMA* 255:3123–3127.

Kolata G. 1985. Debate over colon cancer screening (in Research News). *Science* 229:636–637.

Kottmeier PK, Clatworthy HW Jr. 1975. Intestinal polyps and associated carcinomas in childhood. *Am J Surg* 110:709–716.

Leinicke JL, Dodds WJ, Hogan WJ, et al. 1977. A comparison of colonoscopy and roentgenography for detecting polypoid lesions of the colon. *Gastrointest Radiol* 2:125–128.

Lewis RA, Crowder WE, Eierman LA, et al. 1984. The Gardner's syndrome: Significance of ocular features. *Ophthalmology* 91:916–925.

Love RR. 1986. Adenomas as precursor lesions for malignant growth in nonpolyposis hereditary carcinoma of the colon and rectum. *Surg Gynecol Obstet* 162:8–12.

Love RR, Gilchrist KW, Morrissey JF. 1985. Normal mucosal histochemistry and histopathology in familial colorectal cancer. *Dis Colon Rectum* 28:799–803.

Love RR, Morrissey JF. 1984. Colonoscopy in asymptomatic individuals with a family history of colorectal cancer. *Arch Intern Med* 144:2200–2211.

Luk GD, the Colon Neoplasia Work Group. 1986. Colonic polyps and acrochordons (skin tags) do not correlate in familial colonic polyposis kindreds. *Ann Intern Med* 104:209–210.

Lynch HT, ed. 1976. *Cancer Genetics.* Springfield: Charles C. Thomas.

Lynch HT, ed. 1981. *Genetics and Breast Cancer.* New York: V. N. Reinhold.

Lynch HT. 1986. Frequency of hereditary nonpolyposis colorectal carcinoma (Lynch syndromes I and II). *Gastroenterology* 90:486–489.

Lynch HT, Fitzgibbons RJ Jr, Lanspa SJ, et al. In press. Familial polyposis coli and neurofibromatosis in the same patient: A family study. *Ca Genet Cytogenet.*

Lynch HT, Fitzgibbons RJ Jr, Marcus J, et al. 1985c. Colorectal cancer in a nuclear family: Familial or hereditary? *Dis Colon Rectum* 28:310–316.

Lynch HT, Fusaro RM. 1982. *Cancer-Associated Genodermatoses.* New York: V. N. Reinhold.

Lynch HT, Kimberling W, Albano W, et al. 1985b. Hereditary nonpolyposis colorectal cancer, Parts I and II. *Cancer* 56:934–938 and 939–951.

Lynch HT, Krush AJ. 1968. Delay: A deterrent to cancer prevention. *Arch Environ Health* 17:204–209.

Lynch HT, Lanspa SJ, Coffey RJ, et al. In press. Biomarkers, genetics, and gastrointestinal cancer. *Journal of Tumor Marker Oncology.*

Lynch HT, Lynch PM, Albano WA, et al. 1981. The Cancer Family Syndrome: A status report. *Dis Colon Rectum* 24:311–322.

Lynch HT, Rozen P, Schuelke GS. 1985. Hereditary colon cancer: Polyposis and nonpolyposis variants. *CA* 35:95–115.

Lynch HT, Rozen P, Schuelke GS, et al. 1984. Hereditary colorectal cancer review: Colonic polyposis and nonpolyposis colonic cancer (Lynch syndromes I and II). *Survey of Digestive Diseases* 2:244–260.

Lynch HT, Voorhees GJ, Lanspa SJ, et al. 1985a. Pancreatic cancer and hereditary nonpolyposis colorectal cancer: A family study. *Br J Cancer* 52:271–273.

Lynch PM, Lynch HT, eds. 1985. *Colon Cancer Genetics.* New York: V. N. Reinhold.

Lynch PM, Lynch HT, Harris RE. 1977. Hereditary proximal colonic cancer. *Dis Colon Rectum* 20:661–668.

Magee DF, Dalley AF II. 1986. The colon and defecation. In *Digestion and the Structure and Function of the Gut,* DF Magee, AF Dalley II, eds., vol. 8, pp. 256–302. Basel: Karger Continuing Education Series.

Mamazza J, Gordon PH. 1982. The changing distribution of large intestinal cancer. *Dis Colon Rectum* 25:558–562.

Mecklin J, Järvinen HJ. 1986. Clinical features of colorectal carcinoma in cancer family syndrome. *Dis Colon Rectum* 29:160–164.

Mecklin J, Järvinen HJ, Peltokallio P. 1986a. Cancer family syndrome. Genetic analysis of 22 Finnish kindreds. *Gastroenterology* 90:328–333.

Mecklin J, Järvinen HJ, Peltokallio P. 1986b. Identification of cancer family syndrome (letter). *Gastroenterology* 90:1099.

Miller RE. 1974. Detection of colon carcinoma and the barium enema. *JAMA* 230:1195–1198.

Moertel CG, Hill JR, Adson MA. 1970. Surgical management of multiple polyposis: The problem of cancer in the retained bowel segment. *Arch Surg* 100:521–526.

Moore JRL, Lamont JT. 1984. Colorectal cancer: Risk factors and screening strategies. *Arch Intern Med* 144:1819–1823.

Rao BN, Pratt CB, Fleming ID, et al. 1985. Colon carcinoma in children and adolescents. A review of 30 cases. *Cancer* 55:1322–1326.

Reichmann A, Levin B, Martin P. 1982. Human large bowel cancer: Correlation of clinical and histopathological features with banded chromosomes. *Int J Cancer* 29:625–629.

Rickert RR, Auerbach OA, Garfinkel L, et al. 1979. Adenomatous lesions of the large bowel. *Cancer* 43:1847–1857.

Rothberg PG, Spandorfer JM, Erisman MD, et al. 1985. Evidence that c-*myc* expression defines two genetically distinct forms of colorectal adenocarcinoma. *Br J Cancer* 52:629–632.

Rozen P, Fireman Z, Terdiman R, et al. 1981. Selective screening for colorectal tumors in the Tel-Aviv area: Relevance of epidemiology and family history. *Cancer* 47:827–831.

Russell AH, Tong D, Dowson LE, et al. 1984. Adenocarcinoma of the proximal colon. *Cancer* 53:360–367.

Schottenfeld D, Winawer SJ. 1982. Large intestine. In *Cancer Epidemiology and Prevention*, D Schottenfeld, JF Fraumeni, eds., pp. 703–727. Philadelphia: W. B. Saunders.

Schrock TR. 1983. Fiberoptic colonoscopy. In *Gastrointestinal Disease*, MH Sleisinger, JF Fordtran, eds., pp. 1617–1627. Philadelphia: W. B. Saunders.

Shamsuddin AM, Phelps PC, Trump BF. 1982. Human large intestinal epithelium: Light microscopy, histochemistry, and ultrastructure. *Hum Pathol* 13:790–803.

Sherlock P, Lipkin M, Winawer SJ. 1980. The prevention of colon cancer. *Am J Med* 68:917–931.

Silverberg E. 1984. Cancer statistics 1984 (American Cancer Society). *CA* 34:7–23.

Simon JB. 1985. Occult blood screening for colorectal carcinoma: A critical review. *Gastroenterology* 88:820–837.

Snyder DN, Heston JF, Meigs JW, et al. 1977. Changes in site distribution of colorectal carcinoma in Connecticut, 1940–1973. *American Journal of Digestive Diseases* 22:791–797.

Søndergaard JO, Svendsen LB, Witt IN, et al. 1985. Mandibular osteomas in colorectal cancer. *Scand J Gastroenterol* 20:759–761.

Søndergaard JO, Svendsen LB, Witt IN, et al. 1986. Mandibular osteomas in the Cancer Family Syndrome. *Br J Cancer* 52:941–943.

Stevenson JK, Reid BJ. 1986. Unfamiliar aspects of familial polyposis coli. *Am J Surg* 152:81–86.

Sundblad AS, Paz RA. 1982. Mucinous carcinomas of the colon and rectum and their relation to polyps. *Cancer* 50:2504–2509.

Symonds DA, Vickery AL. 1976. Mucinous carcinoma of the colon and rectum. *Cancer* 37:1891–1900.

Tedesco FJ, Waye JD, Raskin JB, et al. 1978. Colonoscopic evaluation of rectal bleeding. *Ann Intern Med* 89:907–909.

Thomas JF, Dockerty MB, Waugh JM. 1948. Multiple primary carcinomas of the large intestine. *Cancer* 1:564–573.

Whitehead R. 1985. Normal appearances in colonic biopsy specimens. In *Major Problems in Pathology, Vol. 3, Mucosal Biopsy of the Gastrointestinal Tract*, JL Bennington, ed., pp. 209–212. Philadelphia: W. B. Saunders.

Williams NS, Johnston D. 1985. The current status of mucosal proctectomy and ileo-anal anastomosis in the surgical treatment of ulcerative colitis and adenomatous polyposis. *Br J Surg* 72:159–168.

Winawer S, Schottenfeld D, Sherlock P. 1985. Screening for colorectal cancer: The issues. *Gastroenterology* 88:841–844.

Annual Clinical Conference on Cancer, Vol. 30
Gastrointestinal Cancer: Current Approaches to Diagnosis and Treatment
© 1988 by The University of Texas System Cancer Center

10. Choosing Endoscopic Alternatives for Diagnosis and Treatment of Colorectal Neoplasia

John R. Stroehlein

When choosing endoscopic alternatives for the diagnosis and treatment of large bowel neoplasia, two fundamental questions must be answered. Should an endoscopic procedure be performed and, if so, what procedure should be selected? Answers to these questions are primarily determined by their clinical context. It is therefore essential to discuss various clinical situations in which one may choose between available endoscopic alternatives.

THE SYMPTOMATIC PATIENT

When a patient has symptoms or signs that suggest the possibility of colorectal cancer, the endoscopic procedure of choice is colonoscopy. This conclusion does not discount the role of air-contrast barium enema in this clinical setting, since careful air-contrast examination carries a very high diagnostic yield (Beggs and Thomas 1983; Dodd 1985). It simply emphasizes the importance of, first, visualizing the entire large bowel if a patient has symptoms or signs that suggest large bowel cancer and, second, being careful not to attribute these symptoms to incidental findings.

The selection of colonoscopy as the endoscopic alternative for the symptomatic patient is based on the high possibility or probability that a lesion is present in this clinical setting, the need to perform a biopsy or remove synchronous tumors if an index lesion is found on sigmoidoscopy or barium enema x-ray examination, and the difficulty of trying clinically to predict the cause of certain signs or symptoms. The latter difficulty is underscored by the result of a study of 145 patients over age 40. Seventeen percent of 63 patients whose primary care physicians clinically considered the source of bleeding to be anal-rectal had disease involving the more proximal rectum or colon. In addition, in 5% of 97 patients who also received specialty consultation and proctoscopy, the source of bleeding was still believed to be anorectal when, in fact, each had a bleeding lesion involving a more proximal portion of the large bowel (Goulston 1986).

Colonoscopy is the endoscopic procedure of choice for the symptomatic patient not only for the above reasons, but also because colonoscopy has, in several studies, been shown to be somewhat superior to a barium enema in identifying carcinoma and polyps (Tedesco et al. 1978; Brand et al. 1980). Colonoscopy, however, is not error free (Miller 1981). When the clinical suspicion or probability of carcinoma is high and either colonoscopy or barium enema is negative, this enhances the possibility that the result is a false-negative. This is because the predictive value of any test is related to the prevalence or probability of a particular disease in a given patient or population. This concept is illustrated by the following example wherein the hypothetical sensitivity and specificity of a test remains constant, but its predictive value varies considerably, depending on the prevalance or probability of disease in the situation being evaluated.

A. Very unlikely (1 : 9) that a condition is present using a test with 80% sensitivity and specificity.

| | Condition | | |
	Present 100	Absent 900	Predictive Value (PV)
Test Pos	80	180	31% (Pos PV)
Test Neg	20	720	97% (Neg PV)

B. Very likely that a condition is present using the same test.

| | Condition | | |
	Present 900	Absent 100	Predictive Value (PV)
Test Pos	720	20	97% (Pos PV)
Test Neg	180	80	31% (Neg PV)

This example emphasizes the importance of taking into account the clinical probability of disease before trying to determine the predictive value of any test. When a barium enema is nondiagnostic or shows only diverticula, colonoscopy may reveal additional abnormalities (Tedesco et al. 1978, Brand et al. 1980). When colonoscopy is negative and the clinical probability of carcinoma is high, the study may be falsely negative and additional studies be required to establish a diagnosis.

When barium enema and colonoscopy are negative in this context, the sigmoid colon is a major anatomic site of missed diagnosis. This is due to the technical difficulties of visualizing all portions of the sigmoid. Muscular hypertrophy and diverticular disease (Baker and Alterman 1985, Boulos et al. 1985) may compromise the roentgenographic examination. In addition to the technically caused errors produced by the anatomic configuration of the sigmoid and diverticular disease, an interpretive error of equal significance results from attributing occult or overt bleeding to diverticular disease simply because diverticula are present. Admittedly, hemorrhage may occur from diverticular disease; however, the source and pattern of bleeding in this situation is usually acute and of arteriolar origin (Meyers et al. 1976). Quantitative determination of gastrointestinal blood loss has shown that fecal hemoglobin concentration is within normal limits in patients who have diverticulosis (Ahlquist et al. 1985). Consequently, the presence of diverticulosis identified by barium enema examination should not produce a false sense of security that this is indeed the cause of occult bleeding. Overt rectal bleeding admixed with bowel movements or streaked on the stool should not be attributed to diverticular disease until other conditions have been excluded. This pattern of bleeding is not characteristic of diverticular disease. The finding of only diverticulosis on contrast examination does not preclude the need for further study in this clinical setting.

FAMILIAL POLYPOSIS SYNDROME

The endoscopic alternative for the group of patients with familial polyposis syndrome should be flexible sigmoidoscopy or colonoscopy, beginning at adolescence. The distal rectum may be spared of adenomas in patients who have familial polyposis or Gardner's syndrome (De Cosse and Bayle 1985). Examination of the more proximal rectum, sigmoid colon, and even the more proximal large bowel may be necessary in order to identify polyposis in all at-risk individuals. This is because of the phenotypic variability of this disease that, in some persons at risk, has evolved into colon cancer associated with virtually no polyps at the time of diagnosis (Lynch et al. 1979).

Although the median age of onset of polyposis is 25 years, some patients who have this syndrome do not phenotypically manifest the presence of polyps until they are in their fourth to fifth decades of life (Bussey 1975). Since polyps antedate cancer, all patients at risk for familial polyposis need to have an examination of the rectum and sigmoid annually. This should probably be supplemented by full colonoscopy or air-contrast barium enema examination every three years. Once patients are symptomatic from one of these polyposis syndromes, the chance that colon cancer is already present approximates 67% (Bussey 1983). The near certainty that all patients with polyposis will eventually develop cancer and the fact that cancer is already present in two out of three symptomatic patients underscore the importance of surveillance so that premalignant changes may be identified before symptoms develop.

NONPOLYPOSIS INHERITED COLORECTAL CANCER

Nonpolyposis inherited colorectal cancer may be part of the cancer-family syndrome wherein the incidence of adenocarcinoma within a kindred is increased. About 20% of affected persons have a second primary tumor, and over 80% of these have endometrial cancer as another primary lesion (Lynch et al. 1977). Site-specific colorectal cancer involving the colon, stomach, or both has also been described. The endoscopic alternative to choose for nonpolyposis–inherited colorectal cancer is full colonoscopy supplemented by sigmoidoscopy.

The choice of colonoscopy as the endoscopic alternative for this select group of patients is important because the incidence of right-sided colon cancer is more than twice as high in persons who have a familial predisposition to large bowel cancer than in the general population (Anderson and Strong 1974, Lynch, Lynch, and Harris 1977). Colon cancer–prone families who do not have multiple adenomatous polyps, extracolonic signs, or early-onset distal colon cancer appear to have a relatively greater predilection for proximal lesions (Lynch, Lynch, and Harris 1977). Consequently, any surveillance program must involve a technique that, in effect, samples the entire colon. Surveillance must include qualitative or quantitative tests for occult blood in feces.

It is estimated that if one family member has colorectal cancer, the relative risk for others in that kindred is increased about threefold (Woolf 1958). In some kindreds the cumulative incidence of cancer is high and may exceed 50%. Obtaining an accurate and complete pedigree helps in determining the relative risk of cancer for an individual patient and in directing surveillance examinations. Results of a surveillance study of 198 participants who had at least two relatives with colorectal cancer resulted in the detection of five colon cancers; the average detection rate was 3.7 malignancies per 100 examinations for persons over 35 years of age (Anderson and Romsdahl 1977). Although there are no prospective data on when to begin surveillance or what interval to use between surveillance examinations, it appears that the initial examination should be performed when a family member is about 10 years younger than the youngest affected age within a pedigree and should be conducted annually.

CURRENT OR PREVIOUS NEOPLASIA

The development of synchronous or metachronous lesions in the colon should come as no surprise when one realizes that the entire large bowel has been subjected to the same microflora, nutrient metabolites, immunologic status, and biochemical environment. Co-existing cancers occur in at least 1% to 2% of patients who have colon cancer (Moertel, Bargen, and Dockerty 1958). Some investigators have found synchronous cancers in 7% to 8% and at least one synchronous adenoma in almost 50% of patients (Reilly, Rusin, and Theverkauf 1982). Almost 8% of patients who have had colon cancer resected have been reported to eventually develop a new cancer (Reilly, Rusin, and Theverkauf 1982). Over 35% of patients with a single adenoma and over 50% of those with multiple index adenomas develop new polyps (Lambert et al. 1984). These lesions occur in any portion of the large bowel and thus require periodic surveillance of the entire colon and rectum. The endoscopic alternative of choice in this situation is obviously colonoscopy.

The importance of colonoscopic diagnosis of synchronous colorectal neoplasms has been underscored by a study (Pagana et al. 1984) wherein 60 synchronous lesions were found in 157 patients. In 7 of 12 patients who had synchronous cancer, the discovery required alteration of the planned surgical procedure. Metachronous cancers or polyps are no different from initial lesions with respect to the clinical importance of identifying disease before symptoms develop. It is now recognized that metachronous lesions can develop several decades after an original cancer has been resected; two thirds occur after 11 years. Consequently, surveillance has practical implications not only for initial therapy but also for follow-up. The procedure must be continued and needs to include the entire colon because the distribution of metachronous polyps is relatively uniformly distributed and tends to affect the right colon. The reason for an increased incidence of metachronous lesions on the right side is uncertain but parallels observations concerning changes in distribution of all colon cancers studied in a large group of patients at the Mayo Clinic. Investigators identified a 25% increase in lesions proximal to the splenic flexure along with a 16% decrease in lesions involving the colon distal to the splenic flexure (Beart et al. 1983).

ULCERATIVE COLITIS

The endoscopic procedure of choice for surveillance of precancerous lesions associated with ulcerative colitis is colonoscopy. The association of dysplasia and cancer complicating ulcerative colitis has been well established since the first detailed description in 1967 (Morson and Pang 1967). Dysplasia can be identified on rectosigmoidoscopy, and some groups have observed that dysplasia is found as often by rectal biopsies as by colonoscopy (Fochios, Sommers, and Korelitz 1986). Others have found dysplasia on colonoscopic biopsies about three times more often than on rectal biopsy (Hanauer et al. 1984). This discrepancy appears to be related to the nonuniform distribution of dysplasia (Riddell 1983). More important, colonoscopy provides the opportunity to visualize all segments of the colon and to direct biopsies at any plaque or mass lesions, which carry a greater risk for cancers coexisting when the lesions are dysplastic (Blackstone et al. 1981). Although prospective studies have not proved that surveillance enhances survival rates, evidence to date indicates that the endoscopic procedure of choice in this setting is periodic colonoscopy plus biopsies from all segments of the colon. Sigmoidoscopic biopsies may be adjuvant to colonoscopy.

ADENOMAS

The endoscopic procedure of choice for patients who have adenomas is colonoscopy. This is related to the high incidence of synchronous lesions, the therapeutic potential of colonoscopy, and its superior diagnostic yield over barium enema in identifying diminutive polyps (Theoni and Menuck 1977; Hogan et al. 1977; Williams, Macrae, and Bartram 1982). Another consideration in choosing colonoscopy is that it is impossible to establish the histological features of small (less than 5-mm) polyps by their gross appearance. In one study, 209 small lesions were classified as hyperplastic or adenomatous by the endoscopic appearance. Twenty-two percent of those considered to be hyperplastic had to be reclassified, as did 40% of those that were believed grossly to represent adenomas (Kronborg and Haye 1985). The recognition that small polyps may be adenomatous was first appreciated in the proximal colon; however, studies that have correlated the histological type and size of small rectosigmoid lesions have shown that approximately three fourths of small rectosigmoid polyps are in fact neoplastic, and this percentage does not seem to be affected by size (Dubow et al. 1985). Although only a small percentage of adenomas enlarge and become cancerous, which ones will do so cannot be predicted. In view of this fact, the high incidence of synchronous lesions, our inability to predict fully the histological type by size, and the therapeutic potential of colonoscopy make this procedure, at present, the endoscopic procedure of choice for patients who have adenomas.

ROUTINE SURVEILLANCE

The endoscopic procedure of choice for routine surveillance of average-risk, asymptomatic patients is sigmoidoscopy (Bolt 1971; Corman, Coller, and Veidenheimer 1975). Sigmoidoscopy should supplement digital rectal and fecal occult blood tests because small polyps do not bleed enough to be detected by fecal occult blood tests. Their identification depends on direct visualization because (a) the results of guaiac-based stool blood tests are usually negative, (b) mean gastrointestinal blood loss determined by radiolabeled techniques is usually within normal limits, and (c) overt bleeding is unusual for all polyps smaller than 1 cm in diameter (Herzog et al. 1982; Macrae and St. John 1982; Crowley et al. 1983). The difficulty of diagnosing small polyps is supported by quantitative determinations using the Hemo-Quant test, which has confirmed that mean fecal hemoglobin concentration is related to the size of benign lesions and usually remains within normal limits until a lesion measures 2 cm or larger (Ahlquist et al. 1985). Less than 50% of patients with adenomas larger than 1 cm have positive fecal occult blood tests (Norfleet 1986).

Results tend to be positive in patients with polyps of the left colon and those with at least two adenomas (Herzog et al. 1982; Norfleet 1986). Digital rectal examination can only be expected to detect lesions that are within reach of the index finger, and fecal occult blood tests can only be expected to detect lesions that are bleeding. The importance of identifying nonbleeding lesions beyond reach of digital rectal examination and rigid proctosigmoidoscopy is the basis for recommending fiberoptic sigmoidoscopy as the endoscopic alternative in this setting.

The anatomic distribution of polyps in the rectosigmoid and the probability that an index lesion will be present in the lower rectosigmoid and therefore provide an indication for colonoscopic or roentgenographic examination of the entire colon has not been firmly established. The percentage of lesions within reach of the digital rectal examination or rigid sigmoidoscope has decreased over the past 40 years (Rhodes, Holmes, and Clark 1977; Beart et al. 1983). This raises questions as to whether the long 60-cm flexible sigmoidoscope is diagnostically superior to a shorter 35-cm instrument used for surveillance of asymptomatic patients. Many reports compare the total number of polyps or lesions identified by a 60-cm as opposed to a 35-cm sigmoidoscope or rigid proctoscope. The increased yield of the longer scope may appear impressive; however, it is more important to determine the percentage of affected patients who would not be advised to undergo full colonoscopy based on a perfectly normal 35-cm endoscopy and negative fecal occult blood tests. A prospective study indicates that at least 80% of all patients in whom a lesion is identified on 60-cm sigmoidoscopy have at least one abnormality visible with a 35-cm endoscope that would establish the need for full colonoscopy (Dubow et al. 1985).

The role of sigmoidoscopy as a supplement to digital rectal and fecal occult blood tests in asymptomatic persons at average risk is based on an estimated 7% to 10% incidence of polyps in otherwise asymptomatic patients over age 40 (Bold 1971; Corman, Coller, and Veidenheimer 1975). The extent of sigmoidoscopy depends on the spatial distribution of index lesions and should generally include at least the distal 35 cm of the large bowel.

INTERVENTIONAL ENDOSCOPY

Endoscopic procedures can be therapeutic as well as diagnostic. The classic example involves removing adenomas and thus preventing their possible malignant transformation. When polyps contain a focus of cancer, polypectomy may be curative. In this setting, both carcinoma in situ and most tubular adenomas that contain a focus of cancer in the head of a pedunculated polyp are cured by polypectomy because the incidence of residual cancer or nodal metastasis is low (Coutsoftides et al. 1978). Sessile lesions and those that are villous appear to have a higher incidence of residual cancer and may benefit from surgical resection (Christie 1978; Coutsoftides et al. 1978). Indications for resection following endoscopic polypectomy for focally malignant polyps include incomplete polypectomy, positive transection line, invasion of the base or stalk, infiltrative villous lesions, angiomatous or lymphatic invasion, short sessile lesions, and lesions that are highly undifferentiated.

Interventional endoscopy can also be combined with laser therapy (see Faintuch in this volume). The main application of laser therapy for colorectal neoplasia has been to palliate obstructing or bleeding lesions. Applied preoperatively for obstructing disease, patency may be established, thus allowing bowel preparation for a one-stage resection and reanastomosis (Kiefhaber, Kiefhaber, and Huber 1986). Effective palliation of advanced disease eventually is limited by extrinsic compression from extracolonic extension of cancer. Poor accessibility, large lesions, and unfavorable anatomy can be major problems with laser therapy (Mathus-Vliegen 1986). Burt et al. (1985) have described initial successful palliation of 86% of patients who had a variety of gastrointestinal cancers. Since median life expectancy for these patients is approximately three to four months, laser therapy is an endoscopic procedure of choice for this select group. For patients with benign disease, laser phototherapy has been reported to safely and effectively ablate multiple polyps during follow-up after ileorectostomy for familial polyposis (Mathus-Vliegen and Tytgat 1986). Other approaches to the palliative resection of rectal cancer besides laser therapy and electrosurgical fulguration have involved the use of a urologic resectoscope.

During the past 10 years, endoscopic procedures that are capable of examining the entire large bowel have been developed, and their use is now common. As a result, the appropriate endoscopic procedures must be chosen on the basis of their merit and the clinical context in which they are being used.

ACKNOWLEDGMENT

The author wishes to express appreciation to Ms. Wanda Sowders for secretarial assistance.

REFERENCES

Ahlquist DA, McGill DB, Schwartz S, et al. 1985. Fecal blood levels in health and disease. A study using Hemoquant *N Engl J Med* 312:1422–1428.

Anderson DE, Romsdahl MM. 1977. Family history: A criterion for selective screening. In *Genetics of Human Cancer,* JJ Mulvihill, RW Miller, JF Fraumeni Jr., eds., pp. 257–262. New York: Raven Press.

Anderson DE, Strong LC. 1974. Genetics of gastrointestinal tumors. *Proceedings of XIth International Cancer Congress,* Florence, Italy, pp. 267–271. Amsterdam: Excerpta Medica, Series 351.

Baker SR, Alterman DD. 1985. False-negative barium enema in patients with sigmoid cancer and coexistent diverticula. *Gastrointest Radiol* 10:171–173.

Beart RW, Melton LJ III, Maruta M, et al. 1983. Trends in right- and left-sided colon cancer. *Dis Colon Rectum* 26:393–398.

Beggs I, Thomas BM. 1983. Diagnosis of carcinoma of the colon by barium enema. *Clin Radiol* 34:423–425.

Blackstone MO, Riddell RH, Rogers BHG, et al. 1981. Dysplasia-associated lesion or mass (DALM) detected by colonoscopy in long-standing ulcerative colitis: An indication for colectomy. *Gastroenterology* 80:366–374.

Bolt RJ. 1971. Sigmoidoscopy in detection and diagnosis in the asymptomatic individual. *Cancer* 28:121–122.

Boulos PB, Cowin AP, Karamanolis DG, et al. 1985. Diverticula, neoplasia or both? Early detection of carcinoma in sigmoid diverticular disease. *Ann Surg* 202:607–609.

Brand EJ, Sullivan BH, Sivak MV, et al. 1980. Colonoscopy in the diagnosis of unexplained rectal bleeding. *Ann Surg* 192:111–113.

Burt RW, Bowers JH, Hunter JG, et al. 1985. Endoscopic laser surgery. In *Carcinoma of the Large Bowel and its Precursors,* JRF Ingall, AJ Mastromarino, eds., pp. 151–160. New York: Alan R. Liss.

Bussey HJR. 1975. *Familial Polyposis Coli: Family Studies, Histopathology, Differential Diagnosis and Results of Treatment.* Baltimore: Johns Hopkins University Press.

Bussey HJR. 1984. Polyposis syndromes of the gastrointestinal tract. In *Precancerous Lesions of the Gastrointestinal Tract,* P Sherlock, BC Morson, L Barbara, U Veronesi, eds., pp. 43–52. New York: Raven Press.

Christie JP. 1978. Colonoscopic removal of sessile colon lesions. *Dis Colon Rectum* 21:12–14.

Corman ML, Coller JA, Veidenheimer MC. 1975. Proctosigmoidoscopy: Age criteria for examination in the asymptomatic patient. *CA* 25:286–290.

Coutsoftides T, Sivak MV Jr, Benjamin SP, et al. 1978. Colonoscopy and the management of polyps containing invasive carcinoma. *Ann Surg* 188:638–642.

Crowley ML, Freeman LD, Mottel MD, et al. 1983. Sensitivity of guaiac-impregnated cards for the detection of colorectal neoplasia. *J Clin Gastroenterol* 5:127–130.

De Cosse JJ, Bayle JC. 1985. Overview of epidemiology and risk factors associated with colorectal cancer. In *Carcinoma of The Large Bowel and Its Precursors,* JRF Ingall, AJ Mastromarino, eds., pp. 1–12. New York: Alan R. Liss.

Dodd GD. 1985. The air contrast barium enema: Indications and validity. *Prog Clin Biol Res* 186:133–149.

Dubow RA, Katon RM, Benner KG, et al. 1985. Short (35-cm) versus long (60-cm) flexible sigmoidoscopy: A comparison of findings and tolerance in asymptomatic patients screened for colorectal neoplasia. *Gastrointest Endosc* 31:305–308.

Fochios SE, Sommers SC, Lorelitz BI. 1986. Sigmoidoscopy and biopsy in surveillance for cancer in ulcerative colitis. *J Clin Gastroenterol* 8:249–254.

Goulston K. 1986. How important is rectal bleeding in the diagnosis of bowel cancer and polyps? *Lancet* 2:261–265.

Hanauer SB, Levin B, Evans AA, et al. 1984. Location of dysplasia at colonoscopy compared to surgical resection: Inadequacy of rectal biopsy to predict proximal lesions (abstract). *Gastroenterology* 86:1106.

Herzog P, Holtermuller KH, Preiss J, et al. 1982. Fecal blood loss in patients with colonic polyps: A comparison of measurements with 5/chromium-labeled erythrocytes and with the Hemoccult test. *Gastroenterology* 83:957–962.

Hogan WJ, Stewart ET, Geenen JE, et al. 1977. A prospective comparison of the accuracy of colonoscopy vs. air-barium contrast exam for detection of colonic polypoid lesions (abstract). *Gastrointest Endosc* 2:230.

Kiefhaber P, Kiefhaber K, Huber F. 1986. Preoperative neodymium-YAG laser treatment of obstructing colon cancer. *Endoscopy* 18(Suppl 1):44–46.

Kronborg O, Haye E. 1985. Hyperplasia or neoplasia. Macroscopic versus microscopic appearance of colorectal polyps. *Scand J Gastroenterol* 20:512–515.

Lambert R, Sobin LH, Waye JD, et al. 1984. The management of patients with colorectal adenomas. *Ca* 34:167–176.

Lynch HT, Harris RE, Lynch PM, et al. 1977. The role of heredity in multiple primary cancer. *Cancer* 40:1849–1854.

Lynch HT, Lynch PM, Follett KL, et al. 1979. Familial polyposis coli: Heterogeneous expression in two kindreds. *J Med Genet* 16:1–7.

Lynch PM, Lynch HT, Harris RE. 1977. Hereditary proximal colonic cancer. *Dis Colon Rectum* 20:661–668.

Macrae FA, St. John DJB. 1982. Relationship between patterns of bleeding and Hemoccult sensitivity in patients with colorectal cancers or adenomas. *Gastroenterology* 82:891–898.

Mathus-Vliegen EM. 1986. Complications and pitfalls of laser therapy. *Endoscopy* 18(Suppl 1):69–72.

Mathus-Vliegen EM, Tytgat GN. 1986. Laser photocoagulation in the palliation of colorectal malignancies. *Cancer* 57:2212–2216.

Meyers MA, Alonso OR, Gray GF, et al. 1976. Pathogenesis of bleeding colonic diverticulosis. *Gastroenterology* 71:577–583.

Miller RE. 1981. Barium enema vs. colonoscopy. *Gastrointest Endosc* 28:40–41.

Moertel CG, Bargen JA, Dockerty M. 1958. Multiple carcinomas of the large intestine: Review of the literature and a study of 261 cases. *Gastroenterology* 34:85–98.

Morson BC, Pang LSC. 1967. Rectal biopsy as an aid to cancer control in ulcerative colitis. *Gut* 8:423–434.

Norfleet RG. 1986. Effect of diet on fecal occult blood testing in patients with colorectal polyps. *Dig Dis Sci* 31:498–501.

Pagana TJ, Ledesma EJ, Mittleman A, et al. 1984. The use of colonoscopy in the study of synchronous colorectal neoplasms. *Cancer* 53:356–359.

Reilly JC, Rusin LC, Theverkauf FJ. 1982. Colonoscopy: Its role in cancer of the colon and rectum. *Dis Colon Rectum* 25:532–538.

Rhodes JB, Holmes FF, Clark GM. 1977. Changing distribution of primary cancers in the large bowel. *JAMA* 238:1641–1643.

Riddell RH. 1983. Dysplasia in inflammatory bowel disease. In *Pathology of the Colon, Small Intestine and Anus,* HT Norris, ed., pp. 95–97. New York: Churchill Livingstone.

Tedesco FJ, Waye JD, Raskin JB, et al. 1978. Colonoscopy evaluation of rectal bleeding: A study of 304 patients. *Ann Intern Med* 89:907–909.

Theoni RF, Menuck L. 1977. Comparison of barium enema and colonoscopy in the detection of small colonic polyps. *Radiology* 124:631–635.

Williams CB, Macrae FA, Bartram CI. 1982. A prospective study of diagnostic methods in adenoma follow-up. *Endoscopy* 14:74–78.

Woolf CM. 1958. A genetic study of carcinoma of the large intestine. *Am J Hum Genet* 10:42–52.

Annual Clinical Conference on Cancer, Vol. 30
Gastrointestinal Cancer: Current Approaches to Diagnosis and Treatment
© 1988 by The University of Texas System Cancer Center

11. The Management of Familial Colon Cancer in a Special Risk Clinic

Rodger J. Winn, Deborah Coody,
Victor Vogel, Margaret Spitz, and Guy Newell

Primary-care physicians are becoming increasingly concerned with providing cancer screening and prevention counseling to their patients. In the process of these interventions, they are occasionally faced with patients whose family history, occupational exposures, or life-style habits demand a level of clinical investigation or treatment that exceeds their level of knowledge or skills. The University of Texas M. D. Anderson Hospital and Tumor Institute's Special Risk Clinic is a facility to which these patients may be referred.

Designed to provide for the special needs of persons with an extraordinarily high risk of developing cancer, the Special Risk Clinic is staffed by a team of health-care professionals who possess the expertise necessary to evaluate and treat these difficult cases. The Clinic is able to care for such diverse populations as patients with familial breast cancer or dysplastic nevi syndrome, those exposed to asbestos, and those representing geographic and temporal clusters. Based on their local expertise, special risk clinics at other centers may serve a different spectrum of populations.

Familial colon cancer is an ideal entity to be managed in the Special Risk Clinic. Traditionally, patients who have this cancer are seen in one of two settings: a general gastroenterology clinic or practice or a specialized polyposis clinic. The Special Risk Clinic offers a focused approach: it is staffed by a team of medical specialists with the necessary skills but does not require the extensive number of patients needed to justify a single-disease clinic.

Approximately 25% of patients with colorectal cancer have one or more immediate family members with the same disease (Macklin 1960; Lovett 1976). One to five percent of those with colorectal cancer demonstrate family histories that are consistent with autosomally dominant inherited conditions in which 50% of an affected individual's offspring will develop the disease. These inherited entities may be divided into two types: polyposis and nonpolyposis (Lynch, Rozen, and Schuelice 1985). The polyposis type is clinically subdivided into familial, Gardner's, and Turcot's syndromes; the nonpolyposis type includes hereditary site–specific colon cancer, cancer-family syndrome, and Muir-Torre's syndrome.

Since only 1% of all patients with colorectal cancers demonstrate a polyposis history, the majority of familial colon cancers are of the nonpolyposis variety. Lynch et al. (1985b) have elucidated the clinical findings characteristic of nonpolyposis familial colon cancer syndromes: (1) vertical transmission of the disease;

Table 11.1. *Acceptance Criteria for Familial Colon Cancer*

≥ 2 immediate family members with colon cancer
Polyposis
Extracolonic manifestations of polyposis
25+% of immediate family members with heterogeneous tumors
Age < 40 yr with ≥ 2 tumors or 1 right-sided colon carcinoma

(2) a dominant inheritance pattern; (3) an earlier age of onset of tumor (40 years old vs. 60 years old for sporadic cases); (4) an altered anatomic distribution of tumors (right-sided greater than left-sided lesions); (5) occurrence of other tumors in the family, especially endometrial, ovarian, and gastric; and (6) a less aggressive natural history of the tumor.

SCREENING

The first step in accepting a patient for the Special Risk Clinic is screening. Acceptance criteria should be developed that exclude patients with very little chance of having a familial syndrome. Table 11.1 lists the criteria for acceptance at the UT M. D. Anderson Hospital Special Risk Clinic.

Screening can be performed by the Clinic nurse-coordinator. When characteristics are ambiguous, a clinic physician often discusses the case with the referring physician to determine whether the patient's risk fits into a category that justifies the extensive workup of the clinic. Preliminary pedigrees are often elicited to determine the likelihood of the patient's having a true inherited syndrome. Patients with polyposis, osteomas, or cutaneous manifestation of Gardner's syndrome are usually well defined. The acceptance of patients with a 25+% family history of heterogeneous tumors is less automatic, but since it is probable that not all familial clusters have been delineated, patients meeting this criterion are usually accepted. Because the implications of familial colon cancer are profound for younger family members, 40-year-old patients with right-sided lesions or two cancers are accepted, even if their family history is not suggestive, because they actually may represent the first mutation in the pedigree.

WORKUP PROCEDURE

Once accepted, a patient undergoes risk assessment, diagnostic evaluation, and genetic counseling and receives treatment recommendations. The initial clinic visit may require one and one-half to four hours and include visits with a prevention physician and a nurse prevention coordinator, a dental consultation, an ophthalmologic examination, and a gastroenterologic endoscopy session. The clinic administrator generates the necessary forms for soliciting information about pedigrees, recruiting family members, and establishing a surveillance schedule.

Risk Assessment

Risk assessment consists of constructing a modified nuclear pedigree (Lynch et al. 1985a) and then obtaining supportive documentation. A modified nuclear pedigree consists of the index patient's parents, grandparents, aunts and uncles, siblings, and children. Extending the family history to include aunts and uncles is useful because the patient's own generation or that of his children often yields a negative history because of the youth of its members. Documentation can be limited in clear-cut cases such as familial polyposis, where obtaining the records of the patient, his parents, and a sibling can substantiate the familial diagnosis. However, those familial cancer syndromes involving heterogeneous tumors in other generations may require extensive documentation to make possible an accurate risk assessment. Records that must be sought include hospital and physician files, pathology reports, radiological reports, and death certificates. Appropriate authorization for records release is necessary, often making the process drawn out and time-consuming.

After their risk has been assessed, patients are placed in one of three categories: random cluster, probable cancer syndrome, or definite hereditary syndrome. Patients in the first group are reassured and given conventional cancer prevention advice. The Clinic's evaluation continues for those in the last two groups.

Diagnostic Evaluation

The next step is an appropriate diagnostic evaluation. This begins with a complete physical examination, focusing particularly on skin and bone abnormalities. The examination includes a gynecologic evaluation if one has not been performed within one year. An endoscopic evaluation is performed by the Section of Gastroenterology; this includes upper gastrointestinal endoscopy for all patients with Gardner's syndrome. All patients with polyposis receive a routine Panorex X ray of the mandible, looking for osteomata (Bulow et al. 1983), in conjunction with a dental examination. All those with Gardner's syndrome receive an ophthalmologic examination to determine whether there is congenital retinal hyperpigmentation (Lewis et al. 1984).

Recommendations

When the results of these examinations have been analyzed, the patient receives three sets of recommendations: treatment recommendations, genetic counseling, and surveillance recommendations. Table 11.2 diagrams the surgical treatment recommendations of the UT M. D. Anderson Hospital Department of Surgery and Section of Gastroenterology for patients with polyposis. When rectal polyposis is extensive, our approach has been to perform proctectomy because of the high risk of carcinomatous recurrence (Moertel, Hill, and Adson 1971). Specific recommendations for treating polyposis of the duodenum and periampullary areas are not well defined for patients with Gardner's syndrome (Sivak and Jagelman 1984); currently,

Table 11.2. *Surgical Recommendations for Patients with Familial Polyposis*

Colonic Polyps	Procedure	Postoperative Follow-up
< 10 total	Endoscopy removal	Every 6 months
Multiple polyposis with < 20 rectal polyps	Colectomy with ileo-rectal anastomosis or	Every 6 months
	Colectomy with mucosal proctectomy and reservoir ileo-anal anastomosis	Annual
Multiple polyposis with > 20 rectal polyps	Total proctocolectomy with ileostomy	Annual

laser therapy is being investigated. Patients with nonpolyposis syndromes are advised that if a tumor should develop, it is essential that their physicians discuss their care with the Special Risk Clinic so that a decision can be reached jointly about total colectomy versus hemicolectomy and concomitant hysterectomy and oophorectomy.

Probably the most difficult and sensitive activity of the Clinic is genetic counseling. This is provided by the nurse coordinator or a physician. Krush (1983) has described the goals of a counseling session: to inform the patient of the nature of the hereditary process; to help the patient and family understand the implications of the conditions; to enable the family to make the proper treatment decisions; and, most difficult of all, to help the family adapt to the conditions of the disease. In dealing with these families, counselors encounter a broad spectrum of emotional reactions—anger, guilt, fear, anxiety, and denial. The counselor's interventions must be sensitive to such emotions. A sympathetic, sometimes firm, mollifying approach will evolve that is somewhat individualized for each family. The overall objective is to provide the support systems and coping skills necessary for each family to come to grips with the extraordinary demands of this high-risk situation. Polyposis families are urged to write for the polyposis newsletter (*G.I. Polyposis & Related Conditions,* The Moore Clinic, The Johns Hopkins Hospital, Baltimore, MD 21205) for ongoing counseling and support. Often the burden of a familial cancer syndrome leads to broken family patterns or severe internal strains. In these cases, intensive counseling centered around the family dynamics is recommended and appropriate referrals are made.

The final activity of the patient's visit to the Special Risk Clinic is the provision of a surveillance schedule. Surveillance can be carried out at UT M. D. Anderson Hospital in conjunction with annual Special Risk Clinic visits or by the referring physician who is provided with specific surveillance recommendations. Table 11.3 outlines the surveillance recommendations for patients with polyposis. For those with Gardner's syndrome, upper gastrointestinal endoscopies are performed yearly. Annual surveillance for patients with nonpolyposis syndromes does not begin until they reach age 20. Because of the preponderance of right-sided colon lesions found in these patients, yearly colonoscopic examinations are recommended. The need for

Table 11.3. *Surveillance of Persons at Risk for Familial Polyposis*

Age (yr)	Asymptomatic	Symptomatic
≤ 13	None	Flexible sigmoidoscopy
14–19	Annual flexible sigmoidoscopy	Colonoscopy or double-contrast barium enema
20–45	Annual flexible sigmoidoscopy; baseline colonoscopy or double-contrast barium enema at age 20, repeated every third year	Colonoscopy or double-contrast barium enema

women to have an annual pelvic examination is emphasized. If family history suggests that gastric or pancreatic carcinomas are part of the family's tumor constellation, upper gastrointestinal endoscopy or a computerized tomography scan of the abdomen approximately every two years is added to the surveillance schedule.

FAMILY RECRUITMENT

The Special Risk Clinic considers it an obligation to inform family members within the nuclear pedigree about their risk and to provide information about surveillance recommendations. When the identity of family physicians is known, they also are provided with this information. All family members are offered the opportunity to attend the Special Risk Clinic or to telephone for further information. Confidentiality is scrupulously assured. The need for family recruitment becomes obvious when one encounters unfortunate situations where family members were not apprised of the risk by the physician treating the affected family member. The unsuspecting relative who has not been made aware of the family syndrome may not receive screening or may receive the wrong treatment if the disease emerges.

RESEARCH

The last activity of the Special Risk Clinic is research. The familial colon cancer syndromes are prime areas in which to evaluate epidemiologic risk factors, natural history manifestations, treatment modalities, cytogenetic and immunologic implications, and molecular genetic studies (Blattner 1977). Most patients are asked to participate in these studies, and collaborating arrangements have been made with other centers to share research specimens and data.

STAFFING

The personnel required to staff a Special Risk Clinic varies according to the interests and expertise of each clinic. The UT M. D. Anderson Hospital Special Risk Clinic is staffed by medical oncologists and epidemiologists, but similar clinics use surgeons, gastroenterologists, or generalists. A key staff person is a nurse coordinator, responsible for risk assessment, genetic counseling, and family contacts. At UT M. D. Anderson Hospital, this position is filled by a nurse oncologist with a master's degree, but at several other clinics these functions are performed by oncology social workers. Members of the Gastroenterology Service, Dental Service, and Surgical Service are integral members of the clinic team, providing ancillary medical evaluations.

Secretarial and administrative assistance is vital, and one must not underestimate the amount of support necessary to implement the intensive evaluations of a Special Risk Clinic. We are developing a computerized data base to support the Clinic's complex interactions. The components of this data base include administrative and demographic data, clinical data, surveillance monitoring, and follow-up procedures, including scheduling, letter generation, pedigree construction, and statistical analysis capability.

CONCLUSION

The focused approach of a Special Risk Clinic offers those patients who have an extraordinary risk of familial colon cancer the multidisciplinary expertise necessary for successful management of a complex clinical situation. Working with the patient, the family, and the family physician, the Clinic staff tries to arrive at a regimen that will best help the affected person deal with the risk of disease.

REFERENCES

Blattner WA. 1977. Family studies: The interdisciplinary approach. In *Genetics of Human Cancer*, JJ Mulvihill, RW Miller, JF Fraumeni, eds., pp. 269–280. New York: Raven Press.

Bulow S, Søndergaard JD, Witt I, et al. 1983. Mandibular osteomas in familial polyposis coli. *Dis Colon Rectum* 27:105–108.

Krush A. 1983. Counseling for patients and their families with hereditary large bowel cancer. In *Prevention of Hereditary Large Bowel Cancer*, AJ Mastromarino, JRF Ingall, eds., pp. 167–174. New York: Alan R. Liss.

Lewis RA, Crowder WE, Eierman LA, et al. 1984. The Gardner's syndrome: Significance of ocular features. *Ophthalmology* 91:916–925.

Lovett E. 1976. Family studies in cancer of the colon and rectum. *Br J Surg* 63:13–18.

Lynch HT, Fitzgibbons R, Marcus J, et al. 1985a. Colorectal cancer in a nuclear family: Familial or hereditary? *Dis Colon Rectum* 28:310–316.

Lynch HT, Kimberling W, Albano WA, et al. 1985b. Hereditary nonpolyposis colorectal cancer (Lynch Syndromes I and II). *Cancer* 56:934–938.

Lynch HT, Rozen P, Schuelice GS. 1985. Hereditary colon cancer: Polyposis and nonpolyposis variants. *Cancer* 35:95–115.

Macklin MT. 1960. Inheritance of cancer of the stomach and large intestine in man. *JNCI* 24:551–571.

Moertel CG, Hill JR, Adson MA. 1971. Management of multiple polyposis of the large bowel. *Cancer* 28:160–164.

Sivak MV, Jagelman DG. 1984. Upper gastrointestinal endoscopy in polyposis syndromes: Familial polyposis coli and Gardner's syndrome. *Gastrointest Endosc* 30:102–104.

Annual Clinical Conference on Cancer, Vol. 30
Gastrointestinal Cancer: Current Approaches to Diagnosis and Treatment
© 1988 by The University of Texas System Cancer Center

12. Surgical Management of Carcinoma of the Rectum

Robert W. Beart, Jr.

Most physicians would agree that surgery is the mainstay of treatment of carcinoma of the rectum. Although we are aware of the level of sensitivity of rectal cancers to radiation therapy or chemotherapy, at best their efficacy is unpredictable and their role appears to be more for adjuvant than for primary therapy.

LOCAL VERSUS RADICAL RESECTION

Rectal carcinoma can be a complicated problem to treat—complicated by the difficulty of the surgical procedure with its associated significant morbidity and mortality and high risk of local recurrence. The treatment is even more unacceptable to the patient when it necessitates a stoma.

Historically, radical excision has been preferred to local excision because of the aggressive nature of the disease. Therefore, the approach to "take as much as possible" has been the only logical strategy. The abdominoperineal operation as described by Miles in 1908 is the standard with which all other procedures are compared (Miles 1908).

Few would argue with the general principle of wide resection of the tumor with removal of the area of lymphatic drainage. For lesions of the upper and middle rectum, this frequently can be carried out by a low anterior resection, which has associated low morbidity and mortality (Beahrs and Wilson 1976). It is also clear, however, that many patients, particularly those with a Dukes A or B and half of those with Dukes C lesions, would probably fare just as well with local management. Unfortunately, stage cannot be ascertained with certainty until the entire specimen has been removed. Some investigators have attempted through physical characteristics such as size, histology, and mobility to identify lesions that are most likely to be amenable to local management. Size and grade of tumor are objective and easy to duplicate, but the concept of mobility is difficult to describe.

The areas of lymphatic spread of rectal cancer include those lymph-bearing tissues that are lateral, proximal, and 2 cm distal to the tumor. Approximately 10% of patients have tumor that invades adjacent organs or structures. Deep penetration anteriorly into the vagina or into the prostate and bladder may be treated by including these structures in the excised specimen; a cure rate of approximately 30% can be expected in these situations. Lateral extension may be difficult to treat surgically because of the limitations imposed by the lateral pelvic wall and bone. Posterior extension of rectal cancer into the sacrum can occasionally be treated by en bloc resection of the sacrum.

Statistics generated after radical resection reveal mortality rates of 1.3% to 10%, complication rates of 8.1% to 58%, and five-year survival rates of 28% to 52% (Mettlin et al. 1981; Beahrs 1967). Therefore, surgeons have begun to question the true benefit of radical excision and to consider alternative methods of treatment that might yield a lower morbidity and mortality while not sacrificing curability (Rider 1975). Theoretically, local treatment would be adequate in all patients with tumor confined within the bowel. In fact, a number of studies, including those of Morson, Bussey, and Samoorian (1977), Lock et al. (1978), Cuthbertson and Kaye (1978), Deddish (1974), Jackman and Beahrs (1968), and Culp and Jackman (1974), have proved that local excision for certain types of rectal cancer can be an effective and safe alternative to abdominal perineal resection. Unfortunately, variations in age; tumor size, grade, and location; and operation preference in these series have made statistically significant comparisons with other types of therapy difficult. In addition to local excision, electrocoagulation as championed by Strauss et al. in 1935, and more recently by Madden and Kandalaft (1971), Crile and Turnbull (1972) and Eisenstat et al. (1982), has also proved effective but was subject to the same biases. Cryosurgery has been emphasized in some reports, but no large series are available for comparison of its efficacy with that of other techniques.

Radiation in the treatment of rectal carcinoma in studies by Papillon (1982), Sischy et al. (1980), and Syed et al. (1978) has been used in such a select group of patients that interpretation is difficult. Radiation treatment is often limited to patients with polypoid, well-differentiated, superficial small tumors of the mid and lower rectum. Papillon's results strongly support the use of radiation therapy for such lesions. In comparison with other published series, his local recurrence rate of 7.7% is low. This may be attributed to patient selection or to his choice of modality and skill of application.

My colleagues and I conducted a restrospective review of patients with rectal carcinoma who underwent local or radical procedures at the Mayo Clinic from 1956 to 1980. We identified 234 patients who had local treatment that included local excision only in the majority of cases, fulguration, or radiation therapy. For comparison, a group of 511 patients who had been treated with radical resection, were identified. We evaluated both groups by multiple parameters to assess the outcome of therapy and to identify discriminatory parameters.

It is difficult to determine whether these two groups are truly comparable. Patients were frequently selected for local procedures because physical examination suggested that these carcinomas were amenable to such management. In the locally treated group there were no deaths and only a 6% complication rate. One hundred eighty patients never had a recurrence. Five patients had recurrence of disease at distal sites, and 49 had local recurrence, which was subsequently managed by radical resection. At resection, 36 of the 49 patients had localized disease (Dukes A, B, B2). At the time of follow-up, 10 had died of carcinoma of the rectum, 46 had died of other causes, 29 had died of unknown causes, and the rest were free of disease at least five years after treatment.

This experience is not unique. Similar results have been noted in studies by Eisenstat et al. (1982), Papillon (1982), Madden and Kandalaft (1971) and others.

The general guidelines gained from these experiences are that rectal cancers less than 3 cm in diameter and well-differentiated histologically may generally be well managed by local techniques. Radical resection is probably preferable for other lesions and for all nonmobile lesions.

ALTERNATIVES IN SURGICAL APPROACH

The major controversy in the management of carcinoma of the rectum concerns the midrectal region (6–11 cm from the anus). There is little doubt that Miles' procedure of combined abdominoperineal resection should be used for the terminal 5 cm of the rectum: however, the primary problem of this operation is related to the functional and social restrictions of a colostomy. It is appropriate to continue to study the policy of pursuing sphincter preservation in the treatment of carcinoma of the rectum. American College of Surgery data have documented that American surgeons are increasingly avoiding the abdominoperineal resection and choosing to perform low anterior resection or local therapy. In Jones and Thomson's study (1982) of 368 patients who underwent laparotomy for carcinoma of the rectum, 61% had a restorative resection. Operative mortality was 5%. Their basic approach was to undertake restorative anastomosis whenever it appeared to be technically feasible and suited to the patient. The cure rate was somewhat better in the patients in whom intestinal continuity was preserved. This is not surprising because the recurrence rates after abdominoperineal resection for low-lying carcinomas are usually higher than are those for more proximal lesions.

For tumors of the upper rectum and for many in the midrectum, anterior resection with low anastomosis is best. This operation results in acceptable cure, morbidity, and mortality rates as well as completely continent bowel function. After the mesentery of the rectosigmoid is dissected in the normal fashion, the rectum is separated free from the presacral space. If the lesion is very low, the middle hemorrhoidal vessels must be divided and the midrectum mobilized anteriorly, away from the prostate or the vagina. When this has been accomplished, the midrectum should then be sufficiently mobilized so that it can be retracted well out of the pelvis for resection and anastomosis. Traditional wisdom would dictate that at least 5 cm of uninvolved rectum should be obtained below the tumor to assure adequate resection. Beahrs suggested that 2 cm of normal bowel below the tumor would be adequate if measured in the pathology laboratory (Beahrs 1967). Recently, in a study from St. Mark's Hospital, Salt Lake City, it was concluded that 1 cm of normal mucosa in the excised specimen is adequate. Although the surgical margins above and below the lesion are important, the most significant prognostic features of the tumor are lymph node involvement and penetration of the bowel wall (Parks and Percy 1982).

In a retrospective review by Beahrs and Wilson (1976), lesions were classified according to the location from the dentate line. In 346 patients, the tumor was located more than 20 cm from the dentate line; in the remaining 566 patients, the tumor was between 6 and 20 cm distant. A thorough review was undertaken to compare these two groups on the basis of operative mortality and morbidity, including anastomotic complications, 5- and 10-year survivals, and the incidence of local recurrence. In the group of patients undergoing resection of the colon and rectum for cure, 1.9% died after operation. The operative mortality for patients in this group who were more than 70 years old was 3.1%. Causes of death included congestive heart failure (nine), pulmonary failure (four), myocardial infarction (two), and cerebrovascular accident (one). There were no anastomosis-related deaths, although anastomotic complications occurred in 8.1%. There was no difference between high and low anastomoses in terms of overall operative mortality; however, the lower the anastomosis was performed, the greater was the risk of anastomotic complications. A 10% incidence of leakage occurred for anastomoses less than 10 cm from the dentate line. Protective colostomies were rarely used in this series, and it continues to be our experience that unless there is great concern over the integrity of the anastomosis, a diverting colostomy is not necessary.

Actuarial 5-year survival was 72%; for patients at risk, the 10-year survival was 55%. Survival was not compromised by restoration of intestinal continuity deep within the pelvis. Local recurrence alone was found to occur in 7% of patients undergoing a low anterior resection. This is somewhat better than our institutional incidence of 10%. There was very little difference in the overall recurrence rate above the level of 8 cm to the dentate. When the risk of recurrence was related to the length of the distal margin of resection, any margin greater than 2 cm seemed to be associated with an equal risk of local recurrence.

The use of low anterior resection for the treatment of carcinoma of the rectum has been criticized on the basis of an unacceptable recurrence rate, an unacceptable complication rate, and the unacceptable sacrifice of long-term survival in an effort to preserve intestinal continuity. Although anastomotic dehiscence continues to be a significant clinical problem after all colonic anastomoses, an incidence of 7% to 10% would seem to be acceptable, particularly if associated with minimal mortality. Because the lymphatic drainage from the rectum above 5 cm from the dentate line has been demonstrated to be upward along the superior hemorrhoidal system, it is difficult to rationalize removal of the anus on this account for lesions in the midrectum and upper rectum. In addition, there is significant evidence that many of the so-called anastomotic suture line recurrences represent residual pelvic or perirectal disease that has simply invaded the rectum in the area of the anastomosis. In support of this theory are the relatively high rates of pelvic recurrence (9%–25%) after the combined abdominoperineal operation. In Beahrs's experience, tumor margins greater than 2.5 cm did not influence either survival or the incidence of local recurrence. Certainly one should strive to obtain as great a tumor-free margin as possible, but needless sacrifice of the anal sphincters should not be undertaken to achieve this goal.

Survival is the ultimate criterion by which the results of a surgical procedure for cancer must be measured. Virtually all studies within the last decade document similar survival rates for the treatment of midrectal and upper rectal cancers after the Miles procedure and low anterior resection.

An alternative approach to maintaining intestinal continuity is the use of one of the pull-through procedures, but this is rarely necessary. Parks has demonstrated that continence can be preserved with a pull-through (Parks and Percy 1982). Initially, stool frequency is increased since the reservoir capacity of the rectum is compromised. With time, however, the rectum will dilate, the rectal reservoir capacity will be restored, and the patient will resume an acceptable and nearly normal pattern of bowel evacuation (Localio, Eng, and Coppa 1983). This technique could be as curative as an anterior resection, but this has not been proven.

Transsacral and Transsphincteric Approaches

As documented by Localio, Eng, and Coppa's 1983 study, the abdominotranssacral approach to midrectal cancers has gained renewed interest. In this operation, it is possible to perform an anastomosis 2 to 3 cm from the dentate, particularly in the wide pelvis of a female. The anatomy of the anorectal area is complex, with the musculature of the rectum blending with the musculature of the pelvis and perineum. Although drawings of the internal and external sphincter and related musculature are usually fairly clear, many surgeons are uncertain about the relationships between the structures and the complications that manipulation of them would produce. Experience has shown that these structures may be vigorously retracted or divided as long as normal anatomic restitution is made. Incontinence is rare after the transsacral procedure, which leaves the sphincter mechanism intact. There is a little danger of destroying the nerve supply to the rectum if sacral resection is limited to below the third sacral vertebra. The transsphincteric approach can also be safely done without resulting in incontinence if reconstruction is carefully carried out. If the anatomy is grossly distorted by disease, inflammation, or previous surgery, however, proper identification of the various components of the somatic tube is difficult and proper reconstruction unpredictable.

In the above-cited study, Localio and associates reported on 646 patients with primary adenocarcinoma of the rectum treated between 1966 and 1981. Three hundred twenty had an anterior resection, 175 had a resection by the abdominotranssacral approach, and 151 underwent abdominoperineal resection. Patients selected as candidates for the abdominosacral resection included men with lesions 7 to 11 cm from the anal verge and women with lesions 5.5 to 10 cm from the anal verge. For this procedure, patients were placed in the lateral position. In 35 patients, the operation could be completed with anterior resection after mobilization of the rectum. In seven patients, an abdominoperineal resection was necessary. With the abdominotranssacral approach, the operative mortality rate was 2.2% and the anastomotic leak rate was 9.7%. The first 100 patients had a leak rate of 12%, and the subsequent 75 patients had a leak rate of 6.7%. Most of the leaks were from well-controlled posterior fistulas. Leaks occurred more frequently in men (15%) than in women (6.3%) and were highest in men 65 years or younger. This has prompted surgeons to routinely use protective colostomy in this age/sex group. Sphincter function was preserved in all patients undergoing abdominotranssacral resection. Crude survival rates were 66% for patients undergoing anterior resection, 63% for abdominotranssacral resection, and 43% for abdominoperineal resection. In this study by Localio et al., the abdominosacral resection permits direct posterior exposure of the rectum for wide resection, measurement of the distal margin, and sutured end-to-end anastomosis without disturbing the sphincters. This approach obviated much of the blind lateral dissection often necessary in the male pelvis. Localio and associates, however, did not address the long-term implications of the posterior rectal-cutaneous fistula.

Many who consider the transsacral approach are concerned about healing and the risk of fecal fistula. The original Kraske (transsacral) procedure resulted in an unacceptable incidence of fecal fistulas. However, Kraske's operation was developed before the era of proper bowel preparation, antibiotics, and proper drainage principles. If a leak does result after transsacral surgery, it is usually resolved by proper drainage. Posterior resection alone is not recommended as a standard procedure for rectal cancer. This approach is best used in conjunction with anterior resection to allow a low anastomosis (Knight and Griffen 1980).

Sphincter-Splitting

Sphincter-splitting enhances exposure of the distal rectum and can be used for appropriate rectal tumors, rectal prolapse, high fistulas, stenosis, and rectal reconstructions. It can be carried out with regional anesthesia and is well tolerated by the elderly and the infirm. Careful anatomic reconstruction is necessary to preserve continence, but uniformly good results are obtained when attention is paid to the basic surgical principles. Mason (1977) has best described the technique and has carefully documented its success as well as its indication for small malignancies. The concept of completely dividing the rectum and the sphincter mechanism is offensive to some, but in my experience the procedure is simple and provides excellent exposure in those unusual situations not amenable to more conventional techniques. Allgöwer (1983) applied sphincter-splitting in 48 patients and reported no significant complications and good continence. The surgeon who treats patients with lesions of the rectum should become thoroughly familiar with this procedure.

Circular Stapling

Since 1976, circular staplers have become increasingly attractive for the restitution of rectal continuity. Various techniques have been developed by Knight and Griffen (1980) and others that allow one to do an extremely low anastomosis. It should be emphasized that these instruments do not decrease operative time, or create a more secure anastomosis, or shorten hospitalization time; however, they do facilitate restoration of bowel continuity in otherwise difficult situations. Hurst et al. (1982) have raised concern that the use of circular staplers for rectal carcinoma may be associated with a higher risk for local tumor recurrence. In their experience, 11 of 35 patients who underwent low anterior resection followed by stapling experienced disease recurrence at the anastomotic site from 3 to 22 months after resection. They concluded that the stapler should be used for less aggressive and less advanced tumors.

Our experience suggests that midrectal tumors may indeed be more prone to recur locally when the stapler is used. It is difficult to perceive which factors may predispose to increased recurrence, and there is concern that patient selection may have been influenced by our ability to preserve intestinal continuity. By careful evaluation of our experience, we have been able to identify historical and concurrent controls that allow us to control for tumor size, grade, and location; level of anastomosis; sex of patients; distal margin of resection; and surgical technique. It is our impression that those technical factors that predispose to the use of the stapler are likely to be associated with increased local recurrence, and it is unclear whether abdominoperineal resection would decrease this risk.

CONCLUSION

Great advances are not going to be made in salvaging patients with carcinoma of the rectum by removal of greater amounts of perirectal tissue. However, through more refined understanding of the spread of the disease and more adequate techniques for preoperative staging, substantial advances can be made in tailoring procedures to treat the extent of the disease. By doing this, an improved quality of life may be offered to patients. In addition, individuals who perceive that a colostomy is not routinely necessary perhaps would seek treatment at an earlier point in the progression of their disease.

REFERENCES

Allgöwer M. 1983. Sphincter-splitting approach to the rectum. *Am J Surg* 145:5–7.

Beahrs OH. 1967. Low anterior resection for cancer of the rectosigmoid and rectum. *Surg Clin North Am* 47:971–975.

Beahrs OH, Wilson SM. 1976. The curative treatment of carcinoma of the sigmoid, rectosigmoid, and rectum. *Ann Surg* 183:556–563.

Crile G Jr, Turnbull RB Jr. 1972. The role of electrocoagulation in the treatment of carcinoma of the rectum. *Surg Gynecol Obstet* 135:391–396.

Culp CE, Jackman RJ. 1974. Reappraisal of conservative management of certain select cancers of the rectum. In *Surgery of the Gastrointestinal Tract*, JS Najarian, JP Delaney, eds., pp. 511–519. New York: Intercontinental Medical.

Cuthbertson AM, Kaye AH. 1978. Local excision of carcinomas of the rectum, anus, and anal canal. *Aust NZ J Surg* 48:412–415.

Deddish MR. 1974. Local excision. *Surg Clin North Am* 54:877–880.

Eisenstat TE, Deak ST, Rubin RJ, et al. 1982. Five year survival in patients with carcinoma of the rectum treated by electrocoagulation. *Am J Surg* 143:127–132.

Hurst PA, Prout WG, Kelly JM, et al. 1982. Local recurrence after low anterior resection using the staple gun. *Br J Surg* 69:275–276.

Jackman RJ, Beahrs OH. 1968. *Tumors of the Large Bowel.* Major Problems in Clinical Surgery, vol. 8. Philadelphia: W. B. Saunders.

Jones PF, Thomson HJ. 1982. Long term results of a consistent policy of sphincter preservation in the treatment of carcinoma of the rectum. *Br J Surg* 69:564–568.

Knight CD, Griffen FD. 1980. An improved technique for low anterior resection of the rectum using the EEA stapler. *Surgery* 88:710–714.

Localio SA, Eng K, Coppa GF. 1983. Abdominosacral resection for midrectal cancer. A fifteen-year experience. *Ann Surg* 198:320–324.

Lock MR, Cairns DW, Richie JK, et al. 1978. The treatment of early colorectal cancer by local excision. *Br J Surg* 65:346–349.

Madden JL, Kandalaft S. 1971. Electrocoagulation in the treatment of cancer of the rectum. A continuing study. *Ann Surg* 174:530–540.

Mason AY. 1977. Transsphincteric approach to rectal lesions. *Surg Annu* 9:171–194.

Mettlin C, Mittelman A, Natarajan N, et al. 1981. Trends in the United States for the management of adenocarcinoma of the rectum. *Surg Gynecol Obstet* 153:701–706.

Miles WE. 1908. A method of performing abdomino-perineal excision for carcinoma of the rectum and of the terminal portion of the pelvic colon. *Lancet* 2:1812–1813.

Morson BC, Bussey HJR, Samoorian S. 1977. Policy of local excision for early cancer of the colorectum. *Gut* 18:1045–1050.

Papillon J. 1982. *Rectal and Anal Cancers: Conservative Treatment by Irradiation—An Alternative to Radical Surgery*. New York: Springer-Verlag.

Parks AG, Percy JP. 1982. Resection and sutured colo-anal anastomosis for rectal carcinoma. *Br J Surg* 69:301–304.

Rider WD. 1975. The 1975 Gordon Richards Memorial Lecture—Is the Miles operation really necessary for the treatment of rectal cancer? *J Can Assoc Radiol* 26:167–175.

Sischy B, Remington JH, Sobel SH, et al. 1980. Treatment of carcinoma of the rectum and squamous carcinoma of the anus by combination chemotherapy, radiotherapy and operation. *Surg Gynecol Obstet* 151:369–371.

Strauss AA, Strauss SF, Crawford RA, et al. 1935. Surgical diathermy of carcinoma of rectum: Its clinical end results. *JAMA* 104:1480–1484.

Syed A, Pirthawala A, Neblett D, et al. 1978. Primary treatment of carcinoma of the lower rectum and anal canal by a combination of external irradiation and interstitial implant. *Radiology* 128:199–203.

Annual Clinical Conference on Cancer, Vol. 30
Gastrointestinal Cancer: Current Approaches to Diagnosis and Treatment
© 1988 by The University of Texas System Cancer Center

13. Radiotherapy for Early Rectal Cancer

Tyvin A. Rich

Interest is increasing in providing the patient with invasive low rectal cancer an alternative curative treatment to the standard surgical recommendation of combined abdominal-perineal resection and permanent colostomy. The alternatives to radical surgery investigated so far can be broadly categorized by three approaches: (1) locally destructive methods using electrocoagulation (Eisenstat et al. 1982; Gingold, Mitty, and Tadros 1983; Hughes et al. 1982; Madden and Kandalaft 1971) or fulguration (Jackman 1961; Kratzer and Onsanit 1972), or intracavitary irradiation (Papillon 1982); (2) local excision alone (Grigg et al. 1984; Hager, Gall, and Hermanek 1983; Morson, Bussey, and Samoorian 1977) for highly selected patients with small, mobile, superficially invasive lesions usually confined to the muscularis propria; and (3) low segmental excision and reanastomosis (Williams 1984). For these different methods, not surprisingly, there are markedly similar indications for patient selection designed to assure favorable local-control and survival results. An important selection factor is tumor size, commonly described as the maximum tumor diameter at proctoscopy.

LOCAL THERAPY ALONE

A literature review of 10 series using electrocoagulation, fulguration, or local excision demonstrates that about 70% of all patients had tumors smaller than 3 cm and the remainder had tumors measuring between 4 cm and 7 cm (table 13.1). Although primary tumor size in rectal cancer has little prognostic value per se, it is obviously important when determining the appropriateness of local therapy.

Selecting patients for local therapy based on tumor size alone seems reasonable, since the recurrence and survival rates for the patients listed in table 13.1 are similar to those achieved with radical surgery. However, a major criticism of conservative approaches, particularly the locally destructive methods, is the lack of pathological staging and, therefore, the absence of a basis for a direct comparison with radical surgery, where the extent of primary disease and the status of the lymphatics can be pathologically examined. Some of this criticism can be avoided by comparing the local excision information about the depth of tumor invasion with the extent of bowel wall penetration of tumors removed by radical surgery. Since patients treated with local excision alone have predominately T1 or T2 tumors, a comparison with the data of Wood et al. (1979) (table 13.2) illustrates the prognostic utility of the degree of bowel penetration and shows five-year survival rates of 71% to 76% for patients with limited disease.

Table 13.1. *Literature Review of 10 Series Using Conservative Surgical Approaches*

Method/Study	No. of Patients	Tumor Size (cm)						Local Recurrence Rate (%)	5-year Survival Rate (%)[a]
		1	2	3	4	5	6		
Electrocoagulation									
Hughes et al. 1982	39		14	13	8		4	44	69
Eisenstat et al. 1982	29							65	68
Gingold, Mitty, and Tadros 1983	41		6	10	10	5	5	66	32
Madden and Kandalaft 1971	77		48 (>1–<4)				19 (>5–<7)	35	64[b]
Fulguration									
Kratzer and Onsanit 1972	27		14	4	4	4	1	15	64
Jackman 1961	252		170 (>2–<3)		64 (>3–<5)		13 (>5–<7)	4[c]	96
Local excision									
Grigg et al. 1984	16		16 (<3)					6	100
Hager, Gall, and Hermanek 1983	95		95 (<3)					8–17	78–96[d]
Morson, Bussey, and Samoorian 1977	143	13 (<1)	73	26	15	6	5 (>5)	5	83–100
Stearns, Sternberg, and DeCosse 1985	31		4	9	9	5	3 (>5)	39	84
Total	750	13	460 (2–3)	130 (≤4)		70 (>4–≤7)			
Percentage of total known tumor sizes			70% (<3)	29%		10%			

[a] Determinate rate.
[b] Average follow-up, 4 years.
[c] Based on 211 patients.
[d] Ranges based on high-risk and low-risk groups.

Table 13.2. *Survival of Patients with Rectal Cancer According to TNM Categories Established Postsurgically by Pathological Assessment*

TNM Category	No. of Patients	5-year Survival Rate (%)
T1N0M0 Tumor confined to mucosa or submucosa; no metastasis	43	76
T2N0M0 Tumor extension to muscularis but not beyond serosa	210	71
T3N0M0 Tumor extension beyond bowel wall or serosa	124	60

Source: Wood et al. 1979.

Another criticism of the conservative methods is that they provide no information as to the lymph node status. This uncertainty is addressed by some interesting data regarding the cumulative frequency of tumors with positive lymph nodes plotted as a function of increasing tumor size (Spratt 1974) (fig. 13.1). These data, based on 764 pathologically examined cases, show that the cumulative probability of lymph node involvement for rectal cancers no larger than 3 cm is 5% or less. It is not surprising, therefore, to find a low frequency of lymph node metastases or even of subsequent systemic metastasis after purely local methods of treatment when cancers are small and adequately treated.

A few investigators have noted a correlation between circumferential involvement and tumor configuration. The chance for successful local tumor eradication is greatest when tumors involve less than one third of the circumference of the bowel wall (Gingold, Mitty, and Tadros 1983). Patients with exophytic tumors do better than those with tumors clinically described as infiltrative.

Mason (1975) proposed that, in addition to tumor size, a second criterion be employed to select patients for local excision. He performed a digital examination and applied the results to a clinical staging system based on the mobility of the lesion (table 13.3). This clinical staging system has been tested in a prospective trial at St. Mark's Hospital, London, where it was found to be accurate in staging the degree of bowel wall penetration in 89% of the patients treated with radical surgery (Nicholls et al. 1982). This same staging system has been reported to be useful in selecting patients for local excision. In the report of Hager, Gall, and Hermanek (1983), the tumor size was limited to a maximum of 3 cm and only patients with clinical stage I or II tumors were treated. However, Mason (1975) believes that patients whose tumors measure up to 4 cm are suitable for local excision.

The selection of patients for local therapy based on tumor size, clinical assessment of tumor mobility, and invasiveness has been used by several investigators, but few studies have attempted to gauge success as a function of tumor size. For example, Hager, Gall, and Hermanek (1983) limited the selection of patients to those with tumors smaller than 3 cm. They further evaluated the risk of failure by the

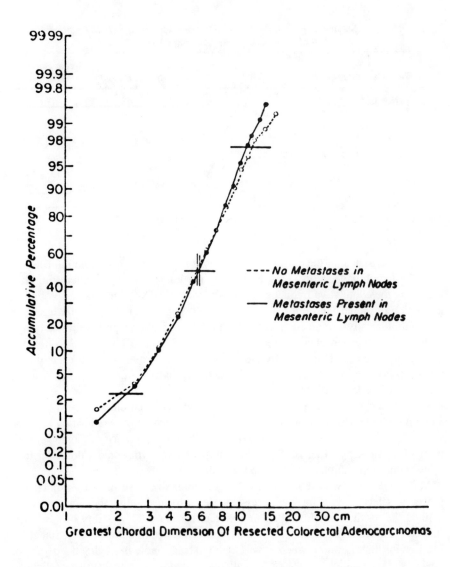

Fig. 13.1. Cumulative frequency of lymph node–negative (42) and positive patients (344) treated with radical surgery at Ellis-Fischel State Cancer Hospital, 1940–1961. Greatest chordal dimensions are recorded. (*Source:* Spratt 1969).

Table 13.3. *Clinical Staging System Used by Mason and Hager to Select Patients for Local Excision*

CS I. TUMOR FREELY MOBILE. The tissue space that allows "free mobility" is the submucosal plane between the muscularis mucosae and the muscle wall of the rectum.

CS II. TUMOR MOBILE. The less-than-free mobility of a cancer invading the muscular wall of the rectum is recognizable.

CS III. TUMOR TETHERED BUT STILL MOBILE. This stage is recognized by the examining finger when growth has transgressed the fascia propria.

CS IV. TUMOR FIXED. Fixity suggests invasion of any adjacent structure, such as the prostate anteriorly or musculoskeletal structures at the back or the sides of the pelvis.

Note: Although tumor size is not mentioned, these authors have rarely used local excision when tumor diameters measure more than 3 or 4 cm.

pathological depth of involvement—into the submucosa versus the muscularis propria. The five-year survival rates were 90% and 78%, respectively. Two other investigative teams specifically looked at the effect of tumor size on rates of local recurrence and survival. Gingold, Mitty, and Tadros (1983), in a study of electro-coagulation, found that a tumor smaller than 3 cm had a three-fold higher chance of cure than a larger tumor. Similarly Papillon (1982), using intracavitary irradiation, found only a small increase in the local failure rate for tumors larger than 3 cm compared to those under 3 cm (7% vs 5%) but a striking, three-fold increase in lymph node relapse (11% vs 4%) for the larger tumors. This degree of nodal failure is predicted by Spratt, whose data indicate that the cumulative probability of lymph node failure can be as great as 15% for lesions between 3 cm and 4 cm (fig. 13.1).

The message of these data is clear: local therapy, regardless of the method, can work for a small group of selected patients with relatively small, mobile tumors. The biological behavior of small cancers (< 3 cm) on this end of the clinical spectrum appears to change quickly as tumor diameter increases; the change may be manifested by an increase in either distant metastasis or local failure rates.

A survey of the literature of local therapy shows that local failures occur regardless of treatment method. The rates of local recurrence range from 8% to 39% for local excision and from 4% to 66% for electrocoagulation or fulguration (table 13.1). The higher rates for the latter techniques are not surprising, given the facts that electrocoagulation or fulguration is less precise and larger lesions are sometimes tackled.

LOCAL THERAPY PLUS ADJUNCTIVE RADIOTHERAPY

Using radiotherapy as an adjunct to conservative surgery to decrease local disease recurrences has both theoretical and actual advantages over surgery alone. For one thing, postoperative radiotherapy allows surgery to be less mutilating. A study from the Joint Center for Radiation Therapy (JCRT) in Boston documents a group of 17 patients with early, low rectal cancers who were treated with postoperative radiation (Rich et al. 1985). Reexamination of the pathological resection specimen revealed that in 65% of those patients, the resection margins were positive. In spite of this highly unfavorable pathological feature, no patient who received an adequate dose of external-beam radiotherapy (> 45 Gy) had a local recurrence (median follow-up was 27 months). Furthermore, only one patient had transient rectal bleeding from the treatment, and all patients retained normal sphincter function.

In this chapter, I describe an additional group of patients who also did well following postoperative radiotherapy after conservative surgical treatment.

Adjuvant Radiotherapy Study: UT M. D. Anderson Hospital

Patient Profile and Irradiation Methods

From January 1978 through June 1986, 15 patients with adenocarcinoma of the low rectum were treated with postoperative radiation at the Department of Radiotherapy at The University of Texas M. D. Anderson Hospital and Tumor Institute at Houston. Five were women and 10 were men; their median age was 58 years. The median tumor location was 3.5 cm (range, 0–8 cm) from the anal verge. The median tumor diameter was 2.5 cm (range, 1.2–6.0 cm). The surgical procedures were: transanal excision, 13; transsphincteric excision, 1; and transanal excision plus multiple fulgurations, 1. Tumors were stage T1 or T2 (tumor extension limited to the mucosa or submucosa) in nine patients, T3 (involvement of perirectal fat) in four, and two were not adequately staged. After excision, three patients had histological evidence of residual tumor.

Every patient received external-beam radiotherapy from megavoltage energy (1.25–25 MV photons). In general, the entire true pelvis was treated with opposed anterior-posterior and lateral field techniques. Boost doses directed to the tumor bed were given with posterior or perineal fields. The total doses of external-beam energy ranged from 30 Gy to 70 Gy (53 Gy median) given over 18 to 50 days in 6 to 35 fractions. In five patients, interstitial iridium-192 delivered an additional 15 Gy to 40 Gy to the tumor site.

Results

One patient experienced local disease recurrence at 41 months after irradiation and was salvaged successfully by radical surgery. The local control rate is 93% (figs. 13.2 and 13.3), and the median follow-up is 48 months. One patient developed liver metastasis at 31 months after radiotherapy and is still living 56 months after radiotherapy. Eight months after radiotherapy, one patient developed mild radiation proctitis, which responded to conservative therapy. All other patients had normal anal sphincter function without evidence of radiation necrosis or symptomatic fibrosis.

DISCUSSION

The use of conservative surgical techniques for low rectal cancer is growing. To date, the proportion of patients considered eligible for local excision has been estimated to be less than 3%. In an effort to offer a greater number of patients a chance to avoid permanent colostomy, the use of combined-modality therapy will probably increase. Two series of patients have now been reported that have shown excellent

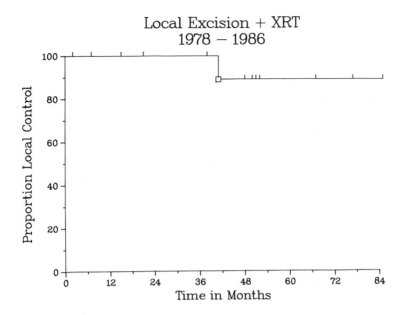

Fig. 13.2. Actuarial local control rates for 15 patients treated with conservative surgery plus postoperative radiation at UT M. D. Anderson Hospital.

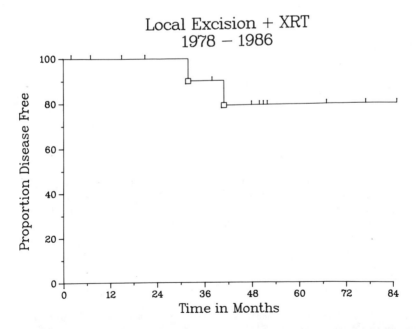

Fig. 13.3. Actuarial disease-free survival rates for 15 patients treated with conservative surgery plus postoperative radiation at UT M. D. Anderson Hospital.

local control from a planned combination of conservative surgery and postoperative irradiation.

The present interest in sphincter-preserving surgery in this age of conservative cancer therapy will undoubtedly cause physicians to ask if limited surgery can be extended to larger numbers of patients. As can be seen from the data presented, the risk of local relapse from either uncontrolled primary or lymph node disease increases with tumor size; therefore, postoperative radiotherapy may play an important role in the management of early, low rectal cancer.

The indications for this treatment, based on our limited experience so far, are twofold.

1. The routine addition of postoperative irradiation appears beneficial for any patient undergoing local excision. The exception may be patients with very small tumors confined to the muscularis mucosa. Patients with deeper levels of invasion (to the submucosa, muscularis propria, and beyond) are at a moderate risk of local relapse and, therefore, could benefit from postoperative irradiation.
2. As larger tumors are treated with local excision, the chance of lymph node metastasis increases. The favorable outcome, so far, is very encouraging: no lymph node failures have been detected in patients treated with radiation. This is not unexpected based on the data from preoperative radiation therapy: in patients so treated, the expected versus observed ratio of lymph node involvement is less than 1 (Kligerman, Urdaneta, and Knowlton 1972; Stevens, Allen, and Fletcher 1976). Moderate doses of radiation ($>45-50$ Gy) are believed to be highly effective in sterilizing microscopic disease in lymph nodes. Thus, the cautious use of combined-modality therapy for patients with tumors larger than 3 cm appears therapeutically warranted.

ACKNOWLEDGMENTS

This work was supported in part by grants CA06294 and CA16672 from the National Cancer Institute, U.S. Department of Health and Human Services.

REFERENCES

Eisenstat TE, Deak ST, Rubin RJ, et al. 1982. Five year survival in patients with carcinoma of the rectum treated by electrocoagulation. *Am J Surg* 143:127–132.
Gingold BS, Mitty WF Jr, Tadros M. 1983. Importance of patient selection in local treatment of carcinoma of the rectum. *Am J Surg* 145:293–296.
Grigg M, McDermott FT, Phil E, et al. 1984. Curative local excision in the treatment of carcinoma of the rectum. *Dis Colon Rectum* 27:81–83.
Hager T, Gall FP, Hermanek P. 1983. Local excision of cancer of the rectum. *Dis Colon Rectum* 26:149–151.
Hughes EP, Veidenheimer MC, Corman ML, et al. 1982. Electrocoagulation of rectal cancer. *Dis Colon Rectum* 25:215–218.
Jackman RJ. 1961. Conservative management of selected patients with carcinoma of the rectum. *Dis Colon Rectum* 4:429–434.
Kligerman MM, Urdaneta N, Knowlton A. 1972. Preoperative irradiation of rectosigmoid carcinoma including its regional lymph nodes. *Am J Radiol* 114:498–503.

Kratzer GL, Onsanit T. 1972. Fulguration of selected cancers of the rectum. *Dis Colon Rectum* 15:431–435.

Madden JL, Kandalaft S. 1971. Electrocoagulation in the treatment of cancer of the rectum. *Ann Surg* 174:530–538.

Mason AY. 1975. Malignant tumors of the rectum. Part II. Local excision. *Gastroenterology* 4:582–593.

Morson BC, Bussey HJR, Samoorian S. 1977. Policy of local excision for early cancer of the colorectum. *Gut* 18:1045–1050.

Nicholls RJ, Mason AY, Morson BC, et al. 1982. The clinical staging of rectal cancer. *Br J Surg* 69:404–409.

Papillon J. 1982. Conservative treatment by irradiation: An alternative to radical surgery. In *Rectal and Anal Cancer,* pp. 77–105. New York: Springer.

Rich TA, Weiss DR, Mies C, et al. 1985. Sphincter preservation in patients with low rectal cancer treated with radiation therapy with or without local excision or fulguration. *Radiology* 156:527–531.

Spratt JS. 1974. Carcinoma of the rectum: Biologic characteristics. *Dis Colon Rectum* 17:591–597.

Stearns MW Jr, Sternberg SS, DeCosse JJ. 1985. Treatment alternatives: Localized rectal cancer. *Cancer* 54:2691–2694.

Stevens KR, Allen CV, Fletcher WS. 1976. Preoperative radiotherapy for carcinoma of the rectosigmoid. *Cancer* 37:2866–2874.

Williams NS. 1984. The rationale for preservation of the anal sphincter in patients with low rectal cancer. *Br J Surg* 71:575–581.

Wood DA, Robbins GF, Zippin C, et al. 1979. Staging of cancer of the colon and cancer of the rectum. *Cancer* 43:961–968.

Annual Clinical Conference on Cancer, Vol. 30
Gastrointestinal Cancer: Current Approaches to Diagnosis and Treatment
© 1988 by The University of Texas System Cancer Center

14. Intraoperative Irradiation for Gastrointestinal Cancers

Leonard L. Gunderson, J. Kirk Martin, Jr., David M. Nagorney,
James A. Martenson, Jennifer Fieck, Robert W. Beart, Jr.,
and Donald McIlrath

Useful palliation can often be achieved when external-beam irradiation and chemotherapy with or without resection are used to treat locally advanced gastrointestinal malignancies. Local control and long-term survival occur in only 5% to 30% of patients, however, due to the limited radiation tolerance of surrounding organs and tissues (Gunderson et al. 1983a, in press[a]). External-beam doses necessary to accomplish such results are 6000 to 7000+ cGy and exceed the radiation tolerance of some organs and structures in the abdomen and pelvis (stomach, small intestine, and spinal cord, 4500–5000 cGy/5–5½ weeks; entirety of both kidneys, 2000–2500 cGy/2–3 weeks). Although portions of the large bowel and bladder can safely receive 6000 to 7000 cGy, the irradiated volume must be small or complications are excessive.

In view of external-beam dose limitations, intraoperative irradiation (IORT) has been employed in an attempt to improve the therapeutic ratio of local control versus complications. The application of IORT has several advantages: (1) all or part of the dose-limiting structures may be excluded by operative mobilization or shielding or by use of variable electron-beam energies, and (2) the volume of the irradiation boost field may be decreased by treating the tumor under direct vision and using appositional placement.

Early investigators employed intraoperative radiation as the sole radiation modality, administering a single dose of 2000 to 4000 cGy with electron beams (Abe et al. 1971; Abe and Takahashi 1981; Goldson 1978, 1981). Supplemental external-beam irradiation was administered only infrequently. Later investigators preferred to use IORT electrons as a "boost" dose in conjunction with conventional fractionated external-beam radiation and, where feasible, resection (Gunderson et al. 1981, 1983b, 1984).

Advantages of a combined external-beam–IORT approach over IORT alone include: (1) improvement in local-regional control because of a decreased risk of marginal recurrence and the radiobiologic advantages of fractionated irradiation and (2) less risk of normal-tissue necrosis. The excellent long-term results achieved with several external-beam-plus-boost techniques for head and neck, breast, and gynecologic malignancies support the concept of this approach, since good local control has been achieved with relatively low morbidity to dose-limiting normal tissues. The only difference is in the method of delivering the boost dose (i.e., head and neck and breast—interstitial; gynecologic—intracavitary; intraabdominal, pelvic, or thoracic—intraoperative electrons).

An IORT dose of 1000 to 2000 cGy has been combined with fractionated external-beam doses of 4500 to 5000 cGy in 180-cGy fractions in pilot studies from Massachusetts General Hospital (MGH) and Mayo Clinic (Gunderson et al. 1981, 1984). Subtotal or gross total resection of disease is also performed, when feasible, for gastric and colorectal lesions but not for initially unresectable pancreatic or biliary duct primaries. The biologic effectiveness of single-dose IORT is considered equivalent to two to three times that quantity of fractionated external-beam treatment (Suit 1973). The effective dose in the IORT boost field, when added to the 4500 to 5000 cGy delivered in 180-cGy fractions with external-beam techniques, is 6500 to 8000 cGy for an IORT dose of 1000 cGy, 7500 to 9500 cGy with a 1500-cGy boost, and 8500 to 11,000 cGy with a 2000-cGy IORT dose.

In this chapter, we discuss the indications for and potential of aggressive combined techniques that include IORT. Results obtained with external-beam techniques alone or with chemotherapy and resection are presented by site to demonstrate the need for higher doses of radiation. Finally, we discuss technical considerations of IORT and results of its use.

UPPER GASTROINTESTINAL MALIGNANCIES

Gastric Cancer

External-Beam Irradiation + 5-Fluorouracil

External-beam irradiation combined with 5-fluorouracil (5-FU) has been shown to have good palliative and occasional curative potential in patients with residual disease after resection or with unresectable lesions. In a randomized Mayo Clinic trial comparing radiation and 5-FU with radiation alone, mean and overall survivals were improved in the combined-modality arm (13 vs. 5.9 months and 3/25 or 12% vs. 0/23 5-year survival) (Holbrook 1974). The Gastrointestinal Tumor Study Group found that a combination of irradiation and 5-FU followed by maintenance with 5-FU-methyl CCNU (MECCNU) was statistically superior to 5-FU-MECCNU alone for long-term survival, producing a plateau of a 20% survival rate between the second and third years of follow-up ($p < .05$) (Schein and Novak 1982).

Intraoperative Irradiation

The only substantial series documenting IORT for gastric cancer come from Japan. Abe and Takahashi (1981) delivered single doses of 2800 to 4000 cGy to the tumor bed and major nodal sites after gastrectomy. In a prospective study, 110 patients were treated by surgery alone and 84 patients by surgery plus IORT; the treatment method was chosen on the basis of day of hospitalization. Although there is a suggestion of a survival advantage in the IORT group for patients with both stage II (78% vs. 55%) and stage III (45% vs. 37%) disease, the most impressive difference is for those with stage IV who had residual disease without distant metastases (19.5% vs. 0%).

Formal randomized trials are indicated to determine whether IORT would be more effective than conventional external-beam irradiation plus chemotherapy or whether a combination of both irradiation modalities would be even more effective. The long-term survival rate of 20% seen with external-beam and chemotherapy in the Gastrointestinal Tumor Study Group trial and with IORT in the Japanese experience closely parallels the incidence of local regional failure as the only pattern of progression of patients with gastric cancer who undergo curative resection (Gunderson and Sosin 1982). These patients frequently experience disease relapses in the liver or peritoneal cavity despite attempts to prevent it with combined-drug chemotherapy, and long-term results will not improve beyond 20% to 30% until effective abdominal treatment is developed.

Pancreatic Cancer

External-Beam Irradiation Plus Chemotherapy

For unresectable lesions, definite palliation and occasional cures can be obtained using external-beam irradiation plus chemotherapy. The duration of palliation appears to increase as the radiation dose increases from 4000 cGy in four to six weeks to 6000 to 6500 cGy in seven to ten weeks (table 14.1). Even at the highest doses, local failure was documented in at least two thirds of the patients (Whittington et al. 1984).

Intraoperative Irradiation ± External-Beam Irradiation

Specialized radiation therapy techniques, including IORT, have been used in an attempt to increase the radiation dose to the tumor volume without increasing normal tissue morbidity (Abe and Takahashi 1981; Goldson 1981; Sindelar et al. 1983; Shipley et al. 1984; Gunderson et al. 1987). Results from Japan for IORT alone (Abe and Takahashi 1981) parallel the Mayo Clinic "no-treatment" or "low-dose external" arms (Moertel et al. 1969). Japanese investigators now more routinely combine external-beam irradiation with IORT, and some prefer to give the entire external-beam component prior to IORT.

The combination of intraoperative and external-beam irradiation has resulted in a lower incidence of local failure in the series from both MGH (Shipley et al. 1984; Wood et al. 1982) and Mayo (Gunderson et al. 1984, 1987), and, in the MGH trial, has improved the median survival over that of conventional external-beam irradiation (table 14.1). It is uncertain whether this improvement is due to superior treatment or patient selection. Although the combination methods deliver a much higher effective dose of radiation than external-beam alone, prospective randomized trials are needed to determine if a therapeutic gain results from the more aggressive techniques.

Table 14.1. *Cancer of the Pancreas: Comparison of Results*

Series	No. of Patients	Median Survival (mo)			Local Failure in Evaluable Patients	
		Total Group	RT	RT + CT	No.	%
Radical operation—MGH (26 postoperative survivors)	31	10.5	—	—	13/26	50
Regional, unresectable (external ± 5-FU)						
1. Mayo Clinic external-beam (Moertel et al. 1969)						
Untreated	67	6.0	—	—	—	—
35 Gy/4 wk ± 5-FU	64	—	6.3	10.4	—	—
2. GITSG (1979; Moertel et al. 1981[a])						
40 Gy/6 wk + 5-FU	79	—	—	6.9	—	—
60 Gy/10 wk ± 5-FU (RT, 25 pts.; RT + CT, 75 pts.)	100	—	5.1 (5.3)	8.7 (11.4)	—	—
3. Duke Curative Group (Haslam, Cavanaugh, and Stroup 1973)						
60 Gy/10 wk ± CT (RT 9 pts.; RT + CT, 11 pts.)	20	—	8	10	—	—

Regional, unresectable (external ± specialized boost)

4. Thomas Jefferson Univ. (Whittington et al. 1984)						
63–67 Gy/7–9 wk, RT ± CT	55	—	7.3	12.4	36/46	78
RT + 125I implant ± CT[b]	33	—	5.5	11.3	5/26	19
			(7.3)	(12.5)		
5. MGH (Shipley et al. 1980, 1984)						
125I + external (40–45 Gy/4.5–5 wk)	12	12	—	—	4/12	33
External + IORT (45–50 Gy) ± CT	29	16.5	—	—	10/29	34
6. Mayo Clinic external + IORT + CT (Gunderson et al. 1987)						
50 Gy/180 cGy per fraction + 20 Gy IORT	44	12.2	—	—	3/42	7[c]
7. Japanese experience (Abe and Takahashi 1981)						
IORT alone	6	—	—	—	—	—
IORT + 40 Gy external	10	—	—	—	—	—

Abbreviations: RT, radiotherapy; CT, chemotherapy; IORT, intraoperative irradiation; MGH, Massachusetts General Hospital; 5-FU, 5-fluorouracil; GITSG, Gastrointestinal Tumor Study Group.

[a] Median survival durations in open figures are 1979 statistics, calculated from start of treatment; numbers in ( ) are 1981 data, calculated from date of surgery.

[b] Median survival statistics in open figures include early postoperative deaths; numbers in ( ) exclude early deaths.

[c] Incidence is 18% in patients at risk one year, 34% at two years.

Table 14.2. *Pancreatic Cancer: Patterns of Failure, External Beam ± IORT, Mayo Clinic*

| Treatment | No. of Patients at Risk | Site of Failure[a] | | | Local Failure Rate (%) | |
		Abdominal No. (%)	Liver No. (%)	PS No. (%)	1 yr	2 yr
External-beam	122	68 (56)	52 (43)	35 (29)	52	80
External-beam + IORT	37	20 (54)	14 (38)	10 (27)	18	34

Abbreviations: IORT, intraoperative irradiation; PS, peritoneal seeding.
[a] Abdominal = liver and/or peritoneal seeding.

External-Beam Irradiation ± Intraoperative Irradiation, Mayo Clinic

Although slight gains in median survival may be achieved by improving local tumor control, a significant number of distant failures may prevent significant improvements in long-term survival. Between February 1974 and April 1985, 159 patients with unresectable but localized pancreatic cancer, as defined at exploratory laparotomy, were treated with radiation at Mayo Clinic (Roldan et al. in press). Postoperative therapy consisted of either external-beam radiation (XRT) with or without 5-FU (122 patients) or XRT with or without 5-FU plus IORT (37 patients). The median lengths of survival of the two treatment groups (XRT vs. XRT + IORT) were not statistically different (12.6 months vs. 13.4 months). The local control rate at one year was 82% for XRT plus IORT ± 5-FU versus 48% for XRT ± 5-FU; at two years it was 66% versus 20%, respectively ($p = .0005$). Owing to the high incidence of abdominal failure (20 of 37, or 54%, developed liver or peritoneal metastases), the decreased frequency of local progression with XRT plus IORT did not translate into an improved survival rate (table 14.2). The latest analysis of the MGH data also implicates distant failure as a significant problem, occurring in 12 of 29 patients at risk (Shipley et al. 1984).

Biliary Duct

Bile-duct cancer is the best disease model in upper gastrointestinal sites for illustrating local control translated into improved survival. At the time of initial presentation, peritoneal seeding is present in only 5% to 10% of patients, and local-regional failures are the most common cause of death. If the bile duct is surgically violated to obtain tissue for diagnosis, however, the incidence of peritoneal seeding may rise to 33% or higher, and aggressive local treatment techniques become less appropriate (Buskirk et al. 1984, 1986). Therefore, thin-needle percutaneous biopsy may be a preferable method to acquire tissue for diagnosis.

External-Beam Irradiation

Significant palliation can be obtained with external-beam irradiation to doses of 4000 to 6000 cGy in four to seven weeks, but long-term local control is rare. In a series by Kopelson et al. (1977), one-year survival was improved when 5-FU was added to external-beam radiation for advanced primary lesions.

Specialized Radiation Techniques

Several Japanese groups have reported using intraoperative electrons as the sole treatment modality for unresectable lesions. In the series by Todoroki et al. (1980), tumor recurred regionally in four of five patients, and the longest survival time was only 18 months. This suggests that tumor had extended beyond the small volume encompassed by the IORT cones (no external-beam irradiation was used).

Radioactive sources temporarily inserted into transhepatic catheters can deliver localized high-dose radiation. This treatment method is attractive in view of its potentially wide applicability. Published series have shown decent short-term results, but local failures have been excessive when only transcatheter radiation was used.

Both of these specialized techniques have limitations if used as the only method of irradiation. We prefer to deliver 4500 to 5000 cGy in 25 to 28 fractions over 5 to 5½ weeks to the primary lesion plus nodal areas with external-beam radiation and use IORT electrons or transcatheter sources as a boost dose: 1500 to 2000 cGy with intraoperative electrons; 2000 to 3000 cGy at a 0.7- to 1.0-cm radius with transcatheter sources. An intraoperative electron boost is used when feasible, as stomach and duodenum can be displaced out of the boost field. For 12 to 18 months after treatment begins, it is difficult to distinguish between problems related to the indwelling tubes, possibly persistent tumor, or radiation fibrosis. Patients deserve aggressive support, and the radiation oncologist needs to be an active member of the follow-up team. Early results with the combined techniques are encouraging (tables 14.3 and 14.4), but patient numbers are small.

Table 14.3. *Biliary Duct Cancer: Survival and Status by Treatment Method, Mayo Clinic (9/86 Analysis)*

Patient Status	No. of Patients	XRT + resection	XRT ± 5-FU	XRT + [192]Ir	XRT + IORT
Alive					
No disease	2	—	—	1 (52)	1 (16.5)
Disease	1	—	—	—	1 (46.5)
Uncertain	1	—	—	1 (18)[a]	—
Dead					
No disease[a]	1	—	—	—	1 (4)
Disease	23	7 (5.5–39)	11 (5–16)	4 (10–18)	1 (37)
Uncertain	8	—	—	4 (10–15)	4 (6.5–21)
Totals		7	11	10[a]	8

Note: Numbers in ( ) represent survival in months.

Abbreviations: XRT, radiation therapy; IORT, intraoperative irradiation.

[a]One patient lost to follow-up at 18 months, status uncertain.

Table 14.4. *Biliary Duct Cancer: Survival by Treatment Method, Mayo Clinic (9/86 Analysis)*

| | Survival | | | | |
| | 12 mo | 18 mo | 24 mo | 36 mo | ≥42 mo |
Treatment	No. (%)	No. (%)	No. (%)	No. (%)	No. (%)
XRT ± 5-FU (11)	6 (55)	—	—	—	—
XRT + resection (7)[a]	4 (57)	2 (29)	2 (29)	2 (29)	—
XRT + [192]Ir (10)[b]	8 (80)	3 (30)	1 (11)	1 (11)	1 (11)
XRT + IORT (8)[c]	6 (75)	3 (43)	2 (29)	2 (29)	1 (14)

Abbreviations: XRT, radiotherapy; 5-FU, 5-fluorouracil; IORT, intraoperative irradiation.
[a] Subtotal resection in five, total in two.
[b] Nine at risk ≥24 months; 1/9 had subtotal resection.
[c] Seven at risk ≥18 months, none of whom had been resected.

External-Beam Irradiation Alone or with Specialized Boost, Mayo Results

Thirty-six patients with biliary duct carcinoma were treated at Mayo Clinic with radiation delivered with curative intent between January 1980 and March 1985. All
patients received a minimum dose of 4500 cGy in 25 fractions. Surgical exploration
was performed in 32 of the 36 patients, and 7 had a total or subtotal resection of
tumor prior to irradiation.

Three of 18 patients treated with specialized boost techniques (^{192}Ir or IORT) are
alive without evidence of disease 16.5, 46.5, and 52 months after the date of diagnosis. The remaining 33 patients (specialized boost techniques, 15 patients; external-
beam alone, 18 patients) are dead after a median survival duration of 12 months
(range, 4 to 39 months). The immediate cause of death in several patients who had
no evidence of disease progression appeared to be cholangitis; in some cases, it was
associated with sepsis, abscess, or diminished hepatic function owing to obstructed
percutaneous transhepatic drainage tubes. When the length of survival was analyzed
by treatment method, we found that the only patients who survived 18 months or
longer were either those who underwent total or subtotal surgical resection prior to
external-beam radiation (two of seven, or 29%) or those who received specialized
radiation boosts (three of ten, or 30%, with ^{192}Ir; three of seven, or 43%, with
IORT).

Patterns of failure were analyzed in detail. Three patients developed extraabdominal distant metastasis, and one additional patient developed hematogenous
metastasis to the liver. In 7 of 21 patients who had undergone total or subtotal tumor
resection, dilation of the bile ducts with probes, or curettement of the bile ducts
during the surgical procedure, treatment failure occurred by development of either
peritoneal dissemination of disease (five patients) or a recurrence in the surgical scar
(one patient) or both (one patient). One additional patient who had only a biopsy
also developed peritoneal dissemination of disease. Local failure occurred in 10 of
18 patients (56%) who received external-beam irradiation alone or with 5-FU, in 3
of 10 (30%) who had a ^{192}Ir boost, and in 2 of 8 (25%) who had an IORT boost.

COLORECTAL CANCER

Local Failure after Conventional Treatment

External-beam irradiation has been combined with surgical resection, chemo-therapy, immunotherapy, or any combination of these techniques to treat locally advanced disease. In separate series from Princess Margaret Hospital (PMH) (Cummings et al. 1983) and Mayo Clinic (O'Connell et al. 1982), using radiation alone (PMH, Mayo) or combined with immunotherapy (Mayo), the local recurrence rate was 90% or higher in evaluable patients. Although a combination of radiation (± 5-FU) with surgery for residual disease after subtotal resection or for initially unresectable disease produces a local control rate better than that with no resection, the risk of local recurrence still remains too high at 30% to 50% (Gunderson et al. 1983c, 1986).

IORT + External-Beam Irradiation

In an attempt to decrease local recurrence and improve survival, both MGH (Gunder-son et al. 1983a) and Mayo (Gunderson et al. in press[a], 1987) have added an intra-operative electron boost to the fractionated external-beam doses of 4500 to 5000 cGy in 180-cGy fractions, with or without resection. The IORT dose varies from 1000 to 2000 cGy dependent on the amount of disease remaining after an attempt at resection: microscopic residual, 1000 cGy; gross residual less than 2 cm, 1500 cGy; gross residual greater than or equal to 2 cm or unresectable, 1750 to 2000 cGy.

In a published MGH trial of 32 patients who received IORT plus external-beam radiation, local control was improved in the patients who had residual disease or were initially unresectable and received IORT; survival, too, was better in the latter group than in historical controls treated with only preoperative radiation and re-section (Gunderson et al. 1983a). In a subsequent MGH analysis of 53 patients treated with IORT for rectal disease (table 14.5), the four-year actuarial survival rate was approximately 50% for those treated for primary disease and 25% for those with recurrence (the expected long-term survival rate for patients with recurrent le-sions is approximately 5% when treated with standard techniques) (Tepper et al. in

Table 14.5. *Rectal IORT: Actuarial Local Control and Survival Rate,*
Massachusetts General Hospital

Patient Status	No. of Patients	Survival Rate (%)	
		24 mo	48 mo
Local Control			
Primary	31	90	85
Recurrent	22	46	30
Survival			
Primary	—	—	52
Recurrent	—	—	25

press). The poorer survival rate for patients with recurrent rather than primary disease is due to a higher incidence of both local and systemic failure. The incidence of moderate or severe soft-tissue complications has not appeared to increase as a result of the aggressive combined treatments (Tepper et al. 1984).

In a series of 51 patients treated with IORT at Mayo for colorectal cancer, results parallel those achieved at MGH (table 14.6, fig. 14.1) (Gunderson et al. in press[a]). Thirty of 51 (59%) are alive and 22 (43%) are free of disease. All local failures have occurred in patients who presented with recurrence or had gross residual disease after partial resection. In patients at risk for one year or longer, the addition of 5-FU during external-beam irradiation appeared to decrease the risk of local recurrence (1 of 11, or 9%, with 5-FU vs. 6 of 31, or 19%, without); a similar decrease occurs in patients receiving adjuvant radiation therapy plus 5-FU. The incidence of distant metastases was high in patients who presented with recurrence.

In the Mayo analysis, the peripheral nerve and the ureter appeared to be dose-limiting structures. Symptomatic or objective neuropathy occurred in 12 of 37 patients (32%) at risk for 12 months or longer who received pelvic IORT. This was

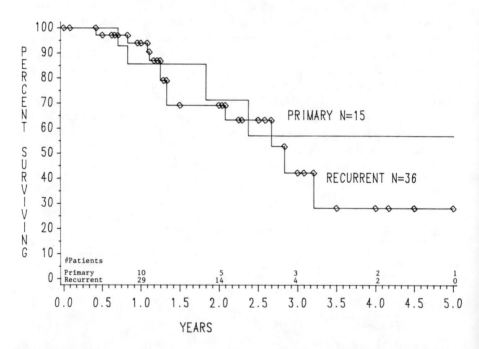

COLORECTAL IORT, MAYO (10/86) ANALYSIS
SURVIVAL – PRIMARY VS RECURRENT

Fig. 14.1. Kaplan-Meier survival curve of 51 patients with locally advanced colorectal cancer treated with external-beam and intraoperative radiation at Mayo Clinic (analysis, October 1986).

Table 14.6. *Colorectal IORT: Incidence and Patterns of Failure, Mayo Clinic (10/86 Analysis)*

Disease Category	Failures		CF			LF			DM			PS		
	No.	%	No.	%	(%)	No.	%	(%)	No.	%	(%)	No.	%	(%)
Total group	24/48+	(50)	1	4	(2)	8	33	(17)	18	75	(38)	4	17	(8)
Primary	6/14	(43)		0		2	33	(14)	4	67	(29)	1	17	(7)
Recurrent	18/ 34[c]	(53)	1	6	(3)	6	33	(18)	14	78	(41)[c]	3	17	(9)[c]

Column group header: Patterns of Failure[a,b] (any component)

Abbreviations: CF, central failure in IORT field; LF, local failure in external beam field; DM, distant metastasis; PS, peritoneal seeding; IORT, intraoperative irradiation.

[a] Three patients died NED ≤ seven months and are excluded from this analysis.
[b] Open numbers indicate percentage of patients who failed; ( ) indicates percentage of the total at risk.
[c] One patient in each group had a solitary liver metastasis resected at IORT—therefore failure in 16/32 (50); DM in 13, PS in 2.

manifested as pain in all 12 (resolved in 5 of 12, severe in 3 of 12), sensory in 8 (none severe), and motor in 7 (resolved in 1 of 7, severe in 1 of 7). The IORT boost included 12 ureters in the 37 patients. Nine ureters were unobstructed prior to IORT, and subsequent hydronephrosis developed in four (44%). Three ureters were initially obstructed by tumor, and hydronephrosis resolved in two.

CONCLUSIONS AND FUTURE POSSIBILITIES

The long-term results of an aggressive local approach for locally advanced gastrointestinal malignancies (initially unresectable, residual after resection, or locally recurrent) are dependent on disease presentation (primary vs. recurrent), the metastatic potential of the treated site, and possibly the sequencing of irradiation and resection (i.e., results appear better for colorectal disease if irradiation precedes resection). In recent trials, irradiation boost techniques using intraoperative electrons or intraoperative or transcatheter brachytherapy (± chemotherapy and resection) have been combined with fractionated external-beam doses of 4500 to 5000 cGy in 180-cGy fractions. For colorectal and biliary cancer, both local control and long-term survival appear to be improved over results achieved with conventional treatment, and continued aggressive local techniques appear to be appropriate. For pancreatic cancer, although local control appears to be improved, median and long-term survivals have not been altered. For partially resected gastric cancer, either IORT used as a single modality or external-beam irradiation plus chemotherapy has yielded five-year survival rates of approximately 20%.

Abdominal failure occurs frequently with resectable as well as unresectable lesions of the pancreas or stomach. Although the aggressive local treatment approaches that combine external-beam irradiation with brachytherapy or intraoperative electron boosts may still be appropriate in the latter sites, treatment of the liver, peritoneal cavity, or both, using intraperitoneal chemotherapy or radiocolloids, infusion chemotherapy, external-beam irradiation, or combinations thereof, may be indicated to try to increase survival rates.

Even with IORT plus external-beam irradiation techniques, central or local failure is excessive. With locally advanced primary or recurrent lesions, or when gross residual disease persists after an attempt at resection, the use of 5-FU during external-beam irradiation and radiation-dose modifiers during IORT needs to be evaluated.

The advent of the aggressive treatment approaches described in this manuscript should make inappropriate a recommendation of therapeutic nihilism for locally advanced gastrointestinal malignancies, because tools now exist for improving the chance of long-term local control or cure. However, because patient symptoms and diagnostic x-ray changes caused by radiation fibrosis can mimic tumor persistence or regrowth, the radiation oncologist needs to be an active member of the follow-up team. Often only time and serial radiographs over a 6- to 12-month period can resolve the issue. Randomized trials by site are needed to determine if the differences observed in prospective nonrandomized IORT trials are real or are the result of differences in patient selection.

ACKNOWLEDGMENTS

The authors appreciate the efforts of Julie Boland and the Mayo Clinic Typing Service for assistance in the preparation of the manuscript.

REFERENCES

Abe M, Takahashi M. 1981. Intraoperative radiotherapy: The Japanese experience. *Int J Radiat Oncol Biol Phys* 7:863–868.

Abe M, Fukada M, Yamano K, et al. 1971. Intraoperative irradiation in abdominal and cerebral tumors. *Acta Radiol* 10:408–416.

Buskirk SJ, Gunderson LL, Adson MA, et al. 1984. Analysis of failure following curative irradiation of gallbladder and extrahepatic bile duct carcinoma. *Int J Radiat Oncol Biol Phys* 10:2013–2023.

Buskirk SJ, Gunderson LL, Nagorney DM, et al. 1986. Analysis of failure following curative irradiation of extrahepatic bile duct cancer. ASTRO Proceedings. *Int J Radiat Oncol Biol Phys* 12(Suppl 1):120.

Cummings BJ, Rider WD, Harwood AR, et al. 1983. External beam radiation therapy for adenocarcinoma of the rectum. *Dis Colon Rectum* 26:30–36.

Gastrointestinal Tumor Study Group. 1979. Comparative therapeutic trial of radiation with or without chemotherapy in pancreatic carcinoma. *Int J Radiat Oncol Biol Phys* 5:1643–1647.

Goldson A. 1978. Preliminary clinical experience with intraoperative radiotherapy. *J Natl Med Assoc* 70:493–495.

Goldson AL. 1981. Past, present and future prospects of intraoperative radiotherapy (IOR). *Semin Oncol* 8:59–65.

Gunderson LL, Cohen AM, Dosoretz DD, et al. 1983a. Residual, unresectable, or recurrent colorectal cancer: External beam irradiation and intraoperative electron beam boost ± resection. *Int J Radiat Oncol Biol Phys* 9:1597–1606.

Gunderson LL, Martin JK, Beart RW, et al. In press (a). External beam and intraoperative electron irradiation for colorectal cancer. *Ann Surg*.

Gunderson LL, Martin JK, Beart RW, et al. In press (b). Intraoperative radiation for colorectal cancer. In *Intraoperative Radiation Therapy,* M Abe, R Dobelbower, eds. Boca Raton: CRC Press.

Gunderson LL, Martin JK Jr, Earle JD, et al. 1984. Intraoperative and external beam irradiation with or without resection: Mayo pilot experience. *Mayo Clin Proc* 59:691–699.

Gunderson LL, Martin JK Jr, Kvols LK, et al. 1987. Intraoperative and external beam irradiation ± 5FU for locally advanced pancreatic cancer. *Int J Radiat Oncol Biol Phys* 13:319–329.

Gunderson LL, Martin JK Jr, O'Connell MJ, et al. 1986. Local control and survival in locally advanced gastrointestinal cancer. *Int J Radiat Oncol Biol Phys* 12:661–665.

Gunderson LL, Shipley WU, Suit HD, et al. 1981. Intraoperative irradiation: A pilot study combining external beam photons with "boost" dose intraoperative electrons. *Cancer* 49:2259–2266.

Gunderson LL, Sosin H. 1982. Adenocarcinoma of the stomach: Areas of failure in a re-operation series (second or symptomatic look): Clinico-pathologic correlation and implications for adjuvant therapy. *Int J Radiat Oncol Biol Phys* 8:1–11.

Gunderson LL, Tepper JE, Biggs PJ, et al. 1983b. Intraoperative ± external beam irradiation. *Curr Probl Cancer* 7:1–69.

Gunderson LL, Tepper JE, Dosoretz DE, et al. 1983c. Patterns of failure after treatment of gastrointestinal cancer. *Cancer Treatment Symposia* 2:181–197.

Haslam JB, Cavanaugh PJ, Stroup SL. 1973. Radiation therapy in the treatment of irresectable adenocarcinoma of the pancreas. *Cancer* 32:1341–1345.

Holbrook MA. 1974. Cancer of the gastrointestinal tract. Radiation therapy. *JAMA* 228:1289–1290.

Kopelson G, Harisiadis L, Tretter P, et al. 1977. The role of radiation therapy in cancer of the extrahepatic biliary system: An analysis of thirteen patients and a review of the literature of the effectiveness of surgery, chemotherapy and radiotherapy. *Int J Radiat Oncol Biol Phys* 2:883–894.

Moertel CG, Childs DS Jr, Reitemeier RJ, et al. 1969. Combined 5-fluorouracil and supervoltage radiation therapy of locally unresectable gastrointestinal cancer. *Lancet* 2:865–867.

Moertel CG, Frytak S, Hahn RG, et al. 1981. Therapy of locally unresectable pancreatic carcinoma: A randomized comparison of high dose (6000 rads) radiation alone, moderate dose radiation (4000 rads + 5-fluorouracil) and high dose radiation + 5-fluorouracil: The Gastrointestinal Tumor Study Group. *Cancer* 48:1705–1710.

O'Connell MJ, Childs DS, Moertel CG, et al. 1982. A prospective controlled evaluation of combined pelvic radiotherapy and methanol extraction residue of BCG (MER) for locally unresectable or recurrent rectal carcinoma. *Int J Radiat Oncol Biol Phys* 8:1115–1119.

Roldan GE, Gunderson LL, Nagorney DM, et al. In press. External beam vs. intra-operative and external beam irradiation for locally advanced pancreatic cancer (abstract). *Cancer.*

Schein PS, Novak J for the Gastrointestinal Tumor Study Group. 1982. Combined modality therapy (XRT-chemo) versus chemotherapy alone for locally unresectable gastric cancer. *Cancer* 49:1771–1777.

Shipley WU, Nardi GL, Cohen AM. 1980. Iodine-125 implant and external beam irradiation in patients with localized pancreatic carcinoma: A comparative study to surgical resection. *Cancer* 45:709–714.

Shipley WU, Wood WC, Tepper JE, et al. 1984. Intraoperative electron beam irradiation for patients with unresectable pancreatic carcinoma. *Ann Surg* 200:289–296.

Sindelar ST, Kinsella T, Tepper J, et al. 1983. Experimental and clinical studies with intra-operative radiotherapy. *Surg Gynecol Obstet* 157:205–219.

Suit HD. 1973. Radiation biology: A basis for radiotherapy. In: *The Textbook of Radiotherapy,* 2nd ed. GH Fletcher, ed., pp. 75–121. Philadelphia: Lea and Febiger.

Tepper JE, Cohen A, Orlow E, et al. In press. Intraoperative irradiation of rectal cancer. In *Intraoperative Radiation Therapy,* M Abe, R Dobelbower, eds. Boca Raton: CRC Press.

Tepper JE, Gunderson LL, Orlow E, et al. 1984. Complications of intraoperative radiation therapy. *Int J Radiat Oncol Biol Phys* 10:1831–1839.

Todoroki T, Iwasaki Y, Okamura T, et al. 1980. Intraoperative radiotherapy for advanced carcinoma of the biliary system. *Cancer* 46:2179–2184.

Whittington R, Solin L, Mohiuddin M, et al. 1984. Multimodality therapy of localized unresectable pancreatic adenocarcinoma. *Cancer* 54:1272–1275.

Wood W, Shipley WU, Gunderson LL, et al. 1982. Intraoperative irradiation for unresectable pancreatic carcinoma. *Cancer* 49:1272–1275.

Annual Clinical Conference on Cancer, Vol. 30
Gastrointestinal Cancer: Current Approaches to Diagnosis and Treatment
© 1988 by The University of Texas System Cancer Center

15. Current Status of Adjuvant Immunotherapy for Human Colorectal Carcinoma

J. Milburn Jessup and George F. Babcock

The advantage of immunotherapy is that it can eliminate the last tumor cell; the disadvantage of immunotherapy is that its efficacy is severely limited by tumor burden. Hanna, McKenzie, and their colleagues (Hanna, Brandhorst, and Peters 1979; Zalcberg et al. 1984) have shown that immunotherapy can destroy established experimental tumors, but with an efficacy limited to a burden of 5 to 10 x 10^6 tumor cells. The smallest clinically detectable malignancies, however, are 1 cm in diameter and contain an average of 1 x 10^9 tumor cells. Further, since a 1-cm primary tumor releases approximately 10^6 cells into the circulation each day and would be present for several years prior to detection, the occult tumor burden at detection would approach 10^9 cells if all shed cells remained viable. Such a burden is too high for an adjuvant immunotherapy program. Yet, when metastases appear, they generally do so at relatively few sites: say, 20 to 30 liver metastases are found. If each metastasis originated from one cell or a few cells, the *effective* or persistent burden of tumor cells with metastatic potential would be less than 10^6 cells. Thus, immunotherapy should be utilized in patients who are rendered free of all gross disease, have a high probability of having residual microscopic metastases, and yet have an effective tumor burden that does not exceed 10^6 malignant cells. Patients with Dukes B2 or C colorectal carcinoma who have undergone potentially curative resection are candidates for adjuvant immunotherapy.

Immunotherapy has four forms: active specific, active nonspecific, passive specific, and passive nonspecific. Active immunotherapy augments or activates the patient's immune response to the cancer. Passive immunotherapy supplements the patient's immune response with an exogenously supplied component of the immune response. Specific immunotherapies are directed to tumor-specific or tumor-associated antigens (TSAs or TAAs, respectively), whereas nonspecific immunotherapies stimulate host immune responses generally, not necessarily just those responses directed to tumor antigens. This review emphasizes the active immunotherapies, since the passive specific and passive nonspecific immunotherapies are reviewed elsewhere in this volume (see Baldwin).

ACTIVE NONSPECIFIC IMMUNOTHERAPY

Nonspecific potentiation or stimulation of host immune responses has had limited success in colorectal carcinoma. The most studied of the immunopotentiators is bacillus Calmette-Guérin (BCG). Mavligit et al. (1977) originally reported that BCG with or without 5-fluorouracil improved the survival of patients with Dukes C colorectal carcinoma compared with matched historical controls who underwent surgery alone. Unfortunately, subsequent randomized prospective trials (Gastro-intestinal Tumor Study Group 1984; Higgins et al. 1984; Panettiere and Chen 1981) could not confirm this finding with BCG, whether it was used alone or in combina-tion with chemotherapy. In fact, the Veterans Administration Surgical Oncology Group study (Higgins et al. 1984) suggested that the addition of the methanol-extraction residue of BCG to 5-fluorouracil and methyl-CCNU may impair survival. Interestingly, the intradermal injection of BCG at a distance from tumor (as is the case when the scarification technique is used) did not inhibit the growth of line 10 hepatoma in inbred guinea pigs (Zbar et al. 1976). Thus, experimental results pre-dicted that nonspecific stimulation with BCG or the methanol-extraction residue of BCG would not enhance control of established micrometastases in patients.

Endogenous Immune Responses to Human Colorectal Carcinoma

There may be other reasons why the nonspecific stimulation of immune responses does not augment immunity to TSAs or TAAs in patients with cancer. The kinetics of clinical cancers are fundamentally different from those of experimental neo-plasms. When animals are inoculated with tumor cells one to seven days before an immunologic manipulation occurs (fig. 15.1), the immunologic "milieu" is unlikely to be the same as that generated during the long latent period during which a cancer in a patient develops from one cell or a few cells into a 1-cm nodule. For instance, guinea pigs injected with the weakly antigenic line 10 hepatoma were not immune to their tumors when subjected to immunotherapy one week after tumor inoculation (Zbar et al. 1976). Thus, patients, unlike animals, may have developed humoral or cell-mediated immunity to their tumors at the time of definitive treatment because their bodies have interacted with the malignancies for a longer time.

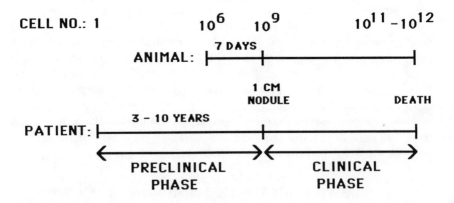

Fig. 15.1. Differences in immune response between clinical and experimental neoplasia are due to the longer preclinical phase in the former tumors.

Table 15.1. *Humoral and Cell-Mediated Immune Responses to Autologous Tumor-Associated Antigens in Patients with Colorectal Carcinoma*

Assay	Antigen	Total	Positive (%)
Antibody	Mucosa	29	6 (21)
	Tumor	31	26 (84)
Delayed-type hypersensitivity	Mucosa	11	2 (18)
	Tumor	11	1 (9)
Mixed lymphocyte– tumor interaction	Mucosa	19	1 (5)
	Tumor	19	6 (32)

We examined in patients with Dukes B2 or C colorectal carcinoma the hypothesis that patients are sensitized to their cancers at the time of diagnosis. Colorectal adenocarcinomas and normal mucosa were excised from surgical specimens and dissociated with enzymes into single-cell suspensions. These cells were then used as targets in an indirect membrane-immunofluorescence assay with the sera from patients to detect autoantibodies to TSAs and TAAs. In addition, the cells were treated with mitomycin C and used as stimulators for a mixed lymphocyte–tumor interaction assay that detects lymphoproliferative responses by the mononuclear cells to autologous TAAs. Finally, irradiated tumor and mucosa cells were injected intradermally into patients after surgery to assess cutaneous delayed-type hypersensitivity responses to autologous TAAs. Eighty-four percent of patients had low titers of antibodies to autologous TAAs, whereas only 37% of patients had a positive lymphoproliferative response to autologous tumor cells, and 9% developed a positive delayed-type hypersensitivity response to their own tumor cells (table 15.1).

Patients develop humoral immune responses to autologous tumor cells, with about a third of patients displaying cell-mediated immunity. However, depletion studies with monoclonal antibodies and complement indicate that many patients may have an OKT8+ suppressor T cell that inhibits the responsiveness of an OKT4+ helper T cell (fig. 15.2). Thus, patients at the time of definitive treatment are immune to their cancers, but the immunity favors humoral immunity, with active suppression of cell-mediated immunity. Since cell-mediated immune responses are considered the major mechanism for tumor rejection, the relatively limited cell-mediated immune responses to TSAs or TAAs suggest that the immune response in patients favors tumor growth rather than inhibition. However, far from being immunologically deficient at the time of treatment, patients are actively producing responses to their tumors, albeit humoral responses. Thus, patients may not benefit from nonspecific stimulation by potent polyclonal activators unless those activators abate the activity of suppressor T cells or alter the balance between humoral and cell-mediated immunity.

Elimination of suppressor cells by low-dose cyclophosphamide is currently under investigation. Berd, Maguire, and Mastrangelo (1984) have demonstrated that the ability to mount de novo or to recall cutaneous hypersensitivity responses is suppressed in patients with advanced cancer. Treatment with cyclophosphamide at 300 mg/m^2 three days prior to sensitization with dinitrochlorobenzene significantly en-

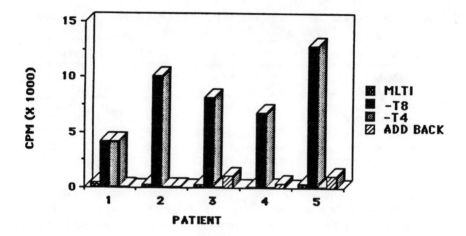

Fig. 15.2. Effects of depletion of T-cell subsets upon lymphoproliferative responses to autologous tumor cells. Peripheral blood mononuclear cells were collected from patients on the morning of surgery and left intact (MLTI, mixed lymphocyte–tumor interaction), depleted of OKT8+ T cells by treatment with OKT8 monoclonal antibody and complement (−OKT8), or depleted of OKT4+ helper cells by treatment with OKT4 antibody and complement (−OKT4). Depletion of OKT8+ T cells increased the proliferative response to autologous tumor cells in four of the five patients. Depletion of the OKT4+ T cells stopped the proliferative response, whereas the addition of the −OKT4 population to the −OKT8 (ADD BACK) population inhibited the proliferative response. These results demonstrate that there was an OKT8+ suppressor T cell that inhibited the proliferative response of an OKT4+ T cell in four of the five patients tested.

hanced the response of patients to the latter substance; the same result was seen with keyhole-limpet hemocyanin sensitization. This work is based on a series of investigations in animals in which low-dose cyclophosphamide inhibited suppressor T cells and augmented the ability of host cells to lyse tumor cells. Thus, low-dose cyclophosphamide may be of use in augmenting responses to tumor-associated antigens by destroying suppressor T cells.

Another nonspecific augmentor of host immune response has also received attention recently. Levamisole is an anthelmintic that has positive immunomodulatory effects. A recent randomized study from Japan (Niimoto et al. 1984) indicates that levamisole significantly enhances survival of patients with lymph node metastases from gastric cancer who receive mitomycin C and tegafur. A Mayo Clinic study published in abstract form (Laurie et al. 1986) demonstrates a similar advantage for patients with Dukes B2 and C colorectal carcinoma who receive levamisole and 5-fluorouracil. Thus, levamisole may be an immunomodulator that should receive further study in colorectal carcinoma, especially if it alters the balance between humoral and cell-mediated immunity.

ACTIVE SPECIFIC IMMUNOTHERAPY

If a patient is responding in an ineffective way to his cancer, can active specific immunotherapy alter the response to favor tumor rejection, say, by increasing cell-mediated immunity to TAAs? Hoover et al. (1984) first showed that patients with Dukes B2 or C colorectal carcinoma who are immunized with their own (autologous) irradiated tumor cells and BCG develop cutaneous delayed-type hypersensitivity reactions to autologous tumor cells without a response to autologous mucosa cells. We (Jessup et al. 1986) confirmed this finding and demonstrated that the autologous tumor cell vaccine must contain 10^7 irradiated tumor cells in each dose. Patients increased their cell-mediated immune responses to autologous TAAs after active specific immunotherapy without much augmentation of the humoral response (Fig. 15.3).

But even if cell-mediated immunity to autologous TAAs is augmented by active specific immunotherapy, is the survival of patients increased? Hoover et al. in 1985 reported preliminary results of a randomized, prospective trial of active specific immunotherapy in patients with Dukes B2 or C disease. Their median follow-up as of that report was 28 months. Twenty patients who received an autologous tumor cell vaccine had a significantly longer disease-free interval and survival compared with 20 patients who only had surgery. Hoover and colleagues have observed, as have we in our work, that the pattern of disease recurrence in immunotherapy patients may be different from that of unvaccinated controls. When disease recurred in the immunotherapy patients of the Hoover et al. study, it did so at fewer sites. No recurrences in the control group had been surgically treatable, whereas all recurrences had been excised in the immunotherapy group. More recent results

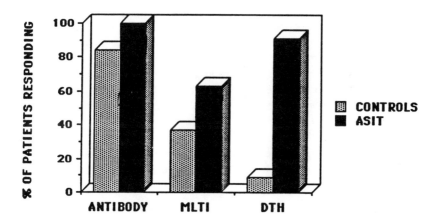

Fig. 15.3. Active specific immunotherapy augments immune responses to autologous colorectal carcinoma. Patients who were not vaccinated (CONTROLS) and patients who received active specific immunotherapy (ASIT) were assessed for cutaneous delayed-type hypersensitivity response to irradiated autologous tumor cells (DTH), and their blood was analyzed for antibody to membrane determinants upon tumor cells (ANTIBODY) and for a lymphoproliferative response to autologous tumor cells (MLTI, mixed lymphocyte–tumor interaction). The results show that the active specific immunotherapy significantly enhanced the delayed-type hypersensitivity responses and augmented the lymphoproliferative response to autologous tumor. The antibody response was also slightly enhanced.

from this pilot study, at a median follow-up of 45 months, were that recurrence had been seen in 43% of the controls as opposed to in 22% of the immunotherapy group, with 23% mortality in the controls and only 6% mortality in the immunotherapy group (Herbert C. Hoover, M.D., Massachusetts General Hospital, personal communication).

Several recently reported or ongoing trials of active specific immunotherapy have supported its efficacy as an adjuvant for surgery in Dukes B2 and C colorectal carcinomas. In a three-way randomization of patients with Dukes C disease (Wunderlich et al. 1985), those who received either a vaccine of neuraminidase-treated human colorectal carcinoma cells or chemotherapy (5-fluorouracil, mitomycin C, β-cytosine arabinoside) showed significant improvement in survival time and significantly fewer distant metastases and liver metastases compared with patients who only received surgery. Similarly, early results from a randomized trial of neuraminidase-treated autologous tumor cells injected along with BCG into patients with Dukes B and C colorectal carcinoma demonstrated a 15% improvement in disease-free survival, which was not, however, significant (Gill 1981). The Eastern Cooperative Oncology Group is currently conducting a confirmatory phase III randomized, prospective trial of active specific immunotherapy with autologous tumor cell vaccine and BCG in patients with Dukes B2 and C colon cancer.

Antiidiotype vaccines represent another promising approach to active specific immunotherapy. Koprowski and associates (DeFreitas et al. 1985; Herlyn et al. 1985) have observed that injection of mouse monoclonal antibody to the TAA on colorectal carcinoma cells into colorectal carcinoma patients induces formation of anti-antibodies, some of which are internal images of the antigen. Immunization with such internal-image antiidiotypic antibody produces anti-anti-antibodies that bind the original antigen. Antiidiotypes are important because immunization with soluble protein antigens usually provides only weak, transient immunity. However, immunization with antiidiotypes bypasses the usual antigen-processing mechanisms and directly stimulates B-cell responses. Thus, one may utilize antiidiotype antibodies to vaccinate against tumor antigens. The validity of such an approach has been recently demonstrated in animal models for hepatitis (Kennedy et al. 1986). Herlyn, Ross, and Koprowski (1986) have also shown that immunization with a goat antiidiotypic antibody to cancer antigen 17-1A induces in mice and rabbits the production of antibodies that bind to colorectal carcinoma cells. This observation opens the possibility of antiidiotypic immunization in man, quite possibly even as a colorectal carcinoma *preventive*.

PASSIVE NONSPECIFIC IMMUNOTHERAPY

Such immunorestorative agents as interferon, interleukin-2, tumor necrosis factor, macrophage-activating factor, and other lymphokines are used in passive nonspecific immunotherapy. Clinical trials with interferons in colorectal cancer have not been successful to date. Trials with the other lymphokines are too preliminary to comment on, although tumor necrosis factor and macrophage-activating factor offer some promise. Fidler et al. (1986) have demonstrated that monocytes from colorectal carcinoma patients in whom chemotherapy and radiotherapy have failed are activated in vitro by liposome-encapsulated macrophage-activating factor to a tumoricidal state that lyses tumor cells but not normal cells. A multiinstitutional phase I trial of this modality is now beginning.

PASSIVE SPECIFIC IMMUNOTHERAPY

Monoclonal antibodies may be therapeutic agents. As potential "magic bullets," they may deliver radioisotopes or drugs or link cytotoxic host cells to tumor cells. Monoclonal antibodies to carcinoembryonic antigen, cancer antigen 19-9, and antigen 17-1A are under the most intensive evaluation and are in phase I and II trials (Sears et al. 1986). Animal studies suggest that monoclonal antibodies alone (Herlyn et al. 1980) or conjugated with radioisotopes (Zalcberg et al. 1984; Goldenberg et al. 1981) or drugs (Kanellos, Pietersz, and McKenzie 1985) inhibit growth of established tumor. Murine IgG2A antibodies (Steplewski et al. 1983) cause human monocytes to lyse tumor cells through an antibody-dependent cellular cytotoxicity mechanism. Murine monoclonal IgG2A to antigen 17-1A was demonstrated by Shen et al. (1984) on the cell membranes of colorectal metastases excised one to two days after the intravenous injection of 200 mg of antibody. In that study, unfortunately, metastases excised more than five days after injection of antibody did not contain antibody, although antigen 17-1A was still demonstrable on the cell surface. McKenzie and collaborators (Zalcberg et al. 1984; Kanellos, Pietersz, and McKenzie 1985) have studied this problem in some detail in animal models and suggest that the efficacy of radioiodinated antibodies may be enhanced by blocking deiodinases with propylthiouracil. Thus, future trials of monoclonal antibody therapy may require manipulations to prolong circulation of the cytotoxic antibody.

CONCLUSIONS

Several prospects now exist for the use of adjuvant immunotherapy in patients who have undergone potentially curative surgery. First, active specific immunotherapy in Dukes B2 and C colorectal carcinoma lesions has demonstrated a 20% decrease in recurrences and is currently under evaluation in a phase III trial.

Second, the combination of 5-fluorouracil and levamisole may be an important active nonspecific adjuvant.

Third, monoclonal antibodies alone or conjugated with toxins may inhibit tumor growth and be useful for passive nonspecific immunotherapy.

Fourth, biologic-response modifiers encapsulated in liposomes may supply immunomodulators to patients who are defective in one or more molecules and enhance host defense mechanisms nonspecifically.

Finally, the prospect now exists to create internal-image antiidiotype vaccines that may be used not only for adjuvant immunotherapy but also for immunoprophylaxis against colorectal carcinoma.

ACKNOWLEDGMENTS

This project was supported by grants from Cutter Laboratories, Inc.; the Annual Campaign of The University of Texas System Cancer Center; the National Cancer Cytology Center; and the Department of Health and Human Services (grant RO1 CA42587).

REFERENCES

Berd D, Maguire HC Jr, Mastrangelo MJ. 1984. Potentiation of human cell-mediated and humoral immunity by low-dose cyclophosphamide. *Cancer Res* 44:5439–5443.

DeFreitas E, Suzuki H, Herlyn D, et al. 1985. Human antibody induction to the idiotypic and anti-idiotypic determinants of a monoclonal antibody against a gastrointestinal carcinoma antigen. *Curr Top Microbiol Immunol* 119:75–89.

Fidler IJ, Jessup JM, Fogler WE, et al. 1986. Activation of tumoricidal properties in peripheral blood monocytes of patients with colorectal carcinoma. *Cancer Res* 46:994–998.

Gastrointestinal Tumor Study Group. 1984. Adjuvant therapy of colon cancer—Results of a prospectively randomized trial. *N Engl J Med* 310:737–743.

Gill G. 1981. Immunotherapy. In *Large Bowel Cancer,* JJ DeCosse, ed., pp. 190–204. Clinical Surgery International, vol. 1. New York: Churchill Livingstone.

Goldenberg DM, Gaffar SA, Bennett SJ, et al. 1981. Experimental radioimmunotherapy of a xenografted human colonic tumor (GW-39) producing carcinoembryonic antigen. *Cancer Res* 41:4354–4360.

Hanna MG Jr, Brandhorst JS, Peters LC. 1979. Active specific immunotherapy of residual micrometastasis. An evaluation of sources, doses and ratios of BCG with tumor cells. *Cancer Immunol Immunother* 7:165–173.

Herlyn D, Lubeck M, Sears H, et al. 1985. Specific detection of anti-idiotypic immune responses in cancer patients treated with murine monoclonal antibody. *J Immunol Methods* 85:27–38.

Herlyn D, Ross AH, Koprowski H. 1986. Anti-idiotypic antibodies bear the internal image of a human tumor antigen. *Science* 232:100–102.

Herlyn DM, Steplewski Z, Herlyn MF, et al. 1980. Inhibition of growth of colorectal carcinoma in nude mice by monoclonal antibody. *Cancer Res* 40:717–721.

Higgins GA, Donaldson RC, Rogers LS, et al. 1984. Efficacy of MER immunotherapy when added to a regimen of 5-fluorouracil and methyl-CCNU following resection for carcinoma of the large bowel. A Veterans Administration Surgical Oncology Group report. *Cancer* 54:193–198.

Hoover HC Jr, Surdyke M, Dangel R, et al. 1984. Delayed cutaneous hypersensitivity to autologous tumor cells in colorectal cancer patients immunized with an autologous tumor cell: Bacillus Calmette-Guérin vaccine. *Cancer Res* 44:1671–1676.

Hoover HC Jr, Surdyke MG, Dangel RB, et al. 1985. Prospectively randomized trial of adjuvant active-specific immunotherapy for human colorectal cancer. *Cancer* 55:1236–1243.

Jessup JM, McBride CM, Ames FC, et al. 1986. Active specific immunotherapy of Dukes B2 and C colorectal carcinoma: Comparison of two doses of the vaccine. *Cancer Immunol Immunother* 21:233–239.

Kanellos J, Pietersz GA, McKenzie IFC. 1985. Studies of methotrexate–monoclonal antibody conjugates for immunotherapy. *JNCI* 75:319–332.

Kennedy RC, Eichberg JW, Lanford RE, et al. 1986. Anti-idiotypic antibody vaccine for type B viral hepatitis in chimpanzees. *Science* 232:220–223.

Laurie J, Moertel C, Fleming T, et al. 1986. Surgical adjuvant therapy of poor prognosis colorectal cancer with levamisole alone or combined levamisole and 5-fluorouracil (5-FU) (abstract). *Proceedings of the American Society of Clinical Oncology* 5:81.

Mavligit GM, Gutterman JU, Malahy MA, et al. 1977. Adjuvant immunotherapy and chemo-immunotherapy in colorectal cancer (Dukes' class C): Prolongation of disease-free interval and survival. *Cancer* 40(Suppl 5):2726–2730.

Niimoto M, Hattori T, Ito I, et al. 1984. Levamisole in postoperative adjuvant immuno-chemotherapy for gastric cancer. A randomized controlled study of the MMC + tegafur regimen with or without levamisole. Report I. *Cancer Immunol Immunother* 18:13–18.

Panettiere FJ, Chen TT. 1981. Update on the SWOG colorectal adjuvant study of 620 patients (abstract *C*-82). *Proceedings of the American Society of Clinical Oncology* 22:353.

Sears HF, Herlyn D, Steplewski Z, et al. 1986. Phase II clinical trial of a murine monoclonal antibody cytotoxic for gastrointestinal adenocarcinoma. *Cancer Res* 45:5910–5913.

Shen JW, Atkinson B, Koprowski H, et al. 1984. Binding of murine immunoglobulin to hu-man tissues after immunotherapy with anticolorectal carcinoma monoclonal antibody. *Int J Cancer* 33:465–468.

Steplewski Z, Herlyn D, Maul G, et al. 1983. Hypothesis: Macrophages as effector cells for human tumor destruction mediated by monoclonal antibody. *Hybridoma* 2:1–5.

Wunderlich M, Schiessel R, Rainer H, et al. 1985. Effect of adjuvant chemo- or immuno-therapy on the prognosis of colorectal cancer operated for cure. *Br J Surg* 72(Suppl): S107–S110.

Zalcberg JR, Thompson CH, Lichtenstein M, et al. 1984. Tumor immunotherapy in the mouse with the use of ^{131}I-labeled monoclonal antibodies. *JNCI* 72:697–704.

Zbar B, Ribi E, Kelly M, et al. 1976. Immunologic approaches to the treatment of human cancer based on a guinea pig model. *Cancer Immunol Immunother* 1:127–137.

Annual Clinical Conference on Cancer, Vol. 30
Gastrointestinal Cancer: Current Approaches to Diagnosis and Treatment
© 1988 by The University of Texas System Cancer Center

16. Chemotherapy for Advanced Colorectal Cancer

Michael J. O'Connell

Colorectal cancer is a common malignant disease in our society: in the United States, its current annual incidence is approximately 140,000 cases. Despite efforts to detect the disease early and improvements in diagnostic methods, only 45% to 50% of patients will be cured by surgical resection. Thus, many patients will develop unresectable metastatic malignant disease and become candidates for chemotherapy.

Whereas dramatic improvements have been documented over the past two decades in chemotherapeutic management of a variety of human malignancies, the treatment of advanced colorectal cancer has not improved substantially. In this chapter, I review the developmental history of chemotherapy for colorectal cancer, comment on the state of the art, and highlight current research strategies to improve the treatment of this disease.

HISTORICAL DEVELOPMENT OF CHEMOTHERAPY FOR ADVANCED COLORECTAL CANCER

Single-Agent Chemotherapy

At the Mayo Clinic, more than 40 chemotherapeutic agents have been studied in search of phase II antitumor activity against colorectal cancer (Moertel and Thynne 1982). Table 16.1 summarizes agents that have demonstrated some degree of activity against this disease. Unfortunately, responses with any of these agents tend to be partial rather than complete, be brief in duration (four- to six-month median), and occur frequently at the expense of considerable toxicity.

None of the agents studied over the past 25 years since 5-fluorouracil (5-FU) was introduced into clinical practice has been found to have superior single-agent activity against colorectal cancer. Experience has shown marked differences in reported tumor-response rates for 5-FU in the treatment of colorectal cancer, depending in part on patient selection factors, criteria for judging tumor response, and statistical variation associated with small treatment groups (Moertel and Thynne 1982). Considerable effort has been put forth to examine a variety of dosage-administration schedules of the fluorinated pyrimidines in this setting. In studies performed at the Mayo Clinic (O'Connell 1983), the oral route of administration of 5-FU has been associated with more erratic serum levels and a shorter tumor-response duration than the intravenous route. Prolonging the duration of infusion to two hours or eight hours for five consecutive days offered no therapeutic advantage over rapid intravenous administration (see table 16.2). 5-Fluoro-2'deoxyuridine

Table 16.1. *Single-Agent Chemotherapy for Advanced Colorectal Cancer*

Drug	No. of Patients Treated	Objective Tumor Response (%)
Fluorinated pyrimidines		
5-fluorouracil (5-FU)	359	17
5-fluoro-2'deoxyuridine (FUDR)	147	22
Ftorafur	36	14
Nitrosoureas		
Methyl CCNU (semustine)	38	18
CCNU (lomustine)	75	9
BCNU (carmustine)	69	10
Chlorozotozin	66	8
Antibiotics		
Mitomycin C	69	12
Miscellaneous agents		
Triazinate (Baker's antifol)	29	17
Razoxane (ICRF-159)	25	12

(FUDR) administered systemically in five-day intensive courses was no more active than 5-FU. Prolonged systemic infusions of FUDR (up to 120 hours) were inferior to rapid intravenous administration.

A general principle has emerged from these studies: doses of 5-FU that produced definite, but not severe, clinical toxicity were associated with an optimal opportunity for tumor response. The Central Oncology Group has confirmed this principle in a prospectively randomized trial that demonstrated the superiority of the intensive intravenous method of 5-FU administration over weekly intravenous therapy, a low-dose nontoxic treatment schedule, and an oral schedule (Ansfield et al. 1977).

The results of 5-FU treatment for advanced colorectal cancer must be put into clinical perspective. Only about 20% of patients experience objective tumor response, and 5-FU therapy has had no demonstrable effect on patient survival when compared to matched historical controls (Moertel and Thynne 1982) or, in a pro-

Table 16.2. *Prospectively Randomized Studies of 5-FU and FUDR Infused Intravenously for Advanced Colorectal Cancer (Mayo Clinic)*

Drug Administration Schedules[a]	No. of Patients	Objective Tumor Response	
1. 5-FU (rapid i.v.)	74	12	
5-FU (2-hr infusion)	75	12	
2. 5-FU (rapid i.v.)	45	20	p = NS
5-FU (8-hr infusion)	45	11	
3. FUDR (rapid i.v.)	63	17	p < .05
FUDR (24-hr infusion)	65	6	

Abbreviations: i.v., intravenous; NS, not significant; FUDR, 5-fluoro-2'deoxyuridine.

[a]Treatment for five consecutive days (and up to four additional doses every other day in studies 1 and 2) with courses repeated at intervals of four to five weeks.

spective clinical trial conducted by the Southwest Oncology Group, to patients receiving a variety of inactive phase II agents (Leichman et al. 1983). Although 5-FU administered by rapid intravenous push in a dose of 500 mg/m^2 for five consecutive days with courses repeated every five weeks is reasonable to use for a control arm against which to assess new treatments in phase III clinical trials, 5-FU alone, given by any method, is not a satisfactory or effective treatment for advanced colorectal cancer.

Empirical Combination Chemotherapy

Experience with diseases such as diffuse histiocytic lymphoma, Hodgkin's disease, and a variety of pediatric malignancies suggested that combining several chemotherapeutic agents together could result in a marked improvement in therapeutic effect over that of a single agent. The key element of successful combination chemotherapy was the availability of several agents that had (a) established activity against the type of cancer in question, (b) different mechanisms of antitumor action, and (c) different (nonoverlapping) dose-limiting toxicities. This strategy has been of no substantial value in managing advanced colorectal cancer, however, probably because of the low order of antitumor activity of the available chemotherapeutic agents.

Early controlled studies suggested higher objective tumor-response rates for fluorouracil-nitrosourea combinations than for single-agent 5-FU (Moertel et al. 1975). However, further experience in our own practice has indicated an overall response rate of 27% in 150 patients for the combination of 5-FU + methyl CCNU + vincristine, and the Eastern Cooperative Oncology Group recently observed only 10 responses in 92 patients (11%) with advanced colorectal cancer treated with 5-FU + methyl CCNU + vincristine (Engstrom et al. 1982). Likewise, the addition of either razoxane (ICRF-159) or triazinate (Baker's antifol) to 5-FU plus methyl CCNU has not improved the treatment effect over that of 5-FU combined with methyl CCNU and vincristine (Schutt et al. 1982). None of the trials of empiric chemotherapy combinations has demonstrated any survival improvement for patients with advanced colorectal cancer.

In summary, the current treatment of advanced colorectal cancer is unsatisfactory. Empirical combination chemotherapy has not improved the therapeutic ratio over that of single-agent intensive-course 5-FU—any improvement in objective tumor-response rate has been overshadowed by drug toxicity. No controlled clinical trial has identified a treatment regimen that improves the survival rate of patients with advanced colorectal cancer.

CURRENT RESEARCH STRATEGIES

Two general investigational approaches are presently being pursued to improve the systemic therapy of advanced colorectal cancer. One is in the area of drug development wherein a variety of cytotoxic agents and biologic-response modifiers are being studied. Another research strategy is aimed at new methods of enhancing the effectiveness of the fluorinated pyrimidines, including prolonged intravenous infusions, intraarterial administration for liver metastases, and biochemical modulation.

New Drug Development

Cytotoxic Agents

To date, the search for new cytotoxic agents with activity against colorectal cancer has been disappointing. Unfortunately, the available animal model tumor systems have not been successful in identifying agents with significant activity against human colorectal cancer. Perhaps a panel of human tumor cell lines grown in soft agar (DeVita 1985) will provide a better model for screening compounds.

In our experience, a soft agar clonogenic cell assay based on the method developed by Hamburger and Salmon (1977) to assess chemotherapy sensitivity of individual patients' colon cancers to a panel of chemotherapeutic agents has not been clinically successful. Several reasons explain this lack of success: the difficulty of reliably growing the tumor cells in culture, the low degree of cytotoxicity of most agents tested against human colorectal cancer, and the frequent inaccessibility, short of an open surgical procedure, of malignant tissue for a biopsy. This technique may become useful in the future if new agents with greater activity against colorectal cancer can be identified and the laboratory assay can be further improved.

Biologic-Response Modifiers

The biologic-response modifiers constitute a potentially promising approach to cancer treatment. These agents, by definition, have the capacity to modulate host immune response. Substantial alterations of cellular immune function have been documented in patients with advanced gastrointestinal cancer (O'Connell et al. 1980); this provides a rationale for using these agents to alter immune response with the aim of effecting regression of tumor. Although studies to date have demonstrated no significant effect in advanced colorectal cancer for either interferon alpha or interferon gamma given as single agents, regressions of metastatic colorectal cancer have been reported for interleukin-2 and lymphokine-activated killer cells in a small group of patients (Rosenberg et al. 1985). However, these results are very preliminary, require confirmation, and occurred at the expense of severe toxicity. The in vivo study of combinations of cytokines and lymphokines (e.g., interferon gamma + interleukin-2, interferon gamma + tumor necrosis factor) and of biologic-response modifiers plus cytotoxic agents has aroused considerable interest, based upon the synergy demonstrated in various in vitro systems. As the function of the human immune system in regulating tumor proliferation becomes better understood and as the mechanisms of action of the biologic-response modifiers become more precisely defined, interest in this area of investigation will increase.

Enhancing the Effectiveness of the Fluorinated Pyrimidines

Prolonged Intraveneous Infusion

One potential way of increasing the action of the fluorinated pyrimidines against advanced colorectal cancer is to use prolonged intravenous infusions of FUDR and

5-FU. The theoretical rationale for administering these agents by prolonged infusion rather than as a bolus is based on their short serum half-life (10–15 minutes following intravenous bolus administration) and the high proportion of malignant cells in human solid tumors that are not undergoing active growth at any one time. The resting cells would be expected to be resistant to the effects of cycle-active antimetabolites such as 5-FU. Longer periods of drug administration, therefore, might result in exposing a greater proportion of the malignant cells to the cytotoxic agent during a sensitive phase of the growth cycle, resulting in an enhanced therapeutic effect.

Phase I studies of continuous intravenous infusion of FUDR (Lokich et al. 1983) and 5-FU (Lokich et al. 1981) via a central venous catheter, using ambulatory infusion pumps, have been reported for periods up to 78 consecutive days. With 5-FU, stomatitis and an unusual symptom complex known as the "hand-foot syndrome"— tender swelling of the fingers and toes frequently associated with paresthesias and dermatitis—have been the dose-limiting side effects. Preliminary experience with this approach in a very small number of patients with advanced colorectal cancer has indicated tumor responses in 31% to 45% of patients (Leichman et al. 1985; Ausman et al. 1985; Belt et al. 1985). The Mid Atlantic Oncology Group has recently completed entering patients into a controlled trial comparing prolonged intravenous 5-FU with intensive-course 5-FU given by rapid intravenous administration (Lokich et al. 1986). The results of this trial will be awaited with interest. At present, no controlled data document an improved therapeutic index for the more demanding and expensive prolonged infusion method.

Biochemical Modulation Studies

A second general area of investigation directed toward improving the efficacy of 5-FU against colorectal cancer employs the principles of biochemical modulation— modifying the metabolism of tumor cells in a manner to enhance the action of a cytotoxic drug to therapeutic advantage. Central to this concept is the *selective* enhancement of antitumor activity to improve therapeutic ratio, not just to increase the potency of the cytotoxic agent. Controlled studies of 5-FU combined with PALA (N-phosphonoacetyl-L-aspartic acid), a potent inhibitor of de novo pyrimidine synthesis that has been shown to increase 5-FU incorporation into tumor RNA in animal model systems, have unfortunately not documented an improved treatment effect over that of 5-FU alone (Buroker et al. 1985). Nor has adding thymidine, an agent that blocks the oxidative metabolism of 5-FU and thereby greatly alters its potency, improved antitumor activity (Buroker et al. 1985) against colorectal cancer.

Currently, investigators are interested in therapy combining folinic acid and 5-FU. The rationale for this treatment is the observation that an excess of intracellular reduced folates enhances 5-FU inhibition of thymidylate synthetase; the presence of this can be achieved by concomitantly administering intravenous folinic acid. A phase II study by Machover et al. (1986) has suggested favorable results for this treatment in patients with advanced colorectal cancer. A number of controlled clinical trials to evaluate this approach clinically are currently in progress.

High-dose methotrexate, used to inhibit purine synthesis and thereby increase cellular levels of phosphoribosyl pyrophosphate, has been shown in murine and cell culture model systems to enhance 5-FU cytotoxicity. Phase II studies have reported favorable results for methotrexate followed by 5-FU and citrovorum rescue in treating a variety of human solid tumors, including colon cancer (Bertino 1984). A randomized trial is in progress (Mayo/North Central Cancer Treatment Group) to determine whether this regimen is more effective than single-agent 5-FU.

At present, biochemical modulation of 5-FU is an appealing investigational concept. However, combination chemotherapy based on sound scientific principles requires data from controlled trials to establish its value in clinical practice. The technology for studying fluorinated pyrimidine metabolism at the cellular level (rather than relying solely on plasma pharmacokinetics) is under development and, it is hoped, will provide additional information about the mechanism of action of these compounds that will lead to their more rational future application in combination regimens.

Intraarterial Infusion for Liver Metastases

Regional (intraarterial) infusion of the fluorinated pyrimidines is a third strategy designed to increase these agents' effectiveness in selected patients who have liver metastases. The fluorinated pyrimidines meet the pharmacokinetic criteria that predict a possible therapeutic advantage for regional administration of a cytotoxic agent: (1) rapid total body clearance as reflected by a short serum half-life when they are given systemically ($T\frac{1}{2}$ 10–15 minutes), and (2) a high extraction ratio for the organ of interest (approximately 95% of FUDR infused into the hepatic arterial circulation is extracted by the liver in the first pass). Although temporary shrinkage of colorectal hepatic metastases was accomplished in a proportion of patients, early studies that employed angiographically placed transcutaneous catheters were associated with high rates of sepsis, catheter dislodgement, and bleeding at the arterial puncture site (Stagg et al. 1984). The only completed controlled evaluation of intraarterial chemotherapy for colorectal cancer metastatic to the liver demonstrated no therapeutic advantage for 5-FU infused by this route for periods of 14 to 21 days over intravenously administered 5-FU (Grage et al. 1979).

More recently, FUDR has been administered by a totally implantable drug-delivery system (Buchwald et al. 1980). This device has been shown to provide a reliable means of drug delivery into the hepatic arterial circulation for prolonged periods with a low rate of infections or vascular complications. Phase II studies (Niederhuber et al. 1984; Balch et al. 1983; Kemeny et al. 1984; Weiss et al. 1983; Shepard et al. 1985) have reported regressions of colorectal hepatic metastases in from as few as 20% to as many as 88% of patients treated (see table 16.3), depending in part on specific response criteria employed. It is possible that the longer median survival times (approaching two years) seen in some of these studies could be due primarily to selection of patients with favorable prognostic features (O'Connell 1984). A major limitation of intraarterial FUDR is its failure to control the extrahepatic malignant disease that becomes clinically apparent in most patients who

Table 16.3. *Phase II Studies of Intraarterial 5-Fluoro-2' deoxyuridine for Colorectal Liver Metastases*

Institution	Study	No. of Patients Treated	Objective Tumor Response (%)
University of Michigan	Niederhuber et al. 1984	93	79
University of Alabama	Balch et al. 1983	81	88
Memorial Sloan-Kettering	Kemeny et al. 1984	41	52
Sidney Farber Cancer Center	Weiss et al. 1983	17	29
University of Chicago	Shepard et al. 1985	40	20

have colorectal liver metastases. Also to be considered is the expense, risk of chemical gastritis or ulceration of the upper gastrointestinal tract, intrahepatic cholestasis, and biliary strictures (Hohn et al. 1985) owing to regional toxic effects of FUDR given over prolonged periods of time. Controlled trials are currently in progress to determine whether intraarterial FUDR causes any real improvement in patient survival or overall therapeutic index when compared with intensive-course intravenous 5-FU (Mayo Clinic/North Central Cancer Treatment Group) or systemic (intravenous) FUDR (Memorial Sloan-Kettering Cancer Center, Northern California Oncology Group, National Cancer Institute). Preliminary results from the Memorial Sloan-Kettering study (Kemeny et al. 1986) have documented a significantly higher objective tumor-response rate associated with intraarterial FUDR, although median patient survival appears not to be affected. The failure of this study to demonstrate any survival improvement may be because patients failing systemic FUDR were then "crossed-over" to treatment with intraarterial FUDR. Patient accrual to the Northern California Oncology Group trial is nearly complete, and the unblinded results of this study should be reported in the near future (personal communication, Dr. David Hohn, Associate Professor of Surgery, University of California [San Francisco], October 1986).

SUMMARY

Currently, only a minority of patients with advanced colorectal cancer derive any clinically meaningful benefit from cytotoxic chemotherapy. Empirically derived combination chemotherapy regimens have not prolonged patient survival. Although appealing from a pharmacologic standpoint, neither intraarterial chemotherapy for patients with hepatic metastases nor prolonged intravenous infusions of the fluorinated pyrimidines have demonstrated an improved therapeutic index over that achieved by intensive-course 5-FU administered as an intravenous bolus. In addition to these approaches, the study of biochemical modulation of the fluorinated pyrimidines and the development of entirely new cytotoxic agents or biologic-response modifiers appear to represent the most hopeful research strategies at the present time.

REFERENCES

Ansfield F, Klotz J, Nealon T, et al. 1977. A phase III study comparing the clinical utility of four regimens of 5-fluorouracil. *Cancer* 39:34–40.

Ausman R, Caballero G, Quebbeman E, et al. 1985. Response of metastatic colorectal adenocarcinomas to long term continuous ambulatory intravenous infusion of 5-fluorouracil (abstract). *Proceedings of the American Society of Clinical Oncology* 4:86.

Balch, CM, Urist MM, Soong SJ, et al. 1983. A prospective phase II clinical trial of continuous FUDR regional chemotherapy for colorectal metastases to the liver using a totally implantable drug infusion pump. *Ann Surg* 198:567–573.

Belt RJ, Davidner ML, Myron MC, et al. 1985. Continuous low dose 5-fluorouracil for adenocarcinoma: Confirmation of activity (abstract). *Proceedings of the American Society of Clinical Oncology* 4:90.

Bertino JR. 1984. Sequential use of methotrexate and 5-fluorouracil in the treatment of solid tumors. In *Fluoropyrimidines in Cancer Therapy,* K Kimura, S Fujii, M Osama, GP Bodey, P Alberto, eds., pp. 251–260. New York, Amsterdam: Excerpta Medica.

Buchwald H, Grage TB, Vassilopoulos PP, et al. 1980. Intra-arterial infusion chemotherapy for hepatic carcinoma using a totally implantable infusion pump. *Cancer* 43:866–869.

Buroker TR, Moertel CG, Fleming TR, et al. 1985. A controlled evaluation of recent approaches to biochemical modulation or enhancement of 5-fluorouracil therapy in colorectal carcinoma. *J Clin Oncol* 3:1624–1631.

DeVita VT Jr. 1985. Principles of chemotherapy. In *Cancer: Principles and Practice of Oncology,* 2 ed., VT DeVita Jr, S Hellman, SA Rosenberg, eds., p. 272. Philadelphia: J. B. Lippincott.

Engstrom PF, MacIntyre JM, Douglass HO Jr, et al. 1982. Combination chemotherapy of advanced colorectal cancer utilizing 5-fluorouracil, semustine, dacarbazine, vincristine, and hydroxyurea: A phase III trial by the Eastern Cooperative Oncology Group. *Cancer* 49:1555–1560.

Grage TB, Vassilopoulos PP, Shingleton WW, et al. 1979. Results of a prospective randomized study of hepatic artery infusion with 5-fluorouracil versus intravenous 5-fluorouracil in patients with hepatic metastases from colorectal cancer: A Central Oncology Group study. *Surgery* 86:550–555.

Hamburger AW, Salmon SE. 1977. Primary bioassay of human tumor stem cells. *Science* 197:461–463.

Hohn D, Melnick J, Stagg R, et al. 1985. Biliary sclerosis in patients receiving hepatic infusions of floxuridine. *J Clin Oncol* 3:98–102.

Kemeny N, Daly J, Oderman P, et al. 1984. Hepatic artery pump infusion: Toxicity and results in patients with metastatic colorectal carcinoma. *J Clin Oncol* 2:595–600.

Kemeny N, Reichman B, Oderman P, et al. 1986. Update of randomized study of intrahepatic vs systemic infusion of fluorodeoxyuridine (FUDR) in patients with liver metastases from colorectal carcinoma (abstract). *Proceedings of the American Society of Clinical Oncology* 5:345.

Leichman L, Fabian C, O'Bryan R, et al. 1983. Evaluation of 5-FU versus a phase II drug in metastatic adenocarcinoma of the large bowel. Southwest Oncology Group (SWOG) study 7940 (abstract). *Proceedings of the American Society of Clinical Oncology* 2:120.

Leichman L, Leichman CG, Kinzie J, et al. 1985. Long term low dose 5-fluorouracil (5FU) in advanced measurable colon cancer: No correlation between toxicity and efficacy (abstract). *Proceedings of the American Society of Clinical Oncology* 4:86.

Lokich J, Bothe A, Fine N, et al. 1981. Phase I study of protracted venous infusion of 5-fluorouracil. *Cancer* 48:2565–2568.

Lokich J, Gillings D, Gullo J, et al. 1986. Bolus versus infusion 5-fluorouracil: A randomized trial in advanced measurable colorectal cancer (abstract). *Proceedings of the American Society of Clinical Oncology* 5:83.

Lokich JJ, Sonneborn H, Paul S, et al. 1983. Phase I study of continuous venous infusion of floxuridine (5-FUDR) chemotherapy. *Cancer Treat Rep* 67:791–793.

Machover D, Goldschmidt E, Chollet P, et al. 1986. Treatment of advanced colorectal and gastric adenocarcinoma with 5-fluorouracil and high-dose folinic acid. *J Clin Oncol* 4:685–696.

Moertel CG, Thynne GS. 1982. Large bowel. In *Cancer Medicine,* JF Holland, E Frei, eds., pp. 1830–1858. Philadelphia: Lea and Febiger.

Moertel CG, Schutt AJ, Hahn RG, et al. 1975. Therapy of advanced colorectal cancer with a combination of 5FU, methyl-1,3-cis (2-chlorethyl)-1-nitrosourea, and vincristine. *JNCI* 54:69–71.

Niederhuber JE, Ensminger W, Gyves J, et al. 1984. Regional chemotherapy of colorectal cancer metastatic to the liver. *Cancer* 53:1336–1343.

O'Connell MJ. 1983. Clinical overview of chemotherapy for gastrointestinal tumors at Mayo Clinic. In *Fluoropyrimidines in Cancer Therapy,* K Kimura, S Fujii, M Ogawa, GP Bodey, P Alberto, eds., pp. 350–358. Amsterdam, New York: Excerpta Medica.

O'Connell MJ. 1984. Gastrointestinal cancer. In *Current Hematology and Oncology,* vol. 3, VF Fairbanks, ed., pp. 417–445. New York: John Wiley and Sons.

O'Connell MJ, Moertel CG, Ritts RE Jr, et al. 1980. Gastrointestinal carcinoma. *Clin Immunother* 6:129–153.

Rosenberg SA, Lotze MT, Muul LM, et al. 1985. Observations on the systemic administration of autologous lymphokine-activated killer cells and recombinant interleukin-2 to patients with metastatic cancer. *N Engl J Med* 313:1485–1492.

Schutt AJ, Scott M, Moertel CG, et al. 1982. Combination chemotherapy in advanced colorectal cancer (abstract). *Proceedings of the American Society of Clinical Oncology* 18:101.

Shepard KV, Levin B, Karl RC, et al. 1985. Therapy for metastatic colorectal cancer with hepatic artery infusion chemotherapy using a subcutaneous implanted pump. *J Clin Oncol* 3:161–169.

Stagg RJ, Lewis BJ, Friedman MA, et al. 1984. Hepatic arterial chemotherapy for colorectal cancer metastatic to the liver. *Ann Intern Med* 100:736–743.

Weiss GR, Garnick MB, Osteen RT, et al. 1983. Long-term hepatic arterial infusion of 5-fluorodeoxyuridine for liver metastases using an implantable infusion pump. *J Clin Oncol* 1:337–344.

Annual Clinical Conference on Cancer, Vol. 30
Gastrointestinal Cancer: Current Approaches to Diagnosis and Treatment
© 1988 by The University of Texas System Cancer Center

17. Biologic Perspectives and New Treatment Approaches for Hepatic Metastases of Colorectal Carcinoma

Glenn Steele, Jr., and Peter Thomas

Although much ado has been made recently in the medical literature concerning resection of isolated liver metastases from colon and rectal carcinoma, only a minute fraction of patients who experience recurrence or metastases from their primary colorectal cancers will benefit from such an approach. Of 140,000 new cases of colon and rectal carcinoma diagnosed each year, about 60,000 patients will eventually die of the disease. "Raw" five-year survival is still about 40% to 50%, with a slightly better survival for colon and a slightly worse survival for rectal carcinoma. Analyses of patients who have died with recurrent colon and rectal carcinoma have shown that a large majority of such patients have hepatic metastases as part of their failure pattern (Pestana et al. 1964). For prophylaxis or treatment of isolated site-specific metastases, however, the important question concerns the kinetics of failure. Is there a time when portal watershed disease or early hepatic metastasis is an isolated event and not part of an overall systemic failure pattern?

When patterns of failure are examined in prospective or in well-analyzed retrospective single- or multi-institutional studies, it becomes apparent that no more than 10% to 20% of patients who experience disease recurrence after resection of high-risk colon and rectal carcinomas (Dukes/Kirklin classifications B2, C1, C2) will have recurrences only in the liver (Lessner et al. 1984; Holyoke et al. 1985). Thus, the ability to apply site-specific therapy in an adjuvant setting, whether it be portal vein infusion of 5-fluorouracil (5-FU) after resection of primary lesions in the colon and rectum (Taylor 1981) or of systemic 5-FU combined with external-beam irradiation to the liver (Gastrointestinal Tumor Study Group [GITSG]), is not likely to show a significant benefit in improving disease-free or overall survival unless two requisites are met. First, the chemotherapy given must be effective in most patients who have advanced colon and rectal carcinoma. Second, because many patients who have liver-only or liver-predominant recurrence may also have insidious systemic disease, adjuvant therapy as regional prophylaxis must also have a systemic effect. In fact, if the recent National Surgical Adjuvant Breast and Bowel Project (NSABP) trial reproducing the Taylor (1981) data confirms the benefit of adjuvant portal vein infusion of 5-FU for high-risk colorectal carcinoma patients, the effect may not necessarily be regional but rather the result of cytotoxicity of the chemotherapeutic agent as tumor cells pass through the portal watershed or of systemic distribution of the drug.

In addition to the severe biologic selection of patients whose liver-only recurrence from colon and rectum cancer primaries is not a part of systemic failure, another significant biologic selection occurs when one looks at patients whose liver-only metastases are surgically resectable. Foster and Adson and their colleagues (Foster and Berman 1977; Wilson and Adson 1976) alluded to the probability that no more than 10% to 15% of all patients referred for surgery of hepatic metastasis are found to have resectable metastases. Several single-institution studies and one multi-institutional prospective study provided some quantitation of this second level of biologic exclusion. Steele et al. (1984), Cady and McDermott (1985), and current GITSG prospective hepatic metastasis resection protocol show that despite preoperative computerized tomography scans, ultrasonography, liver-spleen scans, and most recently magnetic resonance imaging, all with reasonable resolution capacity of the liver, one third of patients predicted to have liver-only resectable metastases will be found at surgery to have previously unsuspected extrahepatic recurrence or to have a multiplicity of liver-only metastases not amenable to surgical resection. These studies clearly show the benefit of surgical staging and underscore the need for additional regional and systemic therapy options for patients entering metastasis resection protocols. Once the surgical staging identifies systemic or intraperitoneal as well as liver recurrence despite preoperative predictions of resectable liver-only metastases, our own institutional contingency includes triage of patients to a systemic Leucovorin/5-FU protocol (GITSG 1987). Other possible systemic or regional treatment plans we have considered include continuous intravenous infusion of 5-FU, intraperitoneal 5-FU or floxuridine (FUDR), and a variety of biologic-response modifier approaches. The availability of these fallback plans (designed to enable us to establish benefit to the patient as well as patterns of subsequent failure) helps us to justify exploration despite the unfortunate fact that a third of patients operated on do not undergo liver resection because of extrahepatic disease, multiplicity of liver metastases, or particular location of an isolated liver metastasis not amenable to resection.

IMPROVED INTRAOPERATIVE TECHNIQUES

Several technical additions to the surgical armamentarium may expand the regional treatment potential even when previously unsuspected multiple liver metastases are found. One example is intraoperative ultrasound used to monitor cryosurgical ablation of multiple metastases. Intraoperative ultrasound has increased our resolution capacity to diagnose previously nonvisualized and nonsurgically palpated liver metastases that are located in the depths of the right or the left liver lobe. This technique gives us more data on patients who earlier would not have been suspected of having residual disease in the liver after resection. Our own group and several European investigators have recently applied intraoperative ultrasound technology routinely at operative staging and have found that at least 15% to 20% of patients believed to have three or fewer liver metastases have more than three (Onik et al. in press). No more than three liver metastases can be resected with good chance of long-term survival benefit. Although this rule is empiric, data from multiple retrospective studies, including the hepatic metastasis registry of Hughes et al. (1986), have shown that the more metastases in the liver, the smaller the chance of curing the patient. Presumably, the greater the number of liver metastases one can see and feel, the greater the number of nonvisualizable metastases in the residual non-resected liver. The "rule of three" is based not only on the effectiveness of surgical techniques but also on the physiological cost of doing a major resection when there is a high probability of microscopic residual disease. Intraoperative ultrasonography has increased our capacity to document liver metastases, has aided in defining the intrahepatic anatomy before resection of liver metastases, and has allowed the application of a cryoablative technique that may have less physiological cost to the patient than major resection.

We recently described (Ravikumar et al. 1987) application of cryoablation when patients are found to have more than three metastases or when isolated metastases are located in particularly difficult anatomic situations (on the vena cava or sur-rounding the takeoff of the right hepatic or the middle hepatic vein). Previously, these patients would have undergone exploratory surgery but not resection. Intra-operative ultrasound provides good clinicopathological correlation with appropriate freezing margins.

In our first phase of clinical application, patients who had resectable metastases underwent cryoablation before resection, with the prediction of adequate margins by intraoperative ultrasound substantiated by subsequent pathological examination of the resected specimen. A second trial currently under way includes patients who have four or more metastases, for whom the physiological cost of major resection compared with expected survival benefit does not justify resection but may justify cryoablation (Ravikumar et al. 1987).

BIOLOGIC SELECTION FACTORS

Is palliation an adequate justification for resecting hepatic metastasis in patients found to have extrahepatic disease? The majority of our patients who undergo operation for potential resection of hepatic metastases from colon and rectal carci-noma do not have symptoms. In this setting, there is nothing to palliate. Numer-ous trials including the recent Lund experience (Sweden) from Bengmark's group (S. Bengmark, personal communication) show no survival benefit in patients who have extrahepatic disease at the time of liver metastasis resection. Surgery per-formed for resection of hepatic metastases from colon and rectal cancer should be done only with curative intent.

When the above considerations are analyzed, no more than 4,000 to 6,000 patients per year will have potentially surgically resectable liver metastases from primary colon and rectal carcinoma. When the next level of biologic selection is added (i.e., 20% to 30% of patients are disease-free five years after isolated liver metastasis resection), it is easy to understand that extension of life is provided to very few patients and that the major emphasis for this unique patient population should be on examining new biologic opportunities and problems.

An ideal start to any discussion of the biology of patients with liver-predominant or liver-only metastatic disease would be to delineate which particular subset of patients with primary colorectal cancer is at highest risk of developing liver-only metastasis. Characterization of patients by Dukes/Kirklin class is not good enough. Nor is the use of preoperative single plasma sample carcinoembryonic antigen (CEA) quantitation. Many anecdotal experiences in which, at the time of primary tumor resection, patients found to have unsuspected liver metastases are now noted to have had significant preoperative CEA elevations (usually in the range of 20–50 ng/ml) do not change the fact that preoperative CEA elevation is not sensitive or specific enough to aid in making prospective therapy decisions. However, since most patients with colorectal cancer need to have their primary tumors resected regardless of their disease stage, preoperative diagnosis of liver metastases is a moot point.

In multi-institutional as well as single-institutional prospective studies in which patients are followed up after high-risk primary colon and rectal carcinoma resection, serial CEA has given good early indication of liver-predominant or liver-only recurrence when it was applied appropriately and interpreted carefully (Steele et al. 1980, 1982). Ideally, application of additional monoclonal or polyclonal antibody to defined cell-surface and cytoplasmic markers associated with gastrointestinal cancers will provide an array of serologic determinants that, together, may be more predictive of tumor recurrence and perhaps even site-specific recurrence than any single marker used alone (Novis et al. 1986).

Application of monoclonal antibody technology to define specific antigen epitopes of glycoproteins shed from gastrointestinal tumors has shown that markers such as CEA are composed of numerous related family members. In our laboratory, we have developed monoclonal antibodies to particular subsets of CEA that have differing kinetics of liver clearance—one group that is slow-clearing and a second group that is fast. Clearance mechanisms depend on CEA receptor–specific uptake by Kupffer cells, chemical modification of the CEA, and subsequent hepatocyte breakdown. We noted in many patients that when circulating CEA is elevated and composed of the biochemical fraction defined immunochemically or by clearance studies as slow CEA, few of these patients were found to have liver metastases. We speculate that certain members of the CEA family may not only provide a monitor of site-specific metastasis but may be involved in the mechanism of metastasis itself.

CARCINOEMBRYONIC ANTIGENS

The level of tumor markers in the circulation is influenced by many factors. Input into the circulation depends on production by tumor, and this is related to tumor size, to tumor invasion that allows secreted markers access to the circulation, to presence and site of metastases, and to the secreted marker's rate of clearance from the circulation. CEA is the most studied conventional marker for colorectal cancer, and our interest has focused on the role of hepatic clearance mechanisms in influencing circulating levels of this glycoprotein. We assume that whatever is learned about the metabolism of CEA will be applicable to many other shed gastrointestinal system–associated markers. That circulating levels of glycoprotein are largely controlled by the liver is increasingly evident. We have known for some time that elevated CEA levels are associated with benign liver diseases. The highest CEA levels are found in patients with colon cancer metastatic to the liver, particularly when associated with intrahepatic cholestasis. In initial studies, Shuster, Silverman, and Gold (1973) investigated the fate of circulating CEA in the rabbit and dog while Primus, Hansen, and Goldenberg (1974) studied its metabolism in hamsters bearing CEA-producing GW39 tumors. Thomas and Hems (1975) investigated the clearance rates of both native CEA and asialo CEA using the perfused rat liver. All these studies showed that the liver was the prime organ responsible for CEA clearance. The study by Thomas and Hems showed that CEA clearance by the perfused rat liver was rapid and, when sialic acid was removed from CEA, the clearance increased to about 10 times the rate for the native molecule.

This information was not unexpected since a receptor for asialo glycoproteins on the hepatocyte had been described earlier. However, the native molecule is still cleared rapidly by the liver both in vivo and in vitro, and further investigation showed that the Kupffer cell was responsible. Following Kupffer cell clearance, CEA is transferred to the hepatocyte, where final degradation takes place (Thomas et al. 1977; Toth et al. 1982). Uptake by the Kupffer cell was shown to be by receptor-mediated endocytosis. Binding of CEA to the receptor did not depend on the terminal carbohydrate structure but seemed to depend on binding to part of the protein component of CEA (Toth et al. 1982). After binding and internalization by the Kupffer cell, the CEA is exocytosed, having lost at least some of its sialic acid, which then allows uptake by the hepatocyte by way of the asialo glycoprotein receptor (Toth et al. 1985). A second minor pathway for CEA clearance exists also, and this involves direct passage of CEA from blood to bile by the paracellular pathway (Thomas and Summers 1978; Thomas 1980). This pathway becomes more important in the presence of cholestatic liver disease when junctional complexes within the liver are disrupted (Thomas, O'Neil, and Zamcheck 1982, 1985). The early studies of Shuster, Silverman, and Gold (1973) showed a biphasic clearance curve for CEA from the circulation of both rabbits and dogs. This could be interpreted as rapid clearance caused by an asialo component, followed by the slower clearance representing uptake by the Kupffer cell. Byrn et al. (1985) showed, however, that the type of clearance from the circulation varies among CEA preparations. The very rapid clearance may still be caused by an asialo component, whereas a less rapid clearance curve may represent Kupffer cell uptake. A third component showing much slower clearance is present in some CEA preparations, however. Although the uptake of this material is by the liver, it appears to be different from the Kupffer cell hepatocyte mechanism described.

Certain patients with very high CEA levels produce a type of CEA that consists predominantly of this slower-clearing component (Thomas et al. 1983). This type of CEA species has lower isoelectric points on agarose isoelectric focusing and higher sialic acid content than the more rapidly clearing forms. We found that CEA isolated from liver metastases tends to be the rapidly clearing kind, whereas CEA isolated from ascites of patients with very high circulating CEA levels tends predominantly to be the slower-clearing form. It is noteworthy that patients with high levels who produce this slow-clearing form of CEA tend to have reasonably good performance status, even with CEA levels as high as 100,000 ng/ml, and they rarely have liver metastases except in the terminal stage of the disease. Ascites formation in these patients tends to be the result of peritoneal metastasis. The slow- and fast-clearing forms of CEA can be separated by isoelectric focusing (Saravis, Thomas, and Zamcheck 1986). The CEA moieties can also be separated by gel-permeation high-pressure liquid chromatography (HPLC) on an SW3000 column. The slow-clearing forms tend to have a shorter retention time than the fast-clearing ones (Toth et al., unpublished data). Cleavage of the six disulfide bridges on CEA causes the fast-clearing form to convert to the shorter retention time associated with the slow-clearing form. Although the isoelectric focusing separation is based on charge differences caused by the larger amounts of sialic acid present on the slow-clearing form, the HPLC separations are likely to reflect conformation differences between the two CEA types. Slayter and Coligan (1975; Coligan and Slayter 1979) studied the conformation of CEA isolated from liver metastases by electron microscopy and showed that the majority of the molecules had a compact cruller-type conformation, though a small proportion, about 15%, had a more extended shape. Uptake experiments in Kupffer cells in vitro have shown reduced uptake of the slow-clearing form of CEA comparable to that of performic acid oxidized fast-clearing CEA. One question that arises, therefore, is: Is the difference in carbohydrate composition between these two CEAs the result of altered conformation, or is the altered conformation the result of differences in carbohydrate structure? The former seems the most likely explanation.

We produced a monoclonal antibody that has specificity for the slow-clearing form of CEA. The antibody is of the IgG1 type and reacts by immunofluorescence and immunoperoxidase staining with a number of colon cancer cell lines. Reaction with this antibody against paraffin sections of hepatic metastases of colorectal cancer is poor, which reinforces the idea that hepatic metastases tend to produce mainly the fast-clearing form of CEA. Rule et al. (1979) reported a pH 3 CEA variant for which they obtained a specific polyclonal antiserum. Whether this variant is identical with our slow type of CEA or not remains to be studied. Plasma assays using specific monoclonal antibody to the slow-clearing CEA are being developed with the aim of detecting patients who produce this CEA variant and examining CEA kinetics after resection of hepatic metastases. The CEA decay curves in these patients may be composites of CEA species with different clearance rates.

Some questions still need to be answered. Is there a relationship between the type of CEA produced and the type of morphological differentiation of the tumor? Does therapy affect the type of CEA produced? To date, our studies of the slow-clearing CEA have shown that patients who produce this type of CEA tend to have very well differentiated mucin-producing tumors that seed the peritoneal cavity rather than metastasize to the liver. Treatment of colon cancer cells in vitro with such differentiating agents as sodium butyrate can increase CEA production markedly and can even cause cells that, under normal circumstances, do not produce CEA to produce at least some (Niles et al. 1985). These agents will also inhibit peanut agglutinin–binding to colon cancer cells, perhaps indicating an increase in surface sialic acid

(Thomas et al. 1983; Thomas, Burke, and Zamcheck 1984). Increases in surface sialation may also reflect increases in sialation of secreted proteins such as CEA. If this is the case, maturational agents may be able to convert fast-clearing forms of CEA into the slow-clearing type, assuming that it is increased sialic acid that causes the conformational changes associated with the slow-clearing variant.

Such switches from fast- to slow-clearing CEA moieties may also be produced by chemotherapy and not be correlated with change in tumor volume. We have observed marked falls in CEA levels during combination chemotherapy of colon cancer patients who produce the slow-clearing variant of CEA. Laboratory studies have shown that these declines in plasma CEA levels are associated with changes in CEA from the slow- to the fast-clearing form. In one case, a patient's plasma CEA level fell from 16,000 to 300 ng/ml with no objective change in tumor volume. This fall in CEA was associated with a change in the isoelectric focusing pattern of the patient's CEA to a more basic form; in rats, clearance rates changed from slow to more rapid clearance. This fall in CEA was associated also with a reduction in the total serum sialic acid. What we may have observed in this case was a general phenomenon in which chemotherapy affected complex carbohydrate synthesis and possibly the patient's ability to terminate carbohydrate chains with sialic acid.

We have already pointed out that the highest circulating CEA levels are associated with liver metastasis from colorectal cancer. This seems reasonable since liver metastases can represent large tumor volume at an anatomical site where the tumor can receive a good blood supply and where secreted products have good access to the circulation. Infiltration of tumor into the liver may also impair hepatic function and result in reduced clearance of the secreted glycoproteins. However, another factor may play a part in this phenomenon. We speculate that colorectal cancer cells that secrete CEA, in particular, fast-clearing forms of CEA, are more likely to produce hepatic metastasis. The mechanisms of site-specific metastasis formation are not well understood, but some reports in the literature suggest that macrophages may be involved in this process. We know that the liver macrophage, the Kupffer cell, has on its surface a receptor that recognizes CEA (Thomas and Summers 1978) and that macrophages can be tumoricidal and are capable of lysing tumor cells (Cohen, Salazar, and Nolan 1982; Malter, Friedrich, and Suss 1986). Mercurio and Robbins (1985) also suggested that branched complex oligosaccharides may be involved in the macrophage-tumor cell interaction and that disruption of these oligosaccharides can prevent tumor cell lysis by the macrophage (Mercurio 1986). Tumor cells are characterized by a predominance of tetrantenary oligosaccharides on their surface, unlike normal cells that contain mainly bi- and triantenary structures (Takasaki, Ikehira, and Kobata 1980). Chandrasekaran et al. (1983) reported that CEA contains a large number of tetrantenary asparagine-linked oligosaccharides. It is possible, therefore, that production of CEA, either in secreted form or present on the tumor cell surface, could be involved in tumor cell–macrophage interaction. Giavazzi et al. (1986) studied a number of moderately well differentiated human colon cancer cell lines for their metastatic ability when the cells were injected into the spleens of nude mice. The work showed a correlation between plasma CEA levels in the patients from whom the tumor was taken, the tumor cells' ability to metastasize to the liver, and the size of metastases produced. The higher the CEA level, the more numerous and larger were the metastases found.

We have been investigating the interactions between fixed tissue macrophages and rat colon carcinoma cells with specific patterns of metastasis formation. The W2054 DMH rat colon carcinoma in our minimal residual disease–setting model will recur in the lung 100% of the time. This tumor does not produce liver metastases. We have looked at cytotoxicity of both liver and lung macrophages from the host rats against these cells and have found that the Kupffer cells have a high killing rate for these tumors, whereas tumor cell killing by lung macrophages is much less. Kupffer cells kill these tumors without previous stimulation with endotoxin or gamma-interferon. Other control tumor cell lines such as the mouse melanoma cell line, p815, are not killed by rat Kupffer cells or alveolar macrophages unless they are stimulated with gamma-interferon and endotoxin. Thus, certain cancer cells can be killed by fixed macrophages without stimulation. This could occur in human beings in whom fixed macrophages may work as a surveillance system to remove what are essentially foreign cells from specific organs. When this surveillance system is blocked, metastases formation is likely. If a human colon cancer cell is an active CEA secretor, we postulate that the CEA produced can bind to the fixed macrophages within the liver or lung and prevent their interactions with tumor cells, thus preventing cytotoxic effects. This might allow tumor cell invasion and development of hepatic metastases. Cells that do not produce CEA would be killed by the fixed macrophages of the liver or the lung, since recognition sites for macrophage cytotoxicity on the cell surface are not blocked by circulating CEA. Colon cancer cells that produce slow-clearing CEA would more likely be killed by fixed liver and lung macrophages because slow-clearing CEA does not bind to CEA receptors on fixed macrophages. This postulate is supported by our observations that patients with high levels of slow-clearing CEA tend not to have liver metastases but often show diffuse peritoneal seeding. In this respect, it is noteworthy that peritoneal macrophages, unlike those in liver and lung, do not have a CEA receptor (Toth et al. 1984). Although poorly differentiated or undifferentiated colon cancer cells rarely produce CEA, they are still capable of metastasizing readily to the liver and to many other organs. This may occur by separate mechanisms because these cells have fewer Golgi bodies, and they may not have the correct carbohydrate signals on their cell surface to allow fixed macrophage recognition and cell killing. Thus, the biology of secreted tumor markers such as CEA and related proteins like nonspecific cross-reacting antigen (NCA) may have implications in predicting future site-specific metastases in patients who remain at high risk after primary tumor resection.

CONSIDERATIONS IN THERAPY

Once it has been determined by surgical staging, and perhaps additional application of intraoperative ultrasonography, that a patient is in the uniquely favored and limited subset of patients who have resectable liver-only metastases from colon and rectal carcinoma, one still must ask whether therapy is in fact adding to the patient's disease-free survival or is simply functioning as a biologic selection process. The key data here are the natural histories of patients who fall into this unique and bio-logically advantageous subset and who do not undergo surgical resection. In 1982, our group published a report of the natural history of 125 patients who presented with liver-only or liver-predominant colorectal adenocarcinoma metastases at the Dana-Farber Cancer Institute and the Brigham and Women's Hospital (Goslin et al. 1982). Of this group, a large minority had experienced no debility and no change in life-style. As one would expect, this group of patients had three or fewer liver me-tastases as defined by ultrasound, liver-spleen scan, or computed tomography scan. The median survival of these asymptomatic patients was 24 months. It must be remembered that this group of patients underwent no therapy to account for this survival.

The widely varying response rates ascribed to regional FUDR delivered by the Infusaid pump into the hepatic artery for liver-only or liver-predominant metastases are probably a function of inadequate trial design of most single-institutional series. Thus, the 29% to 30% response rates of the Dana-Farber and University of Chicago series (Weiss et al. 1983) are no different from the expected median survival of non-treated liver-metastasis patients. Contrast this to the 80% to 85% response rates reported by single-institutional studies at the Universities of Michigan, Alabama, and California at San Diego (Balch et al. 1983). Such widely differing response rates more than likely represent biologic selection of completely different groups of patients whose natural history, rather than therapy, determined their response and survival.

Ultimate application of this regional therapy approach in several properly de-signed controlled trials, one performed by the Northern California Oncology Group and the other by Kemeny et al. at Memorial Sloan-Kettering Cancer Center and col-laborating institutions, has confirmed the original work by Grage et al. (1979) showing that regional and systemic 5-FU are comparable. Regional therapy had no advantage over systemic therapy, despite the increased efficiency of drug extraction when FUDR is delivered directly to the liver. Patient benefit through stabilization of liver disease in the regionally infused group was neutralized by increased systemic tumor recurrence. In addition, the increased invasiveness of the regional approach (by surgery, either resective or to place the arterial catheter and pump) and the toxic effects of regional treatment, such as sclerosing cholangitis, preclude any advantage for regional therapy as long as the drugs to be delivered are limited to 5-FU and FUDR. Technological advances, including the Infusaid device, Silastic outflow catheters, and other even more sophisticated continuous-delivery systems whose flow rates can be externally controlled despite total implantation, await more effec-tive substances to deliver before a significant therapeutic benefit can be achieved for patients.

ANALYSIS OF FAILURE

Major criticism of the trial design of hepatic arterial chemotherapy infusion is equally applicable to hepatic resection series. Thus, there would be only one legiti-mate way of differentiating the effect of surgical intervention from biologic selec-tion in the purported increased survival of patients who underwent resection of liver metastases: with a prospective, randomized trial in which patients were randomly allocated to a group who had surgically staged resectable disease but did not undergo resection, compared with those who had surgically staged resectable disease and underwent resection. Naturally, this trial will never occur. In lieu of such a logically clean but ethically unpalatable approach, we chose the tactic of analyzing patterns of failure after resection of isolated liver metastases from colon and rectal carcinoma. Analysis of failure after resection will also help us determine where the next effort should be made in planning any secondary or adjuvant regional or systemic therapy approach for this unusual group of patients. Finally, we attempted to use patients with resectable liver metastases as a resource for testing new serological tumor markers and in screening for in vivo targeting of potentially valuable reagents with diagnostic and potentially therapeutic specificity.

Our analysis of failure as reported in 1984 with an initial group of 50 patients (Steele et al. 1984) was extended to about 150 patients who underwent liver resection for isolated metastases from colon and rectal carcinoma. Our results were substantiated by other single-institutional trials and by several major retrospective reviews of multi-institutional metastectomy registries as reported by Hughes et al. (1986). All these reports, whether multi-institutional or from single institutions, should be interpreted with care because they are retrospective and have selection biases that are not clearly understood. Nevertheless, these analyses have some themes in common. All show that major liver surgery can be done safely. The consensus is that mortality should be less than 5%. All show the benefit of surgical staging. About one third of patients who are predicted to have liver-only metastases that are resectable will be found, at the time of surgery, to have previously unsuspected extrahepatic metastases or a multiplicity of previously unsuspected liver metastases that do not allow resection. All studies show that patients who undergo resection have a chance for long-term, durable, disease-free survival only if resection shows no evidence of extrahepatic disease. Most studies imply an empiric threshold of three or fewer metastases as making resection worthwhile.

These are not hard data, but they certainly make sense because the more disease one can see in the liver, the more likely is the presence of additional, unseen disease that will lead to more rapid failure after major hepatic resection. Whether longer disease-free survival after resection depends on the time between primary tumor resection and diagnosis of metastasis is still an open question. Nor do we know about longer survival after resection of metastases in patients whose primary tumors were at the "lesser" Dukes/Kirklin stages. Interestingly, the question of whether the patient needs to have a significant amount of normal tissue included in the pathologically defined free margin also remains open. The more recent single-institutional studies as well as the multi-institutional retrospective study from the National Cancer Institute all show a plateauing of the survival curve in successfully resected patients at about three to five years. Thus, this more recent experience confirms what Foster and Adson originally reported when they began the vogue of hepatic metastasis surgery some 10 years ago. It seems that about 20% to 30% of patients will be cured if they fall into this biologically select group. Thus, the only conventional potentially curative approach is to resect such patients' hepatic metastases.

In a single prospective randomized trial (the last residue of the Gastrointestinal Tumor Study Group), research groups are attempting to collect, in a prospective manner, all patients whose hepatic metastases were diagnosed and resected synchronously or metachronously after primary colorectal cancer resection. Questions asked in this multi-institutional study include: (1) How many patients who are predicted to have liver-only resectable disease will in fact be found at operation to have resectable liver-only disease? (2) What is the mortality and morbidity of patients who undergo major liver resection? (3) Is a particular pathologically free surgical margin better (i.e., does more free margin give a greater curative potential)? (4) What are the patterns of failure after surgical resection of liver-only metastases? This study reached its goal of 100 patients in 24 months. The kinetics of failure seem to be like those of many of the single-institutional trial reports, and the data will be extraordinarily valuable in confirming or disputing many of the retrospective analyses summarized above. Presumably, this prospective approach will also provide information concerning the next rational therapeutic step.

Finally, in any discussion of this unusual group of patients, the application of markers for both serological studies and tissue-fixed in vivo targeting must be mentioned. These patients belong to a unique population who present with extensive disease, usually easily documentable by computerized tomography scan, ultrasound, magnetic resonance imaging, or liver-spleen scan. Any shed tumor-associated marker that is useful should be elevated before surgery, should rapidly decrease after surgical clearance of gross disease, and in the unfortunate majority of patients who experience recurrence, should rise serially before or at the time of tumor rerecurrence. The natural history of disease in this group of patients is relatively short. Most patients who experience recurrence will do so within a few years. The prototype gastrointestinal cancer marker, CEA, gives us a good framework for applying any new potentially useful serological markers. Their kinetics may be looked at in a manner similar to CEA definition after liver metastasis resection, and predictions concerning elevations of new markers and subsequent documentation may be based on conventional studies of tumor recurrence.

In addition to serological marker screening, these patients present a valuable setting for testing various antibody or other targeting reagents. Patients are infused with the material before surgery. Surgical resection specimens provide both tumor and surrounding contiguous tissue for quantifying actual concentration differences in tumor and nontumor tissue and for selecting patients whose tumors have particularly highly concentrated epitopes, thus giving some support to the use of that particular targeting reagent in subsequent adjuvant therapy. Such studies, under way in our institution, consist of trials using 17-1A monoclonal antibody against a shared colorectal carcinoma cell-surface antigen described by Sears et al. (1982). Other immunoglobulins, either injected alone or conjugated with radiochemicals or natural toxins, can be applied within the same format. Definition of in vivo targeting can be obtained, which is the first step in any potential specific diagnostic or therapeutic application of such reagents.

Finally, the failure patterns in this group of patients and the need to understand the biologic selection process that permits liver resection in such a minority of patients in whom colorectal surgery failed demands that these patients, 70% to 80% of whom will soon experience re-recurrence, be considered for adjuvant therapy after they recover from liver resection. The fact that the patients are surgically staged, the fact that this is an unusual minimal residual disease setting with a very short natural history, the unique opportunity to screen tumor and nontumor contiguous tissues for specific targeting reagents, and the biologic conundrum of a disease that is systemic but has nevertheless remained regionally circumscribable, all point toward the need to move ahead with subsequent therapy trials despite what initially seems to be complete clearance of all liver metastases. These trials should be designed in a prospective fashion. Ideally, patients should be randomized to two arms, in one of which patients receive no further therapy after successful resection, while the other group is treated according to one or another secondary regional or systemic approach. The selection of the therapy regimen, whether it be chemotherapy, biologic response–modifier therapy, or immunologic and specific tumor-targeting therapy, should depend on analysis of failure in the retrospective and the prospective trials detailed above, proof that enough patients are available for a formal trial, and finally on some confidence that the therapeutic agent being tested has an effect against colorectal adenocarcinoma.

REFERENCES

Balch CM, Urist MM, Soong S-J, et al. 1983. A prospective phase II clinical trial of continuous FUDR regional chemotherapy for colorectal metastases to the liver using a totally implantable drug infusion pump. *Ann Surg* 198:567–573.

Byrn R, Medrek P, Thomas P, et al. 1985. Heterogeneity of CEA affects liver cell membrane binding and its kinetics of removal from the circulation. *Cancer Res* 45:3137–3142.

Cady B, McDermott W. 1985. Major hepatic resection for metachronous metastases from colon cancer. *Ann Surg* 201:204–209.

Chandrasekaran E, Davila M, Nixon D, et al. 1983. Isolation and structures of the oligosaccharide units of carcinoembryonic antigen. *J Biol Chem* 258:7213–7222.

Cohen SA, Salazar D, Nolan JP. 1982. Natural cytotoxicity of isolated rat liver cells. *J Immunol* 129:495–501.

Coligan JE, Slayter HS. 1979. Physical, chemical, and immunological characterizations of saline extracted concanavalin A–purified carcinoembryonic antigen. *Mol Immunol* 16:129–135.

Foster JH, Berman MM. 1977. Solid liver tumors. In *Major Problems in Clinical Surgery*, PA Ebert, ed. Philadelphia: W. B. Saunders.

Giavazzi R, Campbell DE, Jessup JM, et al. 1986. Metastatic behavior of tumor cells isolated from primary and metastatic human colorectal carcinomas implanted into different sites of nude mice. *Cancer Res* 46:1928–1933.

Goslin R, Steele G Jr, Zamcheck N, et al. 1982. Factors influencing survival in patients with hepatic metastases from adenocarcinoma of the colon or rectum. *Dis Colon Rectum* 25:749–754.

Grage TB, Vassilopoulos PP, Shingleton WW, et al. 1979. Results of a prospective randomized study of hepatic artery infusion with 5-fluorouracil versus intravenous 5-fluorouracil in patients with hepatic metastases from colorectal cancer: A Central Oncology Group study. *Surgery* 86:550–555.

Holyoke ED, Mittleman A, Panahon A, et al. (Gastrointestinal Tumor Study Group). 1985. Prolongation of disease-free interval in surgically treated rectal carcinoma. *N Engl J Med* 312:1465–1472.

Hughes KS, Simon R, Songhorabodi S, et al. 1986. Resection of the liver for colorectal carcinoma metastases: A multiinstitutional study of indications of resection. *Surgery* 100:278–284.

Lessner HE, Mayer RJ, Ellenberg SE, et al. (Gastrointestinal Tumor Study Group). 1984. Adjuvant therapy of colon cancer—results of a prospectively randomized trial. *N Engl J Med* 310:737–743.

Malter M, Friedrich E, Suss R. 1986. Liver as a tumor cell killing organ: Kupffer cells and natural killers. *Cancer Res* 46:3055–3060.

Mercurio AM. 1986. Disruption of oligosaccharide processing in murine tumor cells inhibits their susceptibility to lysis by activated mouse macrophages. *Proc Natl Acad Sci USA* 83:2609–2613.

Mercurio AM, Robbins PW. 1985. Activation of mouse peritoneal macrophages alters the structure and surface expression of protein bound lactosaminoglycans. *J Immunol* 135: 1305–1312.

Niles R, Thomas P, Wilhelm S, et al. 1985. Effects of butyrate and retinoic acid on growth and CEA production in 3 colon cancer cell lines (abstract). *Proceedings of the American Association of Cancer Research* 26:37.

Novis BH, Gluck E, Thomas P, et al. 1986. Serial levels of CA 19-9 and CEA in colonic cancer. *J Clin Oncol* 4:987–993.

Onik G, Kane R, Steele G Jr, et al. In press. Monitoring hepatic cryosurgery with sonography. *AJR*.

Pestana C, Reitemeier RJ, Moertel CG, et al. 1964. The natural history of carcinoma of the colon and rectum. *Am J Surg* 108:826–829.

Primus FJ, Hansen HJ, Goldenberg DM. 1974. Altered metabolism of carcinoembryonic antigen in hamsters bearing GW-39 tumors. *Nature* 249:837–838.

Ravikumar TS, Kane R, Cady B, et al. 1987. Hepatic cryosurgery with intraoperative ultrasound monitoring for metastatic colon carcinoma. *Arch Surg* 122:403–409.

Rule A, Foote B, Kirch M, et al. 1979. Purification, immunochemical characterization and clinical testing of a pH 3 carcinoembryonic antigen (CEA) variant. In *Carcinoembryonic Proteins*, Vol. II, FG Lehmann, ed., pp. 39–46. New York: Elsevier/North Holland Biomedical Press.

Saravis CA, Thomas P, Zamcheck N. 1986. Demonstration of carcinoembryonic antigen (CEA) associated with a high sialic acid/fucose ratio (abstract). *Proceedings of the American Association of Cancer Research* 27:1.

Sears HF, Atkinson BF, Mattis J, et al. 1982. Phase I clinical trial of monoclonal antibody in treatment of gastrointestinal tumours. *Lancet* 3:762–765.

Shuster J, Silverman M, Gold P. 1973. Metabolism of human carcinoembryonic antigen in xenogeneic animals. *Cancer Res* 33:65–68.

Slayter HS, Coligan JE. 1975. Electron microscopy and physical characteristics of the carcinoembryonic antigen. *Biochemistry* 14:2323–2330.

Steele G Jr, Ellenberg S, Ramming K, et al. (Gastrointestinal Tumor Study Group). 1982. CEA monitoring among patients in multi-institutional adjuvant G.I. therapy protocols. *Ann Surg* 196:162–169.

Steele G Jr, Osteen RT, Wilson RE, et al. 1984. Patterns of failure after surgical "cure" of large liver tumors—a change in the proximate cause of death and a need for effective systemic adjuvant therapy. *Am J Surg* 147:554–559.

Steele G Jr, Zamcheck N, Wilson RE, et al. 1980. Results of CEA-initiated "second-look" surgery. *Am J Surg* 139:544–548.

Takasaki S, Ikehira H, Kobata A. 1980. Increases of asparagine-linked oligosaccharides with branched outer chains caused by cell transformation. *Biochem Biophys Res Commun* 92:735–742.

Taylor I. 1981. Studies on the treatment and prevention of colorectal liver metastases. *Ann R Coll Surg Engl* 63:270–276.

Thomas P. 1980. Studies on the mechanisms of biliary excretion of circulating glycoproteins: The carcinoembryonic antigen. *Biochem J* 192:837–843.

Thomas P, Birbeck MSC, Cartwright P. 1977. A radioautographic study of the hepatic uptake of circulating carcinoembryonic antigen by the mouse. *Biochem Soc Trans* 5:312–313.

Thomas P, Burke B, Zamcheck N. 1984. Differing effects of sodium butyrate and DMF on poorly differentiated human colon cancer cells (abstract). *Proceedings of the American Association of Cancer Research* 25:42.

Thomas P, Byrn RA, Saravis CA, et al. 1983. Changes in a surface PNA binding glycoprotein of human colon cancer cells treated with DMF. *J Cell Biol* 97:67A.

Thomas P, Hems DA. 1975. The hepatic clearance of circulating native and asialo carcinoembryonic antigen by the rat. *Biochem Biophys Res Commun* 67:1205–1209.

Thomas P, O'Neil PF, Zamcheck N. 1982. Inhibition of specific Kupffer cell clearance of carcinoembryonic antigen from the serum of rats with bile duct ligation. *Biochem Soc Trans* 10:459–460.

Thomas P, O'Neil P, Zamcheck N. 1985. The effects of colchicine and vinblastine on the biliary excretion of carcinoembryonic antigen. *Hepatology* 5:207–210.

Thomas P, Summers JW. 1978. The biliary excretion of circulating asialoglycoproteins in the rat. *Biochem Biophys Res Commun* 80:335–339.

Thomas P, Toth CA, Byrn RA, et al. 1983. Five patients with markedly elevated CEA blood levels and impaired clearance of circulating CEA. *Clin Res* 31:696A.

Toth CA, Thomas P, Broitman SA, et al. 1982. A new Kupffer cell receptor mediating plasma clearance of carcinoembryonic antigen by the rat. *Biochem J* 204:377–381.

Toth CA, Thomas P, Broitman SA, et al. 1984. Receptor mediated endocytosis of carcinoembryonic antigen by rat alveolar macrophages *in vitro*. *Fed Proc* 43:2046.

Toth CA, Thomas P, Broitman SA, et al. 1985. Receptor mediating plasma clearance of carcinoembryonic antigen by rat liver Kupffer cells. *Cancer Res* 45:392–397.

Weiss GR, Garnick MB, Osteen RT, et al. 1983. Long-term hepatic arterial infusion of 5-fluorodeoxyuridine for liver metastases using an implantable pump. *J Clin Oncol* 1:337–344.

Wilson SM, Adson MA. 1976. Surgical treatment of hepatic metastases from colorectal cancers. *Arch Surg* 111:330–334.

Annual Clinical Conference on Cancer, Vol. 30
Gastrointestinal Cancer: Current Approaches to Diagnosis and Treatment
© 1988 by The University of Texas System Cancer Center

18. Bilateral Iliac Artery Infusion of 5-Fluorouracil and Mitomycin C for Palliation of Pelvic Recurrence in Colorectal Cancer

Yehuda Z. Patt, Chusilp Charnsangavej, Marilyn Soski,
and Laura Claghorn

A limited number of therapeutic options are available to patients with metastatic or recurrent colorectal carcinoma localized to the pelvis after radiotherapy or conventional intravenous chemotherapy has failed, since response to phase I drugs is usually minimal. Obstruction of urinary and fecal outflow may be surgically alleviated, but pain caused by pelvic tumors represents a major therapeutic challenge. We have previously observed a high response rate to hepatic arterial infusion of mitomycin C and fluoropyrimidines (Patt et al. 1981, 1983). We decided, therefore, to extend our experience by delivering mitomycin C and 5-fluorouracil (5-FU) into the iliac arteries to treat pelvic metastases or disease recurrence refractory to conventional therapy (Patt et al. 1985).

MATERIALS AND METHODS

Twenty-one patients with metastatic or recurrent colorectal cancer in the pelvis refractory to radiation, systemic chemotherapy, or both, received bilateral iliac arterial chemotherapy infusion. The regimen consisted of 10 mg/m² of mitomycin C given over two hours and 600 mg/m² per day of 5-FU given by continuous infusion daily for five days. Approximately 10,000 U/m² of heparin was added to the therapy to prevent vascular and catheter clotting. To prevent dermatitis over the infused area, hydrocortisone at a dosage of 200 mg per 24 hours was delivered simultaneously, either intraarterially mixed with the 5-FU or intravenously. Arterial catheterization and chemotherapy were repeated every four to five weeks until treatment failed or toxicity became unacceptable.

Under fluoroscopic guidance, catheters were percutaneously placed in both internal iliac arteries by the Seldinger technique. Whenever possible, the vessel supplying the tumor was selectively catheterized. We attempted to assess the percentage of blood flow to the tumor from each side and to deliver a corresponding fraction of the total dosage of chemotherapy into the appropriate artery while delivering the remaining fraction through the contralateral iliac vessel. The patients were confined to bed for the duration of arterial infusion.

Characteristics of the patients are shown in table 18.1. In 17 of the 21 patients,

Table 18.1. *Patient Characteristics: Pelvic Arterial Chemotherapy*

Parameter	Patients ($N = 21$)		
		No.	(%)
Median age in years	54		
(range)	(16–77)		
Interval in months			
From primary to recurrence	24		
(range)	(0–187)		
From recurrence to treatment	8		
(range)	(0–94)		
Sex: male		16	(76)
female		5	(24)
Prior treatment			
Irradiation		5	(24)
Chemotherapy		3	(14)
Irradiation and chemotherapy		12	(57)
None		1	(5)
Presenting symptoms			
Pain		8	(38)
Pain + hydronephrosis		10	(48)
Hydronephrosis		1	(5)
Hematuria		1	(5)
Rectal mass		1	(5)

radiation therapy had failed, and in 15, chemotherapy had failed. Only one patient had never been exposed to chemotherapy or radiation.

Response to Treatment

Definite response or partial remission (PR) was defined as a greater than 50% reduction in the serum level of carcinoembryonic antigen (CEA) when the pretreatment value exceeded 10 ng/ml. Such an elevation was present before treatment in 12 patients. Pre- and post-treatment levels were evaluable, however, in only 11 of the patients. A decrease of greater than 50% in the product of two perpendicular diameters of a tumor mass measurable by computerized tomography (CT), ultrasonography, or arteriography was also considered a PR. Antimass effect was evaluable by CT, ultrasound, or angiography in 10 patients.

Urologic Manifestations

Some urologic manifestations of pelvic tumors were present in most of the patients. Eleven of the 21 had evidence of hydronephrosis visible by CT, ultrasound, or intravenous pyelography. Response to the treatment could be evaluated in 7 of those 11 patients. Five patients had elevated levels of serum creatinine and 12 had hematuria, both of which could be used as indicators of response.

Pain Control

We considered pain relief to be possible evidence of antitumor response to chemotherapy. To quantify pain relief, we devised the scoring system described in table 18.2. During the first and last treatments, each patient was assigned a pain score depending on dose, potency, frequency, and route of administration of pain medication required. In addition, the patients' subjective feeling about their pain, which could not be quantified by this scoring system and yet was classified by them as improved or not, was assigned a class sign under a special column in the results section. Unacceptable high toxicity, objective evidence of disease progression, and lack of pain relief in the absence of objective evidence of improvement were considered indications to remove the patient from the study. To test the significance of differences between the first and last treatments, we used the Wilcoxon signed rank test.

RESULTS

After pelvic arterial chemotherapy in 17 patients, the median carcinoembryonic antigen (CEA) level dropped from 24 to 14 ng/ml ($p < .05$). A greater than 50% drop in the CEA level was observed in 5 of the 11 patients (45%) in whom it was evaluated. A mass effect was visible on the CT scan or angiogram in 10 of those patients, but in only 2 (20%) was a PR observed. In addition, in two patients biopsies were performed in areas where a pelvic mass had been, and no tumor could be detected in those regions.

An evaluation of the effect of pelvic arterial chemotherapy on urologic manifestations showed improvement of hydronephrosis in five of seven patients (71%) in whom it could be evaluated before and after therapy. Modes of evaluation included CT, ultrasound, and intravenous pyelography. In one of five patients (20%) the serum creatinine level decreased more than 30%. Of the 12 patients who had hematuria, 10 (83%) had either a partial or complete clearance of red blood cells from the urine.

Using the scoring system developed for determining severity of pain (table 18.2)

Table 18.2. *Scoring System for Severity of Pain*

Medications Required for Pain Relief	Score
None	0
Oral analgesics:	
acetylsalicylic acid, acetaminophen, propoxyphene hydrochloride	1
Oral schedule II < 4 times a day	2
Oral schedule II ≥ 4 times a day	3
Oral + i.v. or i.m. schedule II < 4 times a day	4
Oral + i.v. or i.m. schedule II ≥ 4 times a day	5

Abbreviations: i.v., intravenously; i.m., intramuscularly.

Table 18.3. *Complications in 45 Cycles of Iliac Arterial Infusion of 5-Fluorouracil and Mitomycin C (21 Patients)*

Complication	Treatment Cycles[a]	
	No.	(%)
Dermatitis over area of infusion	12	(27)
Peripheral neuropathy	8	(18)
Mucositis	3	(7)
Bleeding at arteriotomy	4	(9)
Neutropenia ($<1 \times 10^3/\mu l$)	1	(2)
Thrombocytopenia ($<1 \times 10^3/\mu l$)	1	(2)
Vascular complications	5	(11)
Urinary tract infection	7	(16)
Infection at catheter site	4	(9)

[a] No. and percentage associated with complication.

after pelvic arterial chemotherapy in 18 patients, we noted that 6 patients had a pretherapy score of 4–5, and only 3 had that high a score following therapy. The pain score was zero in three patients before treatment and in six after treatment. The mean pain score before therapy was 2.4, and after arterial chemotherapy it dropped to 1.7 ($p < .05$, Wilcoxon signed rank). No post-treatment pain information was available for 2 patients, but 8 of the 16 evaluable patients had objective pain relief (decrease in their score). Four additional patients reported subjective pain relief that could not be quantified by a decrease in pain score.

Complications of bilateral iliac artery infusion of 5-FU and mitomycin C are described in table 18.3. The most prevalent side effect of iliac artery infusion was skin toxicity. Every patient had some erythema over one or both buttocks. However, only 12 of 45 treatment cycles (27%) were associated with severe dermatitis accompanied by extensive blistering or pain over the infused area that lasted from five to seven days. Two of 21 patients required dose modification because of dermatitis. Corticosteroids (hydrocortisone, 200 mg per day), when added to the 5-FU and administered intraarterially or intravenously, ameliorated or totally prevented this side effect.

Temporary neurotoxicity related to the chemotherapy was observed in 8 of 45 treatment courses (18%). The incidence of neuropathy increased from 14% in the first course to 18% during the second and 33% during the third. One patient reported unilateral hyperesthesia at the L5 distribution. In three patients, peripheral neuropathy presented as "stocking" numbness of the lower extremities. One additional patient complained of pain in one leg; although this could not be clearly associated with the treatment, it was nevertheless classified as neurotoxicity. Mucositis was associated with 3 of 45 treatment courses (7%) and was observed in two different patients; one required dose modification.

Vascular complications occurred in five patients. In one, the effects of an arterial embolus were transient, leaving no permanent sequelae. Three others developed thrombosis of the femoral or iliac arteries, or both. Intraarterial thrombolytic agents resulted in substantial improvements in pain and motor activity in the affected extremity. In one patient, a mycotic aneurysm developed in the left femoral artery. Neutropenia (an absolute granulocyte count of $0.48 \times 10^3/\mu l$) was associated with 1 of 45 treatment cycles (2%). One treatment cycle was associated with a drop in platelet count to $91,000/\mu l$ (table 18.3). Two patients experienced urosepsis after therapy but were not neutropenic at the time. Seven patients suffered from urinary tract infections; four of those had indwelling catheters during treatment. No patient died as a result of treatment complications.

DISCUSSION

The iliac arterial infusion described here was used for palliative treatment of recurrent colorectal cancer in the pelvis. Fifty percent of the patients had objective pain relief, and an additional 25% reported subjective evidence of decreased pain. In 45% of the patients, the serum CEA level decreased more than 50%; however, a PR was radiographically evident in only 2 of 10 patients. Some improvement in hydronephrosis was observed in 5 of 7 evaluable patients, and hematuria improved in 10 of 12 patients. Although this treatment was not permanently effective and the disease eventually recurred in all patients, arterial infusion of mitomycin C and 5-FU was a valid option for pain control in patients in whom systemic chemotherapy and radiation therapy to the pelvis had failed. The treatment's local toxicity could be ameliorated to a great extent by administering hydrocortisone (200 mg/day).

This treatment was primarily effective in alleviating pain. As a result, we conclude that the appropriate management of refractory pelvic recurrence of colorectal cancer should include, first, surgical relief of intestinal and urologic obstruction, and then, to achieve the most effective palliation of pain in patients refractory to radiation therapy, bilateral iliac artery infusion of 5-FU and mitomycin.

REFERENCES

Patt YZ, Chuang VP, Wallace S, et al. 1981. The palliative role of hepatic arterial infusion and arterial occlusion in colorectal carcinoma metastatic to the liver. *Lancet* 1:349–351.

Patt YZ, Peters RE, Chuang VP, et al. 1983. Effective retreatment of colorectal cancer patients with liver metastases. *Am J Med* 75:237–240.

Patt YZ, Peters RE, Chuang VP, et al. 1985. Palliation of pelvic recurrence of colorectal cancer with intra-arterial 5-fluorouracil and mitomycin. *Cancer* 56:2175–2180.

Annual Clinical Conference on Cancer, Vol. 30
Gastrointestinal Cancer: Current Approaches to Diagnosis and Treatment
© 1988 by The University of Texas System Cancer Center

19. Monoclonal Antibodies in Colorectal Cancer Diagnosis and Therapy

Robert W. Baldwin and Vera S. Byers

Monoclonal antibodies that recognize determinants expressed selectively on colorectal cancer cells are being evaluated for targeting therapeutic agents. Therapeutic effectiveness may be improved through antibody localization and retention in tumors, especially metastatic deposits. Additionally, if normal tissues lack significant expression of the antigens associated with malignant cells, it will be possible to minimize drug toxicity, a major limitation in systemic chemotherapy.

One murine monoclonal antibody designated 791T/36 reacting with a membrane glycoprotein antigen (gp72) expressed on a high proportion of colorectal cancers (Durrant et al. 1986) has been selected for designing drug-antibody conjugates (Baldwin 1985; Baldwin and Byers 1985, 1986a, 1986b). In addition, drug conjugates with monoclonal antibodies reacting with tumor-associated carcinoembryonic antigen (CEA) have been developed, providing the possibility of using cocktails of antibody conjugates for therapy.

TUMOR LOCALIZATION OF MONOCLONAL ANTIBODY 791T/36

Clinical immunoscintigraphy studies with 791T/36 antibody radiolabeled with either ^{131}I or ^{111}In have shown localization of antibody in primary, recurrent, and metastatic colorectal cancer (Armitage et al. 1984, 1985a, 1985b; Ballantyne et al. 1986a). In the initial trial, 24 patients with primary colorectal cancer underwent preoperative administration of ^{131}I-labeled antibody and imaging by gamma camera. The primary tumor was imaged successfully in 13 of the 24 patients. If tumors of different parts of the large bowel are considered separately, those within the pelvis (rectum and rectosigmoid) were only detected in 5 of 13 patients (42%), principally because of technical difficulties (^{131}I was excreted through the urinary tract and bladder). In comparison, tumors of 8 of 11 patients (67%) were successfully imaged when the tumor was outside the pelvis. Consistent imaging was also obtained in patients with recurrent or metastatic colorectal cancer. In all, 26 sites of metastasis were examined, and of these, 21 (85%) were positively identified using ^{131}I-labeled 791T/36 for gamma camera imaging (Armitage et al. 1984, 1985a).

Using ^{111}In to label monoclonal antibody 791T/36 has several advantages over using [131]I. [111]In has gamma energy (172–247 keV) making it more suitable for detection by a standard gamma camera and allowing higher count rates both for planar imaging and emission tomography. Its half-life of 2.8 days permits imaging to be delayed until after selective uptake by tumor deposits and clearance from the cir-

Table 19.1. *Immunoscintigraphy with [111] In-Labeled Monoclonal Antibody 791T/36 of Colorectal Cancer*

Site of Primary Carcinoma	Image Result	Site of Metastases or Recurrent Carcinoma	Image Result
—	—	Pelvis	Positive
—	—	Pelvis	Positive
—	—	Right upper abdomen	Positive
—	—	Left upper abdomen Center abdomen	Positive Positive
—	—	Pelvis	Positive
—	—	Pelvis	Positive
—	—	Pelvis	Positive
Rectosigmoid	Positive	Liver	Positive
Sigmoid	Positive	—	Positive
Sigmoid Cecum	Negative Negative	Liver	Negative
Rectosigmoid	Positive	Liver	Negative

Note: Each row represents a case.

culation, but the delay is not excessively long. There is no associated β-particle emission and no significant concentration in the thyroid, gastric mucosa, or the urinary tract. Positive imaging of tumor sites was achieved in all but 1 of 11 colorectal cancer patients (Armitage et al. 1985b). The results of patient imaging are given in table 19.1. All five pelvic and three intraabdominal sites of tumor recurrence produced positive images. Three of the four patients with primary tumors had films that showed positive uptake at the tumor site. Uptake of the radiopharmaceutical in liver limited the detection of liver metastases. Only one of three patients with liver metastases had evidence on film of the metastases, which was observed as uptake increased over 48 hours as defects were filled on the 20-minute image. The films of one patient who had two unresected primary tumors (sigmoid and cecum) and liver metastases showed no increased uptake of labeled antibody. In a few patients, there appeared to be nonspecific activity present in the bowel. One patient had an area of increased uptake on the right side of the abdomen, but a computerized tomography scan showed no evidence of recurrence; the uptake may have been due to bowel activity.

Because of the results of these studies, [131] I- and [111] In-labeled 791T/36 antibody has been prospectively evaluated for the detection of recurrent and metastatic colorectal cancer (Ballantyne et al. 1986a). Patients underwent antibody gamma camera imaging (31 patients with [131] I-labeled antibody; 24 patients with [111] In-labeled antibody). Immunoscintigraphy detected 37 of 58 separate sites of recurrence in 38 patients, the sensitivity with [131] I- and [111] In-labeled antibody being 64% and 61%, respectively (specificity, 67% and 71%, respectively). Liver metastases were detected

Table 19.2. *Radiochemical Analysis of Radioactivity in Resected Tissue from Colorectal Cancer Patients Injected with ^{131}I- or ^{111}In-Labeled 791T/36 Monoclonal Antibody*

Patient	Site of Primary Carcinoma	Distribution of Radioactivity (Tumor:Normal Tissue)
^{131}I Label		
1	Sigmoid	2.2:1
2	Rectosigmoid	5.8:1
3	Rectosigmoid	2.1:1
4	Sigmoid	3.1:1
5	Sigmoid	1.1:1
^{111}In Label		
6	Sigmoid	3.4:1
7	Ascending colon	3.2:1
8	Pelvic recurrence	1.3:1
9	Rectosigmoid	3.4:1

using ^{131}I-labeled antibody in 12 of 18 cases, whereas ^{111}In-labeled preparations were not effective (1 of 6 cases) because of the nonspecific localization of ^{111}In in liver. ^{131}I-791T/36 antibody correctly demonstrated four of nine (44%) sites of pelvic recurrence; with ^{111}In-labeled antibody, uptake was seen in seven of eight (88%) pelvic recurrences.

Resected specimens of tumor and adjacent normal tissue were imaged to measure antibody distribution and the tumor-to-nontumor ratio of radioactivity. In addition, weighed samples of tumor and normal bowel were analyzed radiochemically and a ratio of counts per minute per gram of tissue calculated. Representative samples of the tumor-to-normal tissue ratio (T:N) of radioactivity determined with resected specimens from patients injected with either ^{131}I- or ^{111}In-labeled 791T/36 are summarized in table 19.2. In the five patients injected with ^{131}I-labeled antibody, the T:N ratio ranged from 1.1:1 to 5.8:1. Overall the mean T:N ratio in 29 patients was $2.6 \pm 1.2:1$ in colon carcinomas and $2.4 \pm 0.5:1$ in rectal carcinomas.

In the four patients injected with ^{111}In-labeled antibody, the T:N ratio ranged from 1.33:1 to 3.4:1 (mean, 2.8:1).

MONOCLONAL ANTIBODY TARGETING AND CYTOTOXIC DRUGS

In general, choosing a cytotoxic agent for linking to monoclonal antibody is influenced by a number of factors, including the differential reactivity of antibody with tumor and normal tissue and the requirement to deliver conjugated drug sufficient to produce a therapeutic response. Essentially, therefore, two broad strategies are being pursued for the design of drug-antibody conjugates. On the one hand, highly cytotoxic agents, such as plant and bacterial toxins, are being linked to antibody, since these will produce highly potent immunotoxins (Baldwin and Byers 1986a; 1986b; Vitetta and Uhr 1985). In this case, toxicity for normal tissues has to be carefully evaluated and monitored. The other approach is to select existing chemotherapeutic agents for antibody conjugation, since their toxicity, at least as free drug, is well known. The only important toxicity consideration here is the influence of antibody conjugation. In this case, however, the potency of the chemoimmuno-conjugate is considerably less than that of the immunotoxin, so its efficacy may not be so great (Baldwin 1985; Baldwin et al. 1985).

Immunotoxins

Ribosomal-inhibiting proteins are highly cytotoxic. It has been calculated that one molecule entering the cytoplasm of a cell is sufficient to produce a lethal response. Ricin protein extracted from castor bean is a particularly potent plant toxin, its median lethal dose being about 16 μg/kg body weight (Stirpe and Barbieri 1986). This toxin consists of A and B polypeptide chains. The B chain attaches the toxin to specific cell receptors, and the A chain, the toxic component, exerts its effect following entry into the internal milieu of the cell. To take advantage of these properties, researchers separate ricin into the A and B chain components and link the A chain (RTA) to antibody. This yields immunotoxins in which the binding of the A chain and entry into a cell are dictated by the antibody component (Baldwin and Byers 1985; Vitetta and Uhr 1985).

An immunotoxin (XMMCO-791-RTA) has been constructed by linking monoclonal antibody 791T/36 (XMMCO-791) to ricin A chain, which is specifically cytotoxic for tumor cells, including colorectal cancer cells, which bind this antibody (Embleton et al. 1986). Furthermore, the immunotoxin inhibits growth of human tumor xenografts developing in athymic mice. This is illustrated in figure 19.1, which shows the influence of XMMCO-791-RTA repeated immunotoxin treatment on growth of colon carcinoma xenograft C170.

Biodistribution studies carried out with ^{125}I-labeled RTA coupled to XMMCO-791 indicated that there was an initial rapid clearance of immunotoxin from the blood so that only 22% remained two hours after injection. The majority of this material remained conjugated. The major organ of clearance was the liver, with rapid concentration of immunotoxin in the liver, presumably by the mannose receptors. In the liver, dehalogenation and deconjugation occurred.

Acute and subacute toxicity studies were carried out in rats and mice. Female Sprague-Dawley rats received intravenous injections of the immunotoxin at 1 or 5 mg/kg once a day for 10 consecutive days. Animals were killed and necropsied on days 6, 11, or 17 to assess subacute toxicity and estimate reversibility. There was a significant decrease in body weight from day 3 through day 10 of the study, which was reversible, as evidenced by weight gain through the end of the study. Granulocytosis and a slight decrease in red cells also occurred. Serum albumin levels were significantly depressed but returned to normal one week after cessation of therapy. There was significant hepatomegaly. Histologically, mild hepatic vacuolization was seen, and there was some hepatic necrosis in the high-dose group. Although there was hepatocyte regeneration after cessation of treatment, the hepatic changes persisted through day 17 of the study. There was also mild renal tubular necrosis, but no other histological evidence of toxicity. There was no evidence of cardiac toxicity.

These toxicities were different from those reported with use of either whole ricin

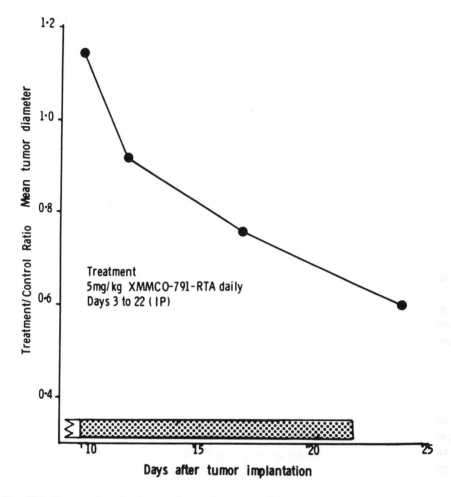

Fig. 19.1. Suppression of colon carcinoma C170 xenografts in athymic mice treated intraperitoneally (*IP*) with immunotoxin XMMCO–791T–RTA.

or RTA. Whole ricin produces lesions in the vascular endothelium and in the reticuloendothelial system, with little or no intestinal damage. In comparison, RTA produces a necrotic lesion in the intestinal crypts, adrenal involution, and protein accumulation in renal tubules. Hepatic necrosis is also seen. Hypoalbuminemia is not a feature of RTA toxicity.

These animal toxicology results were similar to those seen with two other immunotoxins, an antimelanoma antibody and ricin A chain conjugate and an anti–pan T lymphocyte and ricin A chain conjugate. Since the antibodies used to produce these immunotoxins are directed against different antigens, it is most probable that the toxicities will be seen with all immunotoxins, regardless of antibody specificity.

A phase I trial of the antimelanoma immunotoxin has been completed in 22 patients with metastatic melanoma (L. E. Spitler, M.D., personal communication, March 1986). A constellation of transient reversible side effects were noted, including evening temperature elevation with associated fatigue, chills, and myalgias; a fall in serum albumin level with associated weight gain (but no pulmonary edema); a decreased voltage on electrocardiogram without changes in echocardiogram or clinical cardiac symptomatology.

Generally these changes were transient, and they were reversed during completion of therapy. A phase I study of the anticolorectal ricin A chain immunotoxin (XMMCO-791-RTA) is in progress in patients with metastatic colorectal carcinoma. The most prominent side effects noted have been hypoalbuminemia with associated weight gain and decreased voltage on electrocardiogram. The albumin level drop may be precipitous (as much as 50%) and may prove one of the dose-limiting side effects of the immunotoxin. Studies are in progress to determine the etiology of the hypoalbuminemia.

Chemoimmunoconjugates

Antibody conjugates have been constructed with a range of chemotherapeutic agents in clinical use, including methotrexate, Adriamycin, and the vinca alkaloid analogue vindesine (Baldwin 1985; Baldwin et al. 1985). Cytotoxic drugs may be directly linked to antibody through a reactive site that does not compromise drug activity. In this case only a limited number of drug residues can be linked before antibody reactivity is impaired. In order to increase drug-antibody combining ratios, drug carrier systems are being designed. The present design involves a first stage in which a drug is linked to a carrier that has multiple combining sites, and then the drug carrier complex is linked to antibody (Baldwin 1985).

Both these approaches have been used to construct conjugates of methotrexate and monoclonal antibody 791T/36. Direct linkage of methotrexate to antibody produces conjugates containing up to 4 mol of methotrexate for each mole of antibody. Additionally human serum albumin (HSA) has been used as a carrier for methotrexate (fig 19.2). In this case, MTX-HSA conjugates are first constructed and then linked to antibody to produce products (MTX-HSA-791T/36) containing 30 mol to 40 mol of drug per mole of antibody (Garnett and Baldwin 1986). These methotrexate conjugates show greatly enhanced cytotoxicity in vitro for colorectal carcinoma cell lines when compared with free methotrexate (Baldwin et al. 1985; L. G. Durrant, Ph.D., personal communication, 1986). Also, as shown in figure 19.3, when tested against human tumor xenografts that bind the 791T/36 antibody, their therapeutic efficacy is greatly improved (Baldwin 1985).

In view of the cytotoxicity of methotrexate-791T/36 antibody conjugates for colon carcinoma cells, a phase I clinical trial in the treatment of metastatic colorectal cancer is being undertaken. Initially the biodistribution of methotrexate directly linked to monoclonal antibody 791T/36 (MTX-791T/36) was assessed by immunoscintigraphy of ^{131}I-labeled preparations in patients with primary colorectal cancer (Ballantyne et al. 1986b). Gamma camera imaging demonstrated that the biodistribution of the ^{131}I-labeled antibody component of the drug conjugate was similar to that of the unconjugated antibody. Freshly resected tumor and normal

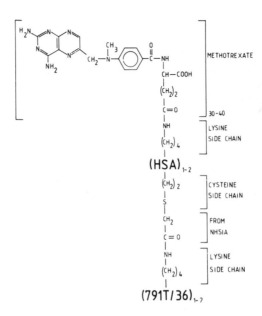

Fig. 19.2. Composition of drug conjugate constructed by linking methotrexate to human serum albumin (*HSA*) and then linking MTX-HSA to monoclonal antibody 791T/36. Reprinted, by permission, from Garnett and Baldwin, 1986.

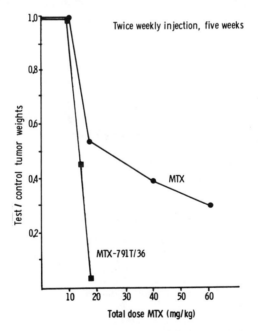

Fig. 19.3. Treatment of tumor 791T xenografts in athymic mice with methotrexate (*MTX*) monoclonal antibody 791T/36 or free methotrexate. Mice were treated twice weekly with either free drug or conjugate for five weeks. Tumor weights in treated and control mice were determined at completion of treatment and the influence of methotrexate (or conjugate) expressed as a test-to-control ratio of mean tumor weights.

colonic tissue were also assayed for radioactivity. Positive tumor localization was measured in 13 of 14 specimens. In six colon tumors the T:N ratio ranged from 2.1–7.9:1, and in eight rectal tumors the ratio ranged from 0.9–6.6:1. The median ratio for both types of tumors was 2.9:1. Tumor localization studies with methotrexate linked to antibody through a human serum albumin carrier are in progress, and these conjugates will be evaluated next in the phase I trial.

CONCLUSIONS

The potential of monoclonal antibodies for targeting cytotoxic drugs in colorectal cancer has been substantiated by extensive in vitro testing with immunotoxins and chemoimmunoconjugates. These antibody conjugates also inhibit growth of human colorectal carcinoma xenografts in athymic mice. These findings together with related toxicology studies now allow clinical trials to be initiated to determine the safety and efficacy of conjugates. Trials will evaluate the efficacy of single antibody conjugates. Colorectal tumors are composed of subpopulations of cells with significant heterogeneity in their biologic properties, including antigen expression (Durrant et al. 1986). It is conceivable, therefore, that cocktails of immunotoxins or drug conjugates may prove even more effective. In this respect, ricin A chain immunotoxins have also been prepared with monoclonal antibodies that react with CEA (Byers et al., unpublished data). These immunotoxins also suppress growth of colorectal carcinoma xenografts so that it is already possible to provide a dual cocktail for therapy. In this context, analysis of antigen expression on colon carcinoma cells derived from primary and metastatic growths has established that a combination of monoclonal antibody 791T/36 and an anti-CEA antibody reacts with more than 91% of tumors, aneuploid tumors showing the strongest reactivity (Durrant et al. 1986 and unpublished data).

ACKNOWLEDGMENTS

These studies were supported by generous grants from the Cancer Research Campaign and Xoma Corporation.

REFERENCES

Armitage NC, Perkins AC, Hardcastle JD, et al. 1985a. Monoclonal antibody imaging in malignant and benign gastrointestinal diseases. In *Monoclonal Antibodies for Cancer Detection and Therapy*, RW Baldwin, VS Byers, eds., pp. 129–158. London: Academic Press.
Armitage NC, Perkins AC, Pimm MV, et al. 1985b. Imaging of primary and metastatic colorectal cancer using an ^{111}In-labeled antitumor monoclonal antibody (791T/36). *Nucl Med Commun* 6:623–631.
Armitage NC, Perkins AC, Pimm MV, et al. 1984. The localisation of an anti-tumour monoclonal antibody (791T/36) in gastrointestinal tumours. *Br J Surg* 71:407–412.
Baldwin RW. 1985. Design and development of drug–monoclonal antibody 791T/36 for cancer therapy. In *Monoclonal Antibody Therapy of Human Cancer*, K Foon, AC Morgan, eds., pp. 23–56. Boston: Martinus Nijhoff.

Baldwin, RW, Byers VS, eds. 1985. *Monoclonal Antibodies for Cancer Detection and Therapy.* London: Academic Press.

Baldwin RW, Byers VS. 1986a. Immunotherapy of cancer. In *Cancer Chemotherapy Annual 8,* HM Pinedo, BA Chabner, eds., pp. 209–223. New York: Elsevier.

Baldwin RW, Byers VS. 1986b. Monoclonal antibody targeting of anti-cancer agents. *Springer Sem in Immunopathol* 9:39–50.

Baldwin RW, Byers VS. In press. Monoclonal antibody targeting of cytotoxic agents for cancer therapy. In *Progress in Immunology VI.* New York: Academic Press.

Baldwin RW, Durrant L, Embleton MJ, et al. 1985. Design and therapeutic evaluation of monoclonal antibody 791T/36-methotrexate conjugates. In *Monoclonal Antibodies and Cancer Therapy,* RA Reisfeld, S Sell, eds., pp. 215–231. New York: Alan R. Liss.

Ballantyne KC, Perkins AC, Armitage NC, et al. 1986a. Comparison of ^{131}I and ^{111}In labeled monoclonal antibody 791T/36 in the detection of recurrent colorectal cancer. *Nucl Med Commun* 7:309.

Ballantyne KC, Perkins AC, Pimm MV, et al. 1986b. Biodistribution and tumour localisation of a monoclonal antibody-drug conjugate (791T/36-methotrexate). *Nucl Med Commun* 7:310.

Durrant LG, Robins RA, Armitage NC, et al. 1986. Association of antigen expression and DNA ploidy in human colorectal tumors. *Cancer Res* 46:3543–3549.

Embleton MJ, Byers VS, Lee HM, et al. 1986. Sensitivity and selectivity of ricin toxin A chain—Monoclonal antibody 791T/36 conjugates against human tumor cell lines. *Cancer Res* 46:5524–5528.

Garnett MC, Baldwin RW. 1986. An improved synthesis of a methotrexate albumin-791T/36 monoclonal antibody conjugate cytotoxic to osteogenic sarcoma cell lines. *Cancer Res* 46:2407–2417.

Stirpe F, Barbieri L. 1986. Ribosome-inactivating proteins up to date. *FEBS Lett* 95:1.

Vitetta ES, Uhr JW. 1985. Immunotoxins. *Annu Rev Immunol* 3:197.

ESOPHAGEAL CANCER

Annual Clinical Conference on Cancer, Vol. 30
Gastrointestinal Cancer: Current Approaches to Diagnosis and Treatment
© 1988 by The University of Texas System Cancer Center

20. Overview of Esophageal Cancer

Stuart Jon Spechler

Cancer of the esophagus is a tumor that is malignant in every sense of the word. It is a disease for which mortality rate and incidence are nearly identical. In the United States during 1985, it is estimated that there were 8,800 deaths owed to esophageal cancer and 9,400 new cases of the disease (Sondik et al. 1985). Cancer of the esophagus is among the most racist and sexist of malignancies in this country, affecting blacks four times as often as whites and men four times as often as women (see table 20.1). For whites, there has been little change in the incidence and mortality for esophageal cancer over the past decade; for blacks during that same period, both incidence and mortality have increased by more than 10% (see table 20.2).

EPIDEMIOLOGY

The epidemiology of esophageal cancer is both fascinating and puzzling. The disease exhibits marked variations in incidence for different geographic regions. Cancer of the esophagus remains a relatively uncommon malignancy in the United States, where it accounts for only about 1% of all cancers (Sondik et al. 1985). In contrast, esophageal cancer is one of the commonest malignant tumors in Curaçao (Freni 1984). Other areas of exceptionally high incidence include the Transkei region of South Africa, northern China, and parts of Iran and the Soviet Union surrounding the Caspian Sea (Kmet and Mahboubi 1972; Gilder 1977; Ying-kai et al. 1982). Paradoxically, areas of high incidence may be found near areas of low incidence. Chinese men in Yangcheng County of Shanxi Province have a mortality rate from esophageal cancer of 169.2/100,000; for men in Yunnan Province, that rate is 1.4/100,000 (Ying-kai et al. 1982). The disease also exhibits striking geographic variations in its male-to-female attack rate. In France, men are affected more than 12 times as often as women (Audigier, Tuyns, and Lambert 1975); in parts of Iran, the incidence is slightly higher in women than in men (Kmet and Mahboubi 1972).

These intriguing epidemiological features have stimulated investigations seeking to identify dietary, cultural, and environmental pathogenetic factors for cancer of the esophagus. Such investigations have found a variety of factors associated with esophageal carcinoma. These include such general dietary factors as poor nutrition or such specific nutritional deficiencies as lack of vitamin A, vitamin C, nicotinic acid, riboflavin, thiamine, iron, magnesium, selenium, and zinc. Also implicated have been the habits of using tobacco, consuming alcohol, and using opium and the environmental factors of high soil salinity and low rainfall. Chronic esophageal irritation associated with achalasia, lye stricture of the esophagus, ingestion of hot foods and liquids, and reflux esophagitis and ingestion of specific carcinogens or

Table 20.1. *Age-Adjusted Incidence and Mortality Rates for Esophageal Cancer*

Group	Incidence (per 100,000)	Mortality Rate (per 100,000)
White males	5.0	4.6
White females	1.5	1.2
Black males	19.9	15.8
Black females	4.0	4.0

Source: Sondik et al. 1985. Incidence and mortality rates are from the National Cancer Institute's Surveillance, Epidemiology, and End Results (SEER) Program for 1983.

Table 20.2. *Ten-Year Trends in Incidence and Mortality Rate for Esophageal Cancer*

Group	Incidence (%)	Mortality Rate (%)
White males	−0.9	+4.2
White females	−5.2	+5.1
Black males	+10.6	+11.5
Black females	+26.2	+10.7

Source: Sondik et al. 1985. Data are from the National Cancer Institute's Surveillance, Epidemiology, and End Results (SEER) Program for 10-year period, 1974–1983.

cocarcinogens (Croton products, nitrosamine compounds, aflatoxin, silica, and asbestos) have also been linked to esophageal cancer. Barrett's esophagus, Plummer-Vinson syndrome, low socioeconomic status, exposure to ionizing radiation, celiac sprue, and tylosis are also associated with esophageal cancer. However, no single risk factor common to all cases has yet been identified. In the United States, there is a strong association between esophageal cancer and the use of alcohol and tobacco (Wynder and Bross 1961). In contrast, alcohol and tobacco do not appear to be important risk factors in Moslem Iran, where the tumor is common. Furthermore, associations are not proof of cause and effect. The pathogenetic mechanisms for cancer of the esophagus remain to be elucidated.

Another remarkable feature of esophageal cancer is its frequent association with other malignancies, particularly those involving the mouth, pharynx, and larynx. In one series from The University of Texas M. D. Anderson Hospital and Tumor Institute, 89 (10.5%) of 850 patients with carcinoma of the esophagus were found to have cancers of the head and neck (Goldstein and Zornoza 1978). In 16 of the 89 cases, the tumors were discovered synchronously. In the remaining 73 cases, the discovery of the esophageal cancer preceded that of the head and neck neoplasm by an average of 46 months. Conversely, in a series of 150 patients with cancers of the head and neck seen at the Boston Veterans Administration Medical Center, 11 (7.3%) had synchronous or metachronous esophageal malignancies (Shapshay et al. 1980). Tobacco use and heavy consumption of alcohol are risk factors shared by cancers of the head and neck and the esophagus; therefore, the association of these tumors may be the result of cigarette smoking and alcohol abuse in affected patients.

Other tumors reported to be associated frequently with esophageal cancer include malignancies of the lung, skin, and stomach (Goodner and Watson 1956; Cahan 1977; Goldstein and Zornoza 1978; Shibuya et al. 1982).

SPECIAL FEATURES OF ADENOCARCINOMA OF THE ESOPHAGUS

There are two important histological types of malignancies subsumed under the rubric "cancer of the esophagus"—squamous cell carcinoma and adenocarcinoma. In most reported series, more than 90% of the patients with esophageal cancer have squamous cell carcinomas (Rosenberg et al. 1985). The epidemiological data discussed so far pertain predominantly to squamous cell tumors of the esophagus. The Surveillance, Epidemiology, and End Results (SEER) Program of the National Cancer Institute does not differentiate between squamous and glandular malignancies when reporting incidence and surveillance data on esophageal cancer. Although it is a common practice to discuss esophageal cancer as if it were one disease, squamous cell carcinoma and adenocarcinoma of the esophagus differ substantially in their epidemiological and clinical features (Wang, Antonioli, and Goldman 1986). Furthermore, there is mounting evidence to suggest that adenocarcinoma of the esophagus is not the rare disease it traditionally has been considered.

Esophageal adenocarcinoma can arise from the sparse glandular elements normally present in the esophagus or from the aberrant glandular epithelium of Barrett's esophagus. Barrett's esophagus is the condition wherein the squamous mucosa that normally lines the distal esophagus is replaced by a columnar epithelium resembling that in the stomach and intestines (Spechler and Goyal 1986). Barrett's epithelium is acquired as the result of chronic reflux esophagitis and can be found in 8% to 20% of patients who have endoscopic examinations for gastroesophageal reflux disease. For unknown reasons, Barrett's esophagus is predominantly a disorder of white males. For patients with Barrett's esophagus, the risk of developing esophageal cancer is increased 30- to 40-fold above that of the general population. It appears that the great majority of adenocarcinomas of the esophagus originate in Barrett's epithelium (Haggitt and Dean 1985).

Morphologically, adenocarcinomas of the esophagus and stomach are indistinguishable, so it may not be possible to determine whether an adenocarcinoma that crosses the gastroesophageal junction originated in esophageal or gastric epithelium. Because adenocarcinoma of the esophagus traditionally has been considered a rare tumor (Bosch, Frias, and Caldwell 1979), glandular neoplasms involving the gastroesophageal junction are often dismissed uncritically as cancers of the gastric cardia that have invaded the esophagus. Strong circumstantial evidence suggests, however, that many so-called cancers of the gastric cardia in fact are esophageal tumors with origins in Barrett's epithelium. In one study from Canada, the clinical features of 51 patients diagnosed as having adenocarcinoma of the gastric cardia were compared with those of 169 patients with cancer elsewhere in the stomach (MacDonald 1972). The investigator found substantial differences in clinical features and suggested that cancer of the gastric cardia may be a different disease than cancer of the body of the stomach. Perhaps it is not merely coincidence that patients

Table 20.3. *Clinical Features of Patients with Cancer of the Gastric Cardia, the Body of the Stomach, and Barrett's Esophagus*

Clinical Feature	Cardia (N = 51)	Stomach (N = 169)	Barrett's (N = 121)
Male:female ratio	7.0:1	2.3:1	5.5:1
Birth where gastric cancer common (%)	6	26	—
Prominent heartburn in past (%)	24	6	64
Hiatus hernia (%)	35	6	71

Source: Cardia and stomach data from MacDonald 1972; Barrett's data from Sjogren and Johnson 1983.

alleged to have cancer of the cardia more closely resemble patients with cancer in Barrett's esophagus than those with stomach cancer in terms of sex and racial characteristics, frequency of symptomatic gastroesophageal reflux, and frequency of hiatus hernia (see table 20.3). It is likely that many patients with esophageal adenocarcinoma arising in Barrett's epithelium mistakenly have been categorized as having cancer of the gastric cardia. Such errors could belie the frequency of adenocarcinoma of the esophagus.

It appears that adenocarcinoma of the esophagus is being diagnosed with increasing frequency. In a series recently reported from the Beth Israel Hospital in Boston, for example, 12 (34%) of 35 esophageal cancers found between 1975 and 1982 were adenocarcinomas; these 12 cases accounted for 60% of the cancers that involved the distal esophagus (Wang, Antonioli, and Goldman 1986). Some of this apparent increase in the frequency of esophageal adenocarcinoma may reflect an increased awareness on the part of clinicians and pathologists of the frequency and importance of Barrett's esophagus. Perhaps fewer Barrett's adenocarcinomas are being mistakenly categorized as cancers of the gastric cardia. Another possible explanation for why adenocarcinoma is being diagnosed with greater frequency is that there has been a true increase in the incidence of this histological type of esophageal cancer. This hypothesis is difficult to prove or disprove because precise data on the incidence of esophageal adenocarcinoma are not readily available. Finally, differences in the prevalence of adenocarcinoma among series of patients with esophageal cancer may reflect differences in the racial characteristics of the patient populations. In striking contrast to squamous cell carcinoma of the esophagus, which has a predilection for blacks, esophageal adenocarcinoma is predominantly a disease of whites (Spechler and Goyal 1986). The ratio of squamous cell to adenocarcinoma of the esophagus would be expected to vary directly with the black-to-white ratio of the patient population.

LYMPHATIC SYSTEM

Regardless of the histological type, esophageal cancer often is disseminated at the time of diagnosis. The extensive lymphatic system of the esophagus is the vehicle for much of this dissemination (Watson et al. 1956). Small lymphatic vessels in the

esophageal mucosa drain into larger submucosal lymph vessels that extend throughout the length of the organ (McCort 1952). Similarly, small lymphatics in the muscularis externa drain into larger vessels that traverse the muscular layers of the
esophagus. These two major groups of esophageal lymphatic channels interconnect
with one another and with vessels supplying adjacent lymph nodes. This intricate
interconnecting lymphatic system provides opportunity for both longitudinal and
lateral spread of esophageal cancer. Thus it is not surprising that intramural microscopic metastases can be found in resected specimens separated from the primary
esophageal tumor by eight or more centimeters (Watson et al. 1956). Furthermore,
it is not unusual to find metastases in the celiac lymph nodes, even in patients with
cancers in the upper one third of the esophagus (Guernsey, Knudsen, and Mark 1970).

The prevalence of lymphatic spread is related imperfectly to the size of the neoplasm. On the basis of an autopsy series it appears that approximately 50% of patients with tumors less than 5 cm in length have lymph node metastases (Fleming
1943). When the tumor length exceeds 5 cm, 90% have metastatic disease. The frequency of extensive lymphatic spread of esophageal cancer explains why simple
segmental resection of the neoplasm often leaves tumor behind and why curative
treatment must include resection or irradiation of wide margins of apparently normal tissue. The frequent longitudinal lymphatic spread of esophageal cancer also is
the rationale for laparotomy to biopsy celiac and gastric lymph nodes before pro-
ceeding with extensive curative surgery. Metastatic involvement of these nodes
would preclude radical surgical resections.

POTENTIAL FOR CURE

For 90% of patients with cancer of the esophagus, dysphagia and weight loss are the
initial symptoms (Rosenberg et al. 1985). Other symptoms are odynophagia, regur-
gitation, and sore throat. Coughing can be caused by aspiration or an esophagotra-
cheal fistula, hoarseness by involvement of the recurrent laryngeal nerve, bleeding
by tumor necrosis or an esophagoaortic fistula, and bone pain by metastases. Sometimes patients develop superior vena cava syndrome. Ordinarily, these symptoms
appear only when the tumor has narrowed the lumen of the esophagus substantially
or has invaded adjacent structures. Therefore, the presence of symptoms suggests
that the patient already has extensive tumor involvement. In one series of 100 patients with symptomatic carcinoma of the esophagus, only 34 were found to have
localized disease at the time of surgery or postmortem examination (Merendino and
Mark 1952). The remaining cases had distant metastases, local invasion of adjacent
structures, local perforations, or fistulas; these complications generally would preclude cure by surgical or radiation therapy. A more recent autopsy series found evidence of metastatic disease in 65 (82%) of 79 cases (Anderson and Lad 1982). In
the absence of a treatment that can eradicate such extensive disease, therefore, cure
does not appear to be possible for a majority of patients with symptomatic cancer of
the esophagus. Furthermore, these patients frequently have severe underlying pulmonary, cardiac, and liver disease that further limits their treatment options. A recent review of 122 reported surgical series that included more than 83,000 patients

found that only 58% of patients evaluated for surgical treatment of esophageal cancer eventually had an operation and that only 39% subsequently had their tumors resected (Earlam and Cunha-Melo 1980a). Stated differently, surgical cure was deemed impossible because of extensive tumor involvement or severe comorbidity in 61% of cases.

Esophageal cancer is a tumor that is clinically silent until it has grown extensively, and most symptomatic patients already have disseminated disease. The median survival after diagnosis is less than six months. There are data to suggest, however, that symptomatic patients have harbored their malignancies for years. Assuming a constant doubling time for squamous cell carcinoma of 56 days, Anderson and Lad (1982) calculate that it would take approximately 4.5 years for an esophageal malignancy to attain a size of 1 cm. Clinical evidence to support this concept of a long symptom-free growth period comes from esophageal cancer surveillance programs in high-incidence areas of China. A recent report from Honan Province describes the results of mass screening for cancer of the esophagus using the technique of esophageal exfoliative cytology (Guanrei et al. 1982). Such screening of more than 28,000 people detected 115 cases of asymptomatic esophageal cancer. Ninety-one of these patients who were not treated with surgery, radiation, or chemotherapy were followed for 19 to 42 months (mean, 35 months). During that time there were two deaths from esophageal cancer, and six other patients developed signs of advanced disease. Eighty-three (91%) of those 91 patients with untreated early esophageal cancers remained asymptomatic. These data suggest that esophageal cancers may grow for years before symptoms develop. Discovery of the tumor during this early asymptomatic phase presumably would improve the chance for cure. Although mass surveillance programs for esophageal cancer are not likely to be cost-effective in this country, where the incidence of the disease in the general population is low, the Chinese experience at least supports the concept of surveillance to detect nascent malignancies for certain high-risk groups such as patients with Barrett's esophagus.

TREATMENT CONSIDERATIONS

Without treatment, cancer of the esophagus appears to be uniformly fatal. Approximately 85% of untreated symptomatic patients die within six months, and none are alive at the end of two years (Roberts 1980). Treatment does improve these grisly statistics, but not dramatically. Despite therapy, only 5% of all patients with cancer of the esophagus are alive five years after the establishment of the diagnosis (Sondik et al. 1985). On the brighter side, cures, though uncommon, do occur. Furthermore, treatment can provide substantial palliation for many patients debilitated by dysphagia and aspiration. Treatment clearly is warranted, but what constitutes the proper treatment for esophageal cancer remains unclear.

Surgical therapy has the advantage of immediate removal of the esophageal tumor, and it can result in both the immediate palliation of symptoms and the prospect for cure. The cost of tumor resection is an operative mortality rate of approximately 30% (with wide variations between individual series), substantial postoperative morbidity, and a distressingly low rate of cure (Earlam and Cunha-Melo 1980a). Unlike surgery, radiation therapy is associated with little acute mortality. Radiotherapy can be directed against the primary tumor and against a wider area of potential microscopic tumor deposits than is practical with surgery (Pearson 1977). The major disadvantages of radiotherapy include the length of time necessary for its completion (often six to eight weeks), the long interval between onset of treatment and any palliation of symptoms (often two to three weeks), radiation damage to normal structures (heart, lungs, spinal cord, esophagus), and a distressingly low rate of cure (Earlam and Cunha-Melo 1980b). Chemotherapy has the potential to eradicate widespread metastatic tumor deposits—an important consideration for a disease that is usually disseminated at the time of diagnosis. The disadvantages of chemotherapy are its substantial associated morbidity and mortality, the frequent failure of the tumor to respond, and the relatively brief duration of the response when it occurs (Kelsen et al. 1984).

The clinician who must recommend therapy for the patient with cancer of the esophagus confronts a bewildering array of treatment options. If operative therapy is chosen, the surgeon must decide on the approach (right or left thoracotomy or no thoracotomy but separate abdominal and cervical incisions), the operation (esophagectomy or bypass, extent of resection), and the reconstructive procedure (esophagogastrostomy, colon interposition, reverse gastric tube, jejunal interposition). If radiation therapy is selected, the radiotherapist must choose the dose, the duration of therapy, the interval between treatments, and the extent of the field. If the option is chemotherapy, the chemotherapist must select the agent or agents, the doses, and the schedule for administration. Furthermore, any of these three treatment modalities can be used alone or in combination with one or both of the others. For example, radiation or chemotherapy or both can be given preoperatively or postoperatively. The number of possible permutations and combinations of these treatment options is formidable.

Since chemotherapy is seldom used as the sole therapeutic modality for esophageal cancer, the clinician's initial treatment decision usually involves a choice between surgery and radiotherapy. This task would be simple if one treatment regimen was clearly superior to the other, but this is not the case. Comparative therapeutic trials are lacking. Most reports merely document an institution's experience with one therapeutic regimen, and the outcomes of such studies are inconclusive. The results of either form of treatment are sadly similar, having cumulative five-year survival rates of approximately 5% (Earlam and Cunha-Melo 1980a, 1980b). The range of reported survival statistics is wide, however, with individual institutions describing five-year survival rates ranging from 1% to more than 40%.

This great disparity in reported survival rates between institutions using similar treatment regimens adds to the difficulty in choosing a therapy. Some of these apparent differences in survival rates are artificial, however, resulting from differences in the patient populations studied and the methods for calculating survival. When interpreting these statistics, therefore, one should consider the following factors that influence survival rates for patients with cancer of the esophagus:

1. Did the study include patients known to have disseminated disease, or was it limited to patients with apparently localized tumors? Survival would be expected to be better for the latter group.
2. In surgical series, were the survival rates estimated for all patients evaluated, only for patients who had operations, or only for patients who had esophageal resections for cure? In radiotherapy series, similarly, did the survival statistics include all patients evaluated, only patients irradiated, or only those irradiated for cure? Ordinarily, curative therapy is attempted only for patients believed to have localized disease who are judged capable of surviving the treatment. Long-term survival rates for such patients would be expected to exceed those of patients deemed incurable because of advanced disease or severe comorbidity.
3. Was the survival rate calculated for all patients who entered the study or only for those who successfully completed therapy? In some series, survival statistics are reported only for patients who survived curative surgery or radiotherapy. Comparisons of such results with those of studies in which survival rates include all patients treated may be misleading.
4. What was the percentage of women in the study population? Survival rates appear to be slightly better for women than for men (Cukingnan and Carey 1978; Sondik et al. 1985); therefore, variations in the percentage of female patients studied could influence the survival statistics.
5. What was the percentage of black patients in the study population? Survival rates are worse for black patients than for white patients (Sondik et al. 1985); therefore, variations in the percentage of black patients studied could influence the survival statistics.
6. Does the study include only patients with squamous cell carcinoma, only those with adenocarcinoma, or both? It is not clear if there are substantial differences in survival rates between patients with these different histological types of esophageal cancer, because data on this issue are contradictory. Nevertheless, it is conceivable that there are such differences in survival rates and that they could alter overall survival statistics if these two are not separated.

Presently, it is difficult to draw meaningful conclusions about what constitutes the "best" treatment for cancer of the esophagus. Prospective, randomized therapeutic trials are sorely needed in this area. In the absence of such studies, a strong case can be made for entry of newly diagnosed patients into well-designed, established research protocols whenever possible. Such an approach eliminates the anguish of choosing among treatments of dubious value, provides clear guidelines for disease management, and offers an opportunity to evaluate the efficacy of the therapy in a systematic and meaningful fashion.

Because esophageal malignancies are frequently disseminated at the time of diagnosis, research efforts directed at refining surgical and radiotherapy techniques to deal with localized tumor may not result in dramatic increases in survival rates. The development of effective systemic therapy for eliminating metastatic tumor deposits may be more productive and should receive higher priority. Research directed at implementing surveillance programs and preventive measures for populations at high risk for developing esophageal cancer might also decrease the unacceptable mortality rate from this devastating disease.

REFERENCES

Anderson LL, Lad TE. 1982. Autopsy findings in squamous-cell carcinoma of the esophagus. *Cancer* 50:1587–1590.

Audigier JC, Tuyns AJ, Lambert R. 1975. Epidemiology of oesophageal cancer in France: Increasing mortality and persistent correlation with alcoholism. *Digestion* 13:209–219.

Bosch A, Frias Z, Caldwell WL. 1979. Adenocarcinoma of the esophagus. *Cancer* 43: 1557–1561.

Cahan WG. 1977. Multiple primary cancers of the lung, esophagus, and other sites. *Cancer* 40:1954–1960.

Cukingnan RA, Carey JS. 1978. Carcinoma of the esophagus. *Ann Thorac Surg* 26:274–286.

Earlam R, Cunha-Melo JR. 1980a. Oesophageal squamous cell carcinoma: I. A critical review of surgery. *Br J Surg* 67:381–390.

Earlam R, Cunha-Melo JR. 1980b. Oesophageal squamous cell carcinoma: II. A critical review of radiotherapy. *Br J Surg* 67:457–461.

Fleming JAC. 1943. Carcinoma of the thoracic oesophagus: Some notes on its pathology and spread in relation to treatment. *Br J Radiol* 16:212–216.

Freni SC. 1984. Long-term trends in the incidence rates of upper digestive tract cancer in the Netherlands Antilles. *Cancer* 53:1618–1624.

Gilder SSB. 1977. Carcinoma of the esophagus. *Ann Intern Med* 87:494.

Goldstein HM, Zornoza J. 1978. Association of squamous cell carcinoma of the head and neck with cancer of the esophagus. *AJR* 131:791–794.

Goodner JT, Watson WL. 1956. Cancer of the esophagus: Its association with other primary cancers. *Cancer* 9:1248–1252.

Guanrei Y, He H, Sungliang Q, et al. 1982. Endoscopic diagnosis of 115 cases of early esophageal carcinoma. *Endoscopy* 14:157–161.

Guernsey JM, Knudsen DF, Mark JBD. 1970. Abdominal exploration in the evaluation of patients with carcinoma of the thoracic esophagus. *J Thorac Cardiovasc Surg* 59:62–66.

Haggitt RC, Dean PJ. 1985. Adenocarcinoma in Barrett's epithelium. In *Barrett's Esophagus: Pathophysiology, Diagnosis, and Management*, SJ Spechler, RK Goyal, eds., pp. 153–166. New York: Elsevier.

Kelsen D, Bains M, Hilaris B, et al. 1984. Combined-modality therapy of esophageal cancer. *Semin Oncol* 11:169–177.

Kmet J, Mahboubi E. 1972. Esophageal cancer in the Caspian littoral of Iran: Initial Studies. *Science* 175:846–853.

McCort JJ. 1952. Radiographic identification of lymph node metastases from carcinoma of the esophagus. *Radiology* 59:691–711.

MacDonald WC. 1972. Clinical and pathologic features of adenocarcinoma of the gastric cardia. *Cancer* 29:724–732.

Merendino KA, Mark VH. 1952. An analysis of one hundred cases of squamous cell carcinoma of the esophagus: Part II. With special reference to its theoretical curability. *Surg Gynecol Obstet* 94:110–114.

Pearson JG. 1977. The present status and future potential of radiotherapy in the management of esophageal cancer. *Cancer* 39:882–890.

Roberts JG. 1980. Cancer of the oesophagus—How should tumour biology affect treatment? *Br J Surg* 67:791–797.

Rosenberg JC, Roth JA, Lichter AS et al. 1985. Cancer of the esophagus. In *Cancer: Principles and Practice of Oncology*, 2 ed., VT DeVita Jr, S Hellman, SA Rosenberg, eds., pp. 621–657. Philadelphia: J. B. Lippincott.

Shapshay SM, Hong WK, Fried MP, et al. 1980. Simultaneous carcinomas of the esophagus and upper aerodigestive tract. *Otolaryngol Head Neck Surg* 88:373–377.

Shibuya H, Takagi M, Horiuchi J, et al. 1982. Carcinomas of the esophagus with synchronous or metachronous primary carcinoma in other organs. *Acta Radiol Oncol* 21:39–43.

Sjogren RW Jr, Johnson LF. 1983. Barrett's esophagus: A review. *Am J Med* 74:313–321.

Sondik EJ, Young JL, Horm JW, et al. 1985. *1985 Annual Cancer Statistics Review*. Bethesda, Md.: National Cancer Advisory Board, National Institutes of Health.

Spechler SJ, Goyal RK. 1986. Barrett's esophagus. *N Engl J Med* 315:362–371.

Wang HH, Antonioli DA, Goldman H. 1986. Comparative features of esophageal and gastric adenocarcinomas: Recent changes in type and frequency. *Hum Pathol* 17:482–487.

Watson, WL, Goodner JT, Miller TP, et al. 1956. Torek esophagectomy: The case against segmental resection for esophageal cancer. *J Thorac Surg* 32:347–357.

Wynder EL, Bross IJ. 1961. A study of etiological factors in cancer of the esophagus. *Cancer* 14:389–413.

Ying-kai W, Guo-jun H, Ling-fang S, et al. 1982. Progress in the study and surgical treatment of cancer of the esophagus in China, 1940–1980. *J Thorac Cardiovasc Surg* 84:325–333.

Annual Clinical Conference on Cancer, Vol. 30
Gastrointestinal Cancer: Current Approaches to Diagnosis and Treatment
© 1988 by The University of Texas System Cancer Center

21. Clinical Trials with Cisplatin, Vindesine, and Bleomycin: Neoadjuvant Chemotherapy for Epidermoid Carcinoma of the Esophagus

Jack A. Roth, Harvey I. Pass, Margaret M. Flanagan,
Geoffrey M. Graeber, Jerry C. Rosenberg,
and Seth M. Steinberg

The results of single-modality treatment for epidermoid carcinoma of the esophagus have not been satisfactory. In general, overall actuarial survival at five years for patients undergoing surgical resection is 10% (Postlethwait 1979; Wang and Chien 1983). The results for radiation therapy used alone are equally disappointing (Beatty, DeBoer, and Rider 1979; Leborgne, Leborgne, and Barlocci 1963; Wara, Mauch, and Thomas 1976). This is not surprising because both surgery and radiation therapy influence local control of the tumor and cannot affect disseminated metastases that may be present at diagnosis. Several autopsy series have demonstrated that, for most patients, tumor is already disseminated at or shortly after diagnosis (Anderson and Lad 1982; Isono et al. 1982). Thus, therapy that is limited to the primary tumor and periesophageal tissue is likely to fail. This has influenced investigators to combine local treatment with systemic chemotherapy in an attempt to control subclinical metastases. In recent studies, chemotherapy has been administered prior to definitive local treatment.

Administration of preoperative neoadjuvant chemotherapy to patients with esophageal carcinoma has several theoretical advantages. One is that reducing the size of the tumor may enable the surgeon to completely resect it. Also, Goldie and Coldman (1984) have advanced the hypothesis that the probability for development of drug-resistant cells correlates positively with tumor burden. Therefore, when metastatic tumor burden is low, preoperative chemotherapy may minimize drug resistance. Preoperative chemotherapy has been shown to be superior to postoperative therapy in some animal models (Fisher, Gunduz, and Saffer 1983; Pendergrast, Drake, and Mardinay 1976). Finally, the true effectiveness of single or combination drug therapy with respect to the primary tumor can be determined if chemotherapy is administered prior to surgery. Because of these theoretical considerations, adjuvant trials have focused on the use of preoperative (neoadjuvant) chemotherapy.

PREVIOUS STUDIES WITH CISPLATIN-CONTAINING COMBINATIONS

The response rate of epidermoid esophageal cancer to single-agent chemotherapy is low (Kelsen 1982). The report of high response rates with cisplatin-based combinations stimulated a number of single-arm feasibility trials involving combination chemotherapy followed by surgery. Three trials have been reported by Kelsen and coworkers. In the first trial (Kelsen et al. 1978), 34 patients with potentially resectable tumors received one cycle of cisplatin-bleomycin prior to surgery (performed on preop day 21). Three to five additional courses of chemotherapy were given postoperatively at six- to eight-week intervals. For the total group of 61 patients, including some with metastatic tumors, the response rate was 15%. Survival following resection in these patients was not different from that of a historical control group.

In a second trial (Kelsen et al. 1983) vindesine was added to the above regimen, and the overall response rate for 68 evaluable patients was 53%. The median survival for 34 patients who underwent surgical exploration was 16.2 months. This survival time was significantly longer than that of the historical control group receiving cisplatin and bleomycin.

In a third study by Kelsen and coworkers (1986), the combination of cisplatin, mitoguazone, and vindesine was studied. The overall response rate was 41% in 42 patients. Toxicity levels and survival rates were similar to those observed with combined cisplatin, vindesine, and bleomycin (DVB).

Schlag and coworkers treated 23 patients with potentially resectable tumors with two cycles of combined cisplatin, vindesine, and bleomycin prior to surgery (Schlag, Hermann, and Fritze 1985). The resection rate was 78%, and the response rate was 44%.

Cisplatin-based combination chemotherapy has also been combined with preoperative radiation therapy. Steiger and coworkers (1981) treated 31 patients with cisplatin and continuous infusion 5-fluorouracil. Twenty-one of those patients underwent esophagectomy. Leichman and coworkers (1984) preoperatively treated 21 patients with combined chemotherapy and radiation therapy. The resection rate was 71%; however, 27% of those patients had treatment-related deaths. The median survival for all patients entered in the trial was 18 months; median survival was 24 months for patients who had no tumor in the resected specimen. Thus, in this study, the addition of preoperative radiotherapy did not improve median survival but did appear to increase treatment-related toxicity.

RANDOMIZED TRIAL OF PRE- AND POSTOPERATIVE CISPLATIN, VINDESINE, AND BLEOMYCIN

The high response rates and prolonged survival for patients receiving preoperative cisplatin-based chemotherapy in phase II trials indicated to us that a randomized trial of preoperative chemotherapy was warranted. The DVB combination was chosen because of the high response rates reported with it in the absence of radio-

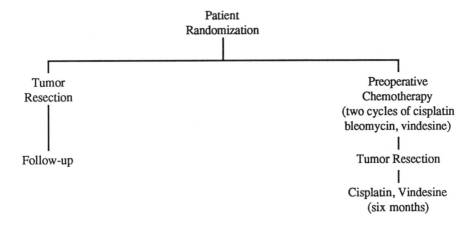

Fig. 21.1. Design of randomized clinical trial to assess the efficacy of pre- and postoperative DVB chemotherapy.

therapy. Postoperative chemotherapy was given for six months because relapses had occurred in a significant number of patients in all phase II studies. The study design is shown in figure 21.1.

PATIENTS AND METHODS

Thirty-nine of 63 patients evaluated for the study were entered into the trials between November 1, 1982, and May 1, 1986. Participating in the cooperative study were the National Institutes of Health, Bethesda, Maryland; Walter Reed Army Medical Center, Washington, D.C.; and Hutzel Hospital, Detroit, Michigan. All patients entered into the study had histological proof of esophageal carcinoma on the preoperative biopsy specimen. In two cases, the diagnosis was undifferentiated carcinoma, and for the remaining cases the diagnosis was epidermoid carcinoma. All tumors originated in the middle or lower third of the thoracic esophagus. Patients were excluded from the study because of the following: extensive local invasion precluding complete surgical resection; lymph node metastases to distant nodal groups; serious concurrent medical disease; biopsy-proven metastases; prior radiation therapy to the thoracic or cervical area; prior major thoracic, gastric, cardiac, or neck surgery; hematologic abnormalities.

The staging system developed by the Union Internationale Contre le Cancer (1982) was used. All patients were initially evaluated with chest roentgenograms, barium swallow and upper gastrointestinal tract series, chest and abdominal computerized tomography scans, bone scans, audiograms, and pulmonary function studies. Bronchoscopy and esophagoscopy were also performed prior to randomization, and all patients signed an informed consent statement. Randomization was done by computer following stratification by tumor location (middle or lower third), sex, and tumor size (by the TNM classification).

Cisplatin (Bristol Laboratories, Syracuse, New York) was administered on day 1 at 3 mg/kg or 120 mg/m^2 (whichever was less) in 3% NaCl with prehydration and a mannitol-induced diuresis. Metoclopramide was given as an antiemetic (Kris et al. 1985). Vindesine (Eli Lilly, Indianapolis, Indiana) (3 mg/m^2) was given on days 1, 8, 15, and 22 of the first two cycles. Bleomycin (Bristol Laboratories, Evansville, Indiana) was given initially in a loading dose of 10 U/m^2 on day 3 followed by an intravenous infusion of 10 U/m^2 over 24 hours for days 4–6. The total dose of bleomycin did not exceed 100 U/m^2. Following the two preoperative cycles and surgery, patients received cisplatin every six weeks and vindesine every two weeks for six months.

Patients were classified as having a complete response only if no tumor was present in the complete resected specimen. Patients classified as having a partial response demonstrated more than 50% reduction in two perpendicular diameters of the tumor as measured by serial radiographic studies. Patients were classified as having progressive disease if there was more than a 25% increase in the size of the primary lesion or if there was development of metastases. Stabilization was indicated when the patient's status failed to qualify for either a response or progressive disease.

The primary tumor was considered to have been completely resected if, in the surgeon's opinion, all local tumor was removed and the histopathological examination of all margins, including the deep margin, was negative for tumor (>2 high-power microscopic fields separating tumor and normal tissue).

Patients were followed at three-month intervals. Studies included a barium swallow, chest roentgenogram, computerized tomograms of the abdomen, and a bone scan.

Survival curves were constructed using the method of Kaplan and Meier. When reported, differences between survival curves were computed using the Mantel-Haenszel method. Tests for association among treatment and response categories and prognostic variables were conducted using Fisher's exact test and two-sided p values for 2 × 2 tables, whereas the chi-square test was used to obtain approximate p values for the 2 × 3 tables.

RESULTS

Thirty-nine patients were randomized in the study. Because of three protocol violations following randomization (one in the surgery only arm and two in the surgery and chemotherapy arm), only 36 patients could be evaluated. An additional 24 patients were initially selected for the study but were not entered because of medical contraindications (10), documented extraesophageal spread (10), ineligible diagnosis (3), or refusal to be randomized (1). The median follow-up for both groups was 30 months.

No statistically significant differences occurred between the two randomized groups for the stratified and nonstratified prognostic factors, including age, percentage of weight loss at diagnosis, administration of total parenteral nutrition, and performance status.

The toxicity of the preoperative chemotherapy was manageable, and no deaths were directly attributable to the chemotherapy. For the 17 patients treated with chemotherapy, 17 had alopecia, 2 had severe nausea and vomiting, 1 had bleomycin pulmonary toxicity, 1 developed sepsis, and 1 had severe neuropathy. Hematologic toxicity was mild with mean nadir values of 1.8 for the white blood cell count, 9.2 for the hemoglobin, and 162 for the platelets. Renal toxicity was also acceptable, and no patients required dialysis. The mean maximum values for blood urea nitrogen and serum creatinine were 25 and 1.4. The mean nadir creatinine clearance was 52. There were two treatment-related deaths, both occurring in the surgery and chemotherapy arm. Both deaths occurred postoperatively during hospitalization. The postoperative complication rate was not increased in the surgery and chemotherapy group. Nine of the 19 patients in the surgery arm (47%) and 5 of the 17 patients in the surgery and chemotherapy arm (29%) had postoperative complications. The differences in complication rates between the two arms of the study were not statistically significant. The incidence of complications related to infections was not increased in the group receiving preoperative chemotherapy.

Administration of the chemotherapy was well-tolerated both pre- and postoperatively. The percentages of the drug dosages specified in the protocol and received by the patients was: cisplatin, 99%; bleomycin, 88%; vindesine, 77%. Myelosuppression and neuropathy were generally the dose-limiting toxic effects for vindesine. Eight of the 17 patients receiving chemotherapy had major responses preoperatively (47%). These included one complete response and seven partial responses. In the remaining patients, there were seven stabilizations and two cases of disease progression. If a patient did not have a response following the first preoperative cycle of chemotherapy, then no response was observed following the second cycle.

There was no statistically significant difference in the resectability rates between the two randomized groups. However, there was a slightly higher percentage of patients in the surgery and chemotherapy arm in whom histological results at the margins were negative following resection (35% vs. 21%).

There was no statistically significant difference between the actuarial survival curves for the two groups of patients. The median survival for both groups was nine months. The estimated actuarial survival at 36 months was 25% for the group receiving chemotherapy and 5% for the surgery only group. However, those patients who had a major response preoperatively to the chemotherapy had a significantly longer actuarial survival than did the patients who did not respond (p2=.008). The survival of the responders was also significantly greater than that of the surgery only group (p2=.05).

Analysis of prognostic factors was then performed to determine whether differences in the distribution of a prognostic factor could completely explain the survival differences between chemotherapy responders and nonresponders. Patient sex, age, and tumor location (middle or lower third) did not correlate with survival. However, those patients with less than a 10% weight loss prior to randomization survived significantly longer than did those patients with a 10% or greater weight loss (p2=.0025). All responding patients had less than a 10% weight loss and thus were in a favorable prognostic group. The median survival for those patients in the surgery only arm who had less than a 10% weight loss was 15 months. The median survival for the chemotherapy responders has not been reached. Thus, it appears that a more favorable pretreatment prognosis is only one factor contributing to the longer survival time of the group of patients responding to chemotherapy.

CONCLUSIONS

Preoperative DVB chemotherapy can be safely given preoperatively to patients with epidermoid carcinoma of the esophagus. Preoperative chemotherapy does not increase the frequency of postoperative complications. Although this study did not conclusively demonstrate a survival benefit for the group receiving preoperative chemotherapy, it is clear that any such benefit would be confined to patients responding to that treatment. The significance of differences between responders and nonresponders remains controversial. The difference observed in our study could not be explained by lead time bias because all patients who responded did so within the first month of treatment and no deaths occurred before one month of treatment had been completed. Thus, it is reasonable to assume that response to therapy was similar to an initial characteristic in that it was determined in all patients prior to any deaths on either arm of the study. However, all responders had less than a 10% weight loss, indicating that they belonged to a favorable prognostic group. This characteristic may influence response to chemotherapy, and the apparent benefit of the chemotherapy to the responders could simply be a reflection of their overall better prognosis. However, the median survival of the chemotherapy responders was still superior to patients with less than a 10% weight loss who did not receive chemotherapy.

Thus, the survival benefits of preoperative DVB chemotherapy appear to be confined to patients with less advanced tumors, and it seems logical to concentrate on this group of patients in future studies. Subsequent studies must also focus on the development of new drug combinations that can produce higher complete response rates.

REFERENCES

Anderson I, Lad T. 1982. Autopsy findings in squamous cell carcinoma of the esophagus. *Cancer* 50:1587–1590.

Beatty JD, DeBoer G, Rider WD. 1979. Carcinoma of the esophagus: Pretreatment assessment, correlation of radiation treatment parameters with survival, and identification and management of radiation treatment failure. *Cancer* 43:2254–2267.

Fisher B, Gunduz N, Saffer EA. 1983. Influence of the interval between primary tumor removal and chemotherapy on kinetics and growth of metastases. *Cancer Res* 43:1488–1492.

Goldie JH, Coldman AJ. 1984. The genetic origin of drug resistance in neoplasms: Implications for systemic therapy. *Cancer Res* 44:3643–3653.

Isono K, Onoda S, Ishikawa T, et al. 1982. Studies on the causes of deaths from esophageal carcinoma. *Cancer* 49:2173–2179.

Kelsen D. 1982. Treatment of advanced esophageal cancer. *Cancer* 50:2576–2581.

Kelsen D, Hilaris B, Coonley C, et al. 1983. Cisplatin, vindesine, and bleomycin chemotherapy of local, regional, and advanced esophageal carcinoma. *Am J Med* 75:645–652.

Kelsen DP, Cvitkovic E, Bains M, et al. 1978. *Cis*-dichlorodiammineplatinum (II) and bleomycin in the treatment of esophageal carcinomas. *Cancer Treat Rep* 62:1041–1046.

Kelsen DP, Fein R, Coonley C, et al. 1986. Cisplatin, vindesine and mitoguazone in the treatment of esophageal cancer. *Cancer Treat Rep* 70:255–259.

Kris MG, Gralla RJ, Tyson LB, et al. 1985. Improved control of cisplatin-induced emesis with high-dose metoclopramide and with combinations of metoclopramide, dexamethasone, and diphenhydramine. Results of consecutive trials in 255 patients. *Cancer* 55:527–534.

Leborgne R, Leborgne JF, Barlocci L. 1963. Cancer of the esophagus: Results of radiotherapy. *Br J Radiol* 36:806–811.

Leichman L, Steiger Z, Seydel HG, et al. 1984. Preoperative chemotherapy and radiation therapy for patients with cancer of the esophagus: A potentially curative approach. *J Clin Oncol* 2:75–79.

Pendergrast WJ, Drake WP, Mardinay MR. 1976. A proper sequence for the treatment of B16 melanoma: Chemotherapy, surgery, and immunotherapy. *JNCI* 57:539–544.

Postlethwait RW. 1979. *Surgery of the Esophagus*. New York: Appleton-Century-Crofts.

Schlag HR, Hermann R, Fritze D. 1985. Pre-operative chemotherapy in localized cancer of the esophagus with cisplatinum, vindesine, and bleomycin. In *Primary Chemotherapy in Cancer Medicine*, D Wagner, G Blijhan, J Smeets, J Wils, eds., pp. 253–258, New York: Alan R. Liss.

Steiger Z, Franklin R, Wilson RF, et al. 1981. Eradication and palliation of squamous cell carcinoma of the esophagus with chemotherapy, radiotherapy, and surgical therapy. *J Thorac Cardiovasc Surg* 82:713–719.

Union Internationale Contre le Cancer 1982. Oesophagus. In *TNM-Atlas, Illustrated Guide to the Classification of Malignant Tumors*, B Spiessl, O Scheibe, G Wagner, eds., pp. 60–69, New York: Springer-Verlag.

Wang PY, Chien KY. 1983. Surgical treatment of carcinoma of the esophagus and cardia among the Chinese. *Ann Thorac Surg* 35:143–151.

Wara WM, Mauch PM, Thomas AN. 1976. Palliation for carcinoma of the esophagus. *Radiology* 121:717–720.

Annual Clinical Conference on Cancer, Vol. 30
Gastrointestinal Cancer: Current Approaches to Diagnosis and Treatment
© 1988 by The University of Texas System Cancer Center

22. Radiotherapy for Esophageal Cancer

Tyvin A. Rich and Jaffer A. Ajani

Until recently, esophageal cancer has not been a favorite discussion topic for either the radiation, medical, or surgical oncologist. The results of radiation treatment, even with modern radiotherapy equipment, have been dismal. The survival data from both radiotherapy and surgical series usually show cure rates of about 5% to 15%.

The collated review of 8,489 patients with esophageal cancer by Earlam and Cunha-Melo (1980) and two large series from The Univeristy of Texas M.D. Anderson Hospital and Tumor Institute at Houston, Texas (MDAH) (Barkley et al. 1981) and from Princess Margaret Hospital, Toronto, Canada (Beatty, DeBoer, and Rider 1979) identify several important factors associating radiotherapy with excellent palliation: younger age, high performance status, female sex, location of lesion (in some series), and absence of distant metastasis. Factors based on surgical staging, such as primary disease extent and lymph node status, may bias the data through treatment selection.

A prospective comparison of radiotherapy versus surgery is lacking, even though some believe that radiotherapy is as effective a treatment for most patients with this highly lethal illness. Although radiotherapy has disadvantages (length of treatment time, acute side effects of esophagitis, or, rarely, pneumonitis), this modality, particularly when used with chemotherapy, can be very effective in achieving palliation and possibly higher cure rates (Beatty, DeBoer, and Rider 1979). Virtually no mortality has been reported with radiotherapy alone or chemoradiation.

In this chapter we focus on recently published studies using chemotherapy and radiotherapy and discuss the preliminary results achieved at MDAH using our combined-modality therapy incorporating systemic therapy and chemoradiation.

RATIONALE OF CHEMOTHERAPY PLUS RADIOTHERAPY

The historical data on failure patterns have demonstrated that a high percentage of patients experience disease recurrence both locally and systemically after "curative" radiotherapy (Beatty, DeBoer, and Rider 1979). In an autopsy series from MDAH, 20 of 24 patients had a component of local failure (Barkley et al. 1980). The incidence of local relapse after radiotherapy is probably related to the initial tumor burden, although one series from the Massachusetts General Hospital showed unacceptable actuarial local failure rates of 50% for patients with T1 tumors and 84% for those with T2 or T3 tumors at two years (Langer et al. 1986). This high local failure rate after radiotherapy alone is an obvious reason for enhancing tumor response by interaction (one hopes synergistic) between the chemotherapeutic agent and radiation, without increasing normal tissue complications unacceptably.

The selection of chemotherapeutic agents to use against esophageal cancer has been empiric and based on information regarding single-agent "response," since survival, per se, has rarely been affected. Beginning in the mid-1970s and continuing until the present, there have been several enthusiastic reports on the use of combination chemotherapy in conjunction with radiation for patients with squamous cell cancers of the esophagus (Coia, Engstrom, and Paul 1986; Richmond et al. 1986). Although some radiation biologists have studied these combinations in vitro, success in guiding the clinician in the choice of drugs, administration schedules, or dosage has been mainly elusive. Recent seminal work from Byfield et al. (1982) on the optimal scheduling of 5-fluorouracil (5-FU) has been derived directly from radiobiologic models in the laboratory.

Combined-modality therapy using chemotherapy and radiation is not a novel idea. In the last MDAH gastrointestinal cancer symposium in 1980, we reported on 27 patients who had been treated between 1970 and 1973 with hydroxyurea and radiation (30 Gy in 10 fractions, Barkley et al. 1980). These patients suffered from severe acute reactions necessitating a reduction in radiation dose and later leading to abandonment of the treatment protocol. Although the local recurrence rate was only 11% (3/27) and survival ranged up to 96 months for one patient, the overall survival duration was poor (7.6 months, median).

Another early report, describing the results with bleomycin and radiation, was a nonrandomized study by Kolaric, Roth, and Dujinovic (1976); radiation doses ranging from 50 to 70 Gy led to a one-year survival rate of 55%. This beneficial result was not confirmed in a randomized study later performed by the Eastern Cooperative Oncology Group (ECOG), which found no difference in median survival duration for patients treated with 50 to 60 Gy and bleomycin versus radiation alone (Earle et al. 1980).

There was, however, interest in preoperative radiotherapy plus bleomycin, especially based on the encouraging results by Fujimaki (1975), who used 30 Gy combined with chemotherapy. Of 76 patients studied, 48 underwent resection; the five-year survival rate was 17% (8/48), but 8 of 27 (30%) at risk for three or more years were still alive (Fujimaki 1975). In another trial by Werner (1979), preoperative radiotherapy (20 Gy) plus methotrexate followed by 36 Gy after resection for selected patients, resulted in a 26-month average survival. Thirty-six patients who did not have surgical resection survived a median of 23 months.

These preliminary data from the 1970s have served as a basis for more intensive combined-modality studies in the last six years that have focused mainly on 5-FU and cisplatin with or without irradiation. Three different approaches have been explored: (1) preoperative chemotherapy with or without postoperative irradiation, (2) preoperative chemotherapy combined with irradiation, and (3) radical chemo-radiotherapy without surgery.

PREOPERATIVE CHEMOTHERAPY WITH OR WITHOUT POSTOPERATIVE IRRADIATION

The use of multiagent preoperative chemotherapy has grown because single-agent therapy yields only marginal response rates of 13% to 40% (see Ajani et al. in this volume). Two important studies from Memorial Sloan-Kettering Hospital, New York, document up to a 63% objective response in the primary tumor after treatment with cisplatin, vindesine, and bleomycin (Kelsen et al. 1984). The highest response rate with this regimen published to date is 76%, including a 20% clinical complete response (CR) (Marsh 1986). Unfortunately, these clinical response rates do not translate into similar pathological CR rates when the surgical specimen is examined miscoscopically. For example, the report by Carey et al. (1986) on cisplatin and 5-FU indicated an objective clinical response rate of 73% (CR + partial response [PR]) and a response evident on endoscopic examination in up to 45% of the patients. However, only 5% (1/24) had a pathological CR. Similar data have been reported by Kelsen et al. (1984), who used cisplatin, bleomycin, and vindesine.

The effect on survival of chemotherapy alone is difficult to assess. The data on single-agent therapy indicate response durations of four to eight months (Marsh 1986). The potential benefits are further obscured by adding preoperative irradiation or surgery. The results of preoperative chemotherapy consisting of cisplatin, bleomycin, and vindesine evaluated in a prospective randomized trial at the National Cancer Institute demonstrated a survival benefit for the responding patients (see Roth et al. in this volume). In summary, the data supporting a survival benefit for chemotherapy in esophageal cancer are not conclusive. Clearly some data indicate drug "activity" on measurable disease and, therefore, presumably on micrometastatic disease as well.

PREOPERATIVE CHEMORADIOTHERAPY

Preoperative radiotherapy alone has been used in many centers in accordance with certain assumptions, such as (1) inoperable cancers may become operable and (2) theoretically, irradiation may reduce the number of viable cancer cells shed into the wound and bloodstream at the time of surgical manipulation, thereby decreasing metastasis. Furthermore, preoperative radiotherapy appears to be a powerful means of pathologically downstaging patients.

Survival rates between 2% and 35% have been reported for preoperative irradiation alone in several large nonrandomized studies (Hancock and Glatstein 1984). In the only randomized study, Launois, Delarue, and Campion (1981) reported a five-year survival rate of 9.5% for radiotherapy alone, which was no different from that of the surgical control arm. At MDAH, 86 patients were treated with preoperative radiation, and 14 patients (25% of those resected) were alive 9 to 66 months later. The median survival duration was 11.6 months. However, an underlying criticism of preoperative radiotherapy is that selection obviously plays a role in the choice of treatment. Since patients who can be made operable by preoperative irradiation may be in a better performance category, the success measured may not necessarily reflect the treatment delivered.

In an effort to increase the proportion of patients whose cancers are operable, Wayne State University began, roughly 10 years ago, pilot studies using preoperative chemoradiotherapy (Steiger et al. 1981a). Based on some encouraging results from combinations of 5-FU and mitomycin C plus concomitant radiotherapy for rectal adenocarcinoma and squamous cell carcinoma of the anus, the investigators examined the radioresponsiveness of squamous cell carcinoma of the esophagus. Their first report (1981a) demonstrated that preoperative chemotherapy (5-FU + mitomycin or cisplatin) and 30 Gy resulted in a 37% (13/37) pathological CR. In this report, the superiority of cisplatin was demonstrated by a lower operative morbidity (25% vs. 52%) in patients receiving cisplatin rather than mitomycin C in conjunction with 5-FU and irradiation. In a second study, the Wayne State group reported a higher pathological CR rate of 47% (7/15) in the primary lesion when cisplatin and 5-FU were combined with irradiation (Leichman et al. 1984). The later study reported a high operative mortality of 26% (5/19); however, more prudent selection of patients for surgical therapy may substantially decrease this mortality, since three of the postoperative deaths reported were of patients with initially unresectable disease.

Survival durations for patients treated with preoperative chemoradiation (5-FU or cisplatin-based regimens) have been reported in the range of 12 to 24 months, and two-year survival rates have been as high as 33% to 44% (Leichman et al. 1984b; Parker et al. 1985; Miller, McIntyre, and Hatcher 1985; Richmond et al. 1986). In one other study, overall survival was significantly higher for the combined-modality group compared to matched historical controls (Popp et al. 1986). The analysis by Leichman et al. (1984b) indicated that among 16 of 42 patients who had a pathological CR after completing all phases of combined therapy, the survival rate was 92% (median duration = 3.5 years). Although these data are very remarkable for the responding patients, the overall value of preoperative chemoradiation cannot be fully understood until prospective trials are completed. Radiation Therapy Oncology Group is presently assessing a phase III trial of preoperative radiotherapy alone versus preoperative chemoradiotherapy.

HIGH-DOSE RADIOTHERAPY AND CONCOMITANT CHEMOTHERAPY—"RADICAL CHEMORADIOTHERAPY"

Reports of several preoperative chemoradiotherapy trials include subgroups of patients whose tumors were not resected because they were unresectable or the patients were medically unfit or refused surgery. This selection process generally means that the unresected group has a worse prognosis than the group resected. Steiger et al. (1981b) reported on "palliative" chemoradiation administered to 25 patients; 11 (44%) achieved local tumor control and were able to swallow until their death. The remaining 14 patients underwent additional palliative surgery because of obstruction or stenoses. The average survival duration for the 25 was 7 months; two lived 9 and 12.5 months, respectively. These poor control figures were not unexpected, since this group was considered for palliative therapy only. Nine patients initially had distant metastases, five had bronchoesophageal fistulas, and medical conditions precluding surgery were found in nine.

Several other reports are more encouraging regarding the "radiocurability" of esophageal cancer by radical chemoradiation. The chemotherapeutic regimens used have varied (table 22.1), but the mainstay of drug therapy has been 5-FU administered either by short (5-day) or protracted (30- to 40-day) infusions. Cisplatin is another agent that appears to be effective when combined with 5-FU and irradiation. Richmond et al. (1986) reported on 17 patients treated with radical radiation (40–60 Gy) given in "conventional" fractions of 2 to 2.5 Gy per day combined with three courses of 5-FU (1,000 mg/m^2 × 4 days) and an intravenous bolus of cisplatin (100 mg/m^2). Nonrandomized comparisons of chemoradiation and radiation alone showed a superior median survival duration (12 vs. 5 months) for chemoradiation and a 2-year survival rate of 37%. Survival differences were not seen between the groups receiving preoperative chemoradiation (30 Gy) and high-dose radiotherapy (40–60 Gy). These data suggest that chemoradiation is better than radiotherapy alone and that surgical therapy may not be necessary when doses of radiation are high ($\geq$ 60 Gy). Further supporting this concept are the data from Memorial Sloan-Kettering Hospital indicating a 22% five-year survival rate for patients treated with high-dose radiation and cisplatin and bleomycin (Coonley, Bains, and Kelsen in press), but these data are based on small numbers (2/9). Two other series with larger numbers of patients from Coia et al. (1984, 1986) and Keane et al. (1985) also substantiate this preliminary optimistic outlook. Both groups administered 5-FU by infusion, 1,000 mg/m^2 over 24 hours for four to five days, plus 10 mg/m^2 mitomycin C at the beginning of planned high-dose radiotherapy. The survival data for both groups are similar; two-year survival rates are 41% and 48%, respectively. The report from the Princess Margaret Hospital, Toronto, demonstrates an actuarial 73% local-control rate at two years, which is significantly better than that of age- and stage-matched historical controls. This study also showed the superiority of continuous irradiation (45–50 Gy) over split-course irradiation (22.5–25 Gy/10 fractions in 2 weeks × 2).

Other investigators have used a slightly different philosophy regarding "radio-sensitization" by chemotherapeutic agents. One agent that has been used repeatedly in the pilot studies described above is 5-FU—a drug that many have considered marginally effective as a single agent against squamous cancer when administered by an intravenous bolus. Experimental data suggest an increased radioenhancement when 5-FU is administered by continuous intravenous infusion and the duration of drug exposure exceeds the tumor cell-cycle time (Byfield, Barone, and Mendelsohn 1980; Byfield et al. 1982). The results of a pilot study using only 5-FU infusion (1,000 mg/m^2/24 hours × four days) and "cyclic" radiotherapy indicated a striking improvement in survival for six patients with squamous cell carcinoma of the esophagus compared with the historical control group treated at the University of California, San Diego (Byfield, Barone, and Mendelsohn 1980).

Table 22.1. Summary of "Radical" Chemoradiation Protocols

Study	Chemotherapy 5-FU	Mitomycin C	Cisplatin	Radiation Dose (Gy/Fractions/ Days)	No. of Patients	Local Control (%)	Survival
Byfield 1980	20–30 mg/kg × 5 days (5–6 cycles)	—	—	50–60/ 20–24/ 70–80	6	83	66%
Steiger 1981	1 g/m² × 4 days (2 cycles)	10 mg/m² × 1	—	50–60/ 30/ 42	25	44[a]	2 pts @ 9 and 12.5 mo
Abitbol 1983	0.8 g/m² × 4 days	—	[b]	60	9	78	30% NED 16–25 mo
Coia 1984	1 g/m² × 4 days (2 cycles)	10 mg/m² × 1	—	60/ 30/ 42–49	13	84	11/13 4–32 mo
Coia 1986	1 g/m² × 4 days (2 cycles)	10 mg/m² × 1	—	—	30	77	62% 1 yr 41% 2 yr 35% 3 yr 27% 5 yr

Study							
Keane 1985	1 g/m^2 × 4 days (1–2 cycles)	10 mg/m^2 × 1 or 2	—	35–50/ 14–20/ 28[c]	15	73	48% 2 yr[e]
				22.5–50/ 9–20/ 56[d]	20	29	13% 2 yr[e]
Coonley 1986	—	—	f	55	9	—	22% 5 yr
Richmond 1986	1 g/m^2 × 4 days (3 cycles)	—	100 mg/m^2 (3 cycles)	40–65/ 33/ 49	17	—	38% 2 yr
Current series	300 mg/m^2 [g] × 30–40 days (protracted infusion with XRT only)	—	g	30–60/ 30/ 42	8	66	88% 6–18 mo

Abbreviations: 5-FU, 5-fluorouracil; NED, no evidence of disease; XRT, radiotherapy.

[a] Percent esophageal cancer palliated.
[b] Cisplatin + methotrexate after 5-FU + irradiation.
[c] Single course.
[d] Split course.
[e] Actuarial survival.
[f] Cisplatin + bleomycin.
[g] All patients treated with 2–6 cycles systemic 5-FU (1 g/m^2/day × 5 days) and cisplatin (20 mg/m^2/day × 5 days) and radiation.

A schedule different from Byfield's short (four to five days) 5-FU infusion is that reported by Rich, Lokich, and Chaffey (1985): protracted intravenous 5-FU infusion (300 mg/m²/24 hr) combined with an entire course of conventionally fractionated irradiation (1.8–2.0 Gy per day) for five to seven weeks. Nine patients with esophageal squamous carcinoma were treated with this combination in the initial report. This group has now reported on a larger group of 12 patients with esophageal cancers, some of whom were treated initially with four to six weeks of continuous-infusion 5-FU alone followed by radiation and protracted 5-FU infusion at a rate of 300 mg/m² for 24 hours (Lokich, Rich, and Chaffey 1986). Tumor responses were seen on a barium swallow test in all patients who had chemotherapy and radiotherapy, and the local control rate was 73%. The median survival duration for the entire group was only six to eight months; however, 25% were alive without disease three years after treatment. Late complications included esophageal stricture in two patients and an esophago-mediastinal fistula in one.

SYSTEMIC CHEMOTHERAPY PLUS RADICAL CHEMORADIOTHERAPY

At MDAH we have combined several aspects of the pilot studies described above. In an effort to attack both distant and local disease, we use systemic chemotherapy first followed by 5-FU-"radiosensitized" radiotherapy with or without surgery. In the subgroup that achieves a clinical CR after only chemotherapy, we perform an esophagectomy. Those patients found to be inoperable for medical reasons or those refusing surgery receive a high dose of radiation (60–65 Gy in seven weeks). We have followed a small group of patients between 6 and 20 months since treatment who have had systemic chemotherapy and radiotherapy with or without 5-FU by protracted infusion. All of these patients presented with advanced or recurrent disease in the esophagus, and one patient had metastatic disease. Seven patients received five or six cycles of 5-FU (1,000 mg/m²/24 hr × five days) and cisplatin (20 mg/m²/day × five days with 5-FU). Radiotherapy was given to the primary tumor and mediastinum in doses of more than 55 Gy (one patient received only 30 Gy plus 5-FU, 300 mg/m² daily infusion). The survival data of these patients are illustrated in figure 22.1 along with our previous results for radiotherapy alone (1970–1979) and radiotherapy plus hydroxyurea (1970–1973). It is apparent that our recent preliminary experience on unselected patients is very encouraging.

The success of several programs using chemoradiation without surgery raises the question of the role of surgery for patients with esophageal cancer. The operative mortality for esophageal cancer ranges from less than 5% to 20% (Hancock and Glatstein 1984). Our data from MDAH showed an operative mortality of 9.5% for preoperative irradiation and 4% to 10% for surgery alone (Barkley et al. 1980). Chemoradiation could offer a reasonable alternative to surgery for most patients. A direct comparison of surgery versus radical chemoradiation is warranted to assess the effectiveness of local control and to determine survival rates. Surgery will still have an important role as salvage therapy and possibly for purposes of staging and evaluating metastatic disease.

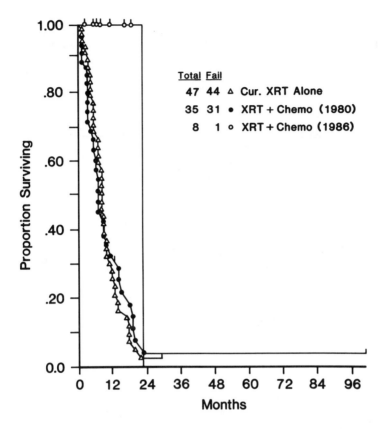

Fig. 22.1. Actuarial survival for a previously reported group of patients with esophageal cancer treated with radiotherapy alone or in combination with hydroxyurea (reported in 1980). The current series treated with radiotherapy (60 Gy) and continuous infusion of 5-FU (300 mg/m²) is shown in comparison.

SUMMARY

Combined-modality programs using systemic chemotherapy and radiotherapy are currently being studied intensively, since pilot studies have consistently shown improvement in one- and two-year survival statistics compared with historical controls. Although the mechanisms of interaction of the most popular chemotherapeutic drugs (5-FU and cisplatin) used with irradiation are not fully understood, the studies so far have indicated an acceptable level of toxicity. Pathological CRs ranging from 37% to 45% have been reported in some series and translate into excellent survival rates for some patient subgroups. The program currently under way at MDAH employs initial aggressive systemic chemotherapy followed by 5-FU-"sensitized" radiotherapy. We are encouraged by our early results, which need to be confirmed by prospective trials.

ACKNOWLEDGMENTS

This work was supported in part by grants CA 06294 and CA 16672 from the National Cancer Institute, Department of Health and Human Services, U.S.A.

REFERENCES

Barkley HT, Hussey DH, Saxton JP, et al. 1981. Radiotherapy in the treatment of carcinoma of the esophagus. In *Gastrointestinal Cancer,* JR Stroehlein, MM Romsdahl, eds. pp. 171–187. New York: Raven Press.

Beatty JD, DeBoer G, Rider WD. 1979. Carcinoma of the esophagus: Pretreatment parameters with survival and identification and management of radiation treatment failure. *Cancer* 43:2284–2287.

Byfield JR, Barone R, Mendelsohn J. 1980. Infusional 5-fluorouracil and x-ray therapy for non-resectable esophageal cancer. *Cancer* 45:703–708.

Byfield JE, Calabro-Jones P, Klisak I, et al. 1982. Pharmacologic requirements for obtaining sensitization of human tumor cells in vitro to combined 5-fluorouracil or Ftorafur and x-rays. *Int J Radiat Oncol Biol Phys* 8:1923–1933.

Carey RW, Hilgenberg AD, Wilkens EW, et al. 1986. Preoperative chemotherapy followed by surgery with possible postoperative radiotherapy in squamous cell carcinoma of the esophagus: Evaluation of the chemotherapy component. *J Clin Oncol* 4:697–701.

Coia L, Engstrom P, Paul A. 1986. Non-surgical management of esophageal cancer (abstract). *Int J Radiat Oncol Biol Phys* 12:119–120.

Coia LR, Engstrom PE, Paul A, et al. 1984. A pilot study of combined radiotherapy and chemotherapy for esophageal carcinoma. *Am J Clin Oncol* 7:653–659.

Coonley C, Bains M, Kelsen DP. In press. *Cis*-platin-bleomycin in the treatment of esophageal carcinoma: A final report. *Cancer.*

Earlam R, Cunha-Melo JR. 1980. Oesophageal squamous cell carcinoma II. A critical review of radiotherapy. *Br J Surg* 67:457–461.

Earle JR, Gelber RD, Moertel CG, et al. 1980. A controlled evaluation of combined radiation and bleomycin therapy for squamous cell carcinoma of the esophagus. *Int J Radiat Oncol Biol Phys* 6:821–826.

Fujimaki M. 1975. Role of preoperative administration of bleomycin and radiation in the treatment of esophageal cancer. *Jpn J Surg* 5:48–50.

Hancock SL, Glatstein E. 1984. Radiation therapy of esophageal cancer. *Semin Oncol* 11:144–168.

Keane TJ, Harwood AR, Elhakin T, et al. 1985. Radical radiation therapy with 5-fluorouracil infusion and mitomycin C for esophageal carcinoma. *Radiother Oncol* 4:205–210.

Kelsen D, Bains M, Hilaris B, et al. 1984. Combined modality therapy of esophageal cancer. *Semin Oncol* 11:169–177.

Kolaric K, Roth A, Dujinovic I. 1984. The value of two combined chemoradiotherapy approaches in the treatment of inoperable esophageal cancer. *Tumori* 70:69–75.

Langer M, Choi NC, Orlow E, et al. 1986. Radiation therapy alone or in combination with surgery in the treatment of carcinoma of the esophagus. *Cancer* 58:1208–1213.

Launois B, Delarue D, Campion JP. 1981. Preoperative radiotherapy for carcinoma of the esophagus. *Surg Gynecol Obstet* 153:690–692.

Leichman L, Steiger Z, Seydel HG, et al. 1984a. Combined preoperative chemotherapy and radiation therapy for cancer of the esophagus: The Wayne State University, Southwest Oncology Group and Radiation Therapy Oncology Group experience. *Semin Oncol* 11:178–185.

Leichman L, Steiger Z, Seydel HG, et al. 1984b. Preoperative chemotherapy and radiation therapy for patients with cancer of the esophagus: A potentially curative approach. *J Clin Oncol* 2:75–79.

Lokich JJ, Rich TA, Chaffey JR. 1986. Protracted infusional 5-fluorouracil in gastro-intestinal malignancy. In *Neo-adjuvant Chemotherapy Colloque INSERM,* vol. 137, John Libbey, ed., pp. 683–689. London: Eurotex Ltd.

Marsh JC. 1986. Management of cancer of the esophagus. *Curr Concepts Oncol* 8(2): 15–22.

Miller JI, McIntyre B, Hatcher CR. 1985. Combined treatment approach in surgical management of carcinoma of the esophagus: A preliminary report. *Ann Thorac Surg* 40:289–293.

Parker EF, Marks RD, Kratz JM, et al. 1985. Chemoradiation therapy and resection for carcinoma of the esophagus: Short term results. *Ann Thorac Surg* 40:121–125.

Popp MB, Hawley D, Reising J, et al. 1986. Improved survival in squamous esophageal cancer. *Arch Surg* 121:1330–1334.

Rich TA, Lokich JJ, Chaffey JT. 1985. A pilot study of protracted venous infusion of 5-fluorouracil and concomitant radiation therapy. *J Clin Oncol* 3:402–406.

Richmond J, Seydel HG, Bae Y, et al. 1986. Comparison of three treatment strategies for esophageal cancer within a single institution (abstract). *Int J Radiat Oncol Biol Phys* 12:119.

Steiger Z, Franklin R, Wilson RF, et al. 1981a. Complete eradication of squamous cell carcinoma of the esophagus with combined chemotherapy and radiotherapy. *Am Surg* 47: 95–98.

Steiger Z, Franklin R, Wilson RF, et al. 1981b. Eradication and palliation of squamous cell carcinoma of the esophagus with chemotherapy, radiotherapy, and surgical therapy. *J Thorac Cardiovasc Surg* 5:713–719.

Werner ID. 1979. The multidisciplinary approach in the management of squamous carcinoma of the esophagus: The Groote Schuur Hospital experience. *Front Gastrointest Res* 5: 130–135.

Annual Clinical Conference on Cancer, Vol. 30
Gastrointestinal Cancer: Current Approaches to Diagnosis and Treatment
© 1988 by The University of Texas System Cancer Center

23. Carcinoma of the Esophagus: Contribution of Chemotherapy

Jaffer A. Ajani, Marion J. McMurtrey, Tyvin A. Rich,
Roxann Blackburn, Eric Chang-Tung, Bernard Levin, Jack A. Roth,
and Clifton F. Mountain

Carcinoma of the esophagus is an aggressive malignancy. In the United States, it accounts for approximately 1.1% to 1.5% of all malignancies, and each year nearly 9,000 deaths from this tumor are reported and between 9,000 and 10,000 new cases are diagnosed. Thus, esophageal cancer, with a five-year survival of only 5% to 20%, appears to be as virulent as pancreatic cancer; in contrast, 30% to 40% of patients with carcinoma of the colon or stomach survive five years or more (Silverberg 1987).

More than 50% of esophageal cancers are of squamous histology. In the past, morbidity due to local disease exceeded that due to the systemic disease; recently, however, better local control has made systemic disease the more frequent cause of both mortality and morbidity. Surgery, radiation therapy, and combinations of these modalities have been used with variable success in the control of the primary tumor. It is clear, however, that treatment strategies directed only toward control of the primary disease have resulted in the low five-year survival. Seventy to eighty percent of all the patients sooner or later develop metastatic disease; most of the patients die of metastatic disease.

Figure 23.1 is a graphic model of esophageal carcinoma. The primary tumor is diagnosed late in the United States: at the time of its detection, metastases are usually already seeded and growing. If a patient receives therapy directed only toward the primary disease, five-year survival cannot be expected to be very high. This model also emphasizes the need to treat the metastatic disease at the outset.

In carcinoma of the esophagus, chemotherapy has been utilized only recently and is evolving as a method of treatment. Although published results of early clinical trials have been interesting and promising, many questions remain unanswered and much research remains to be done. The following summarizes representative chemotherapy trials in esophageal carcinoma, mainly in cases of squamous histology.

SINGLE-AGENT THERAPY

Only a limited number of chemotherapeutic agents have fully been individually investigated in esophageal carcinoma. A low order of activity usually ranging between 15% and 25% has been observed with various agents. The median duration of response has been disappointingly low, approximately three to four months (Marsh

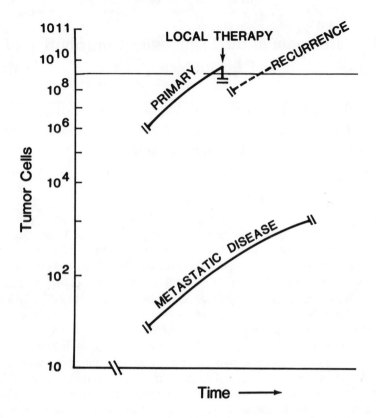

Fig. 23.1. A graphic model of the natural history of esophageal carcinoma. Metastatic disease was present in more than 70% of patients at the time of clinical detection.

1986). The response data of the active single agents in this cancer are summarized in table 23.1 Experience with single agents has been in a miscellaneous group of patients, with those with prior treatment and metastatic disease included.

Cisplatin, one of the most important agents against this disease, has been investigated by two of the major collaborative groups in the United States. The Southwest Oncology Group treated 45 patients with 50 mg/m² of cisplatin on days 1 and 8 every 28 days. Of 35 evaluable patients, 3 achieved a complete remission and 6 a partial remission; the median duration of partial remission was around three months, but the duration of complete remission was longer in 2 patients (Panettiere et al. 1984). The Eastern Cooperative Oncology Group in a randomized study treated 54 patients with cisplatin (50 mg/m² every three weeks) or mitomycin C (20 mg/m² every four weeks × 2, then 10 mg/m²). Cisplatin yielded a response rate of 25% with a median response duration of 16 weeks, and mitomycin C resulted in a 42% response rate for a median of 12 weeks (Engstrom, Lavin, and Klaassen 1983).

Mitoguazone was investigated in an important study conducted at Memorial Sloan-Kettering Cancer Center. Twenty-three patients with disease refractory to

Table 23.1. *Single-Agent Chemotherapy in Carcinoma of the Esophagus:*
Additive Results of Trials

Agent	No. of Patients	Response (%)
Bleomycin	142	22
Cisplatin	102	20
Methotrexate	92	27
Vindesine	87	24
5-Fluorouracil	67	16
Mitomycin C	58	40
Doxorubicin	52	13
Mitoguazone	45	28

Source: Adapted from Marsh 1986.

a cisplatin-containing regimen were treated with mitoguazone on a weekly basis, and four patients (17%) responded, with a median response duration of two months (Kelsen et al. 1982).

Vindesine at 3 mg/m^2 weekly for four weeks followed by monthly maintenance was administered to 53 patients with advanced esophageal cancer (Bezwoda et al. 1984). An objective response was observed in 14 patients (26%).

5-Fluorouracil, methotrexate, bleomycin, doxorubicin, and several other single agents have demonstrated some degree of activity against this cancer, but with a short duration of response. Complete responses have been rare.

COMBINATION CHEMOTHERAPY

The results of several combination chemotherapy trials in esophageal carcinoma have been published in the last few years. Summaries of representative trials are shown in table 23.2. The credit for demonstrating effectiveness of combination chemotherapy in squamous cell carcinoma of the esophagus should go to Kelsen et al., who have done the pioneering work in this area.

The combination of cisplatin (at 3 mg/m^2 on day 1) and bleomycin (at 10 mg/m^2 as loading dose followed by a continuous infusion for three additional days) was given to 70 patients by Coonley et al. (1984). Only 3 of 18 patients with metastatic disease achieved remission; median duration was six months. The median survival of these 18 patients was only four months. Forty-three patients in this series received just one course of chemotherapy for local disease to be resected; only 6 achieved a partial remission upon chemotherapeutic treatment.

The combination of 5-fluorouracil (at 600 mg/m^2 on days 1 and 8), doxorubicin (at 30 mg/m^2 × 1), and cisplatin (at 75 mg/m^2 × 1), repeated every four weeks, was given to 21 patients with advanced measurable disease. Seven patients (33%) responded, with the median survival of all patients being only eight months (Gisselbrecht et al. 1983). Only five patients in this group had received prior radiation therapy.

Perhaps the important trial that established squamous cell carcinoma of the esophagus as a chemotherapy-sensitive tumor was that from Memorial Sloan-Kettering

Table 23.2. *Combination Chemotherapy in Carcinoma of the Esophagus:*
Results of Respective Trials

Combination	Disease Stage	No. of Evaluable Patients	Response (%)
Cisplatin + bleomycin	Local	43	14
	Advanced	18	17
5-Fluorouracil + doxorubicin + cisplatin	Advanced	21	33
Vindesine + bleomycin + cisplatin	Local	45	62
	Advanced	27	30
Cisplatin + vindesine + mitoguazone	Local	19	42
	Advanced	20	40
Vindesine + bleomycin + cisplatin	Advanced	28	25
Bleomycin + cisplatin + methotrexate + mitoguazone	Advanced	14	64
Bleomycin + cisplatin + methotrexate	Advanced	31	26

Cancer Center utilizing vindesine (at 3 mg/m^2 on days 1, 8, 15, and 22), bleomycin (at 10 mg/m^2 by infusion on days 3–6 and 31–34), and cisplatin (at 120 mg/m^2 every six weeks) (Kelsen et al. 1983). Eight of 27 patients with metastatic disease achieved partial remission, with a median response duration of seven months. A higher response rate (62%) was observed with this chemotherapy in patients who had resectable locally advanced disease.

Thirty-two patients treated with the same combination by another group (Dinwoodie et al. 1986) resulted in a much lower response rate (25%). The median survival of all patients was 14 weeks.

Thirty-nine patients treated with a combination of cisplatin (at 100 mg/m^2 every six weeks), vindesine (at 3 mg/m^2 every two weeks), and mitoguazone (at 500 mg/m^2 every two weeks) resulted in a response rate of 41% (Kelsen et al. 1986). The median survival of all patients was 4.8 months. The median duration of response was three months. The dose levels were not escalated in this study.

Combination chemotherapy that would result in higher response rates and longer duration of remissions is necessary to prolong survival in these patients.

COMBINED-MODALITY THERAPY

Therapy utilizing a combination of modalities is a unique method of approaching patients with locally advanced carcinoma of the esophagus. By combining various treatment modalities, one could conceivably maximize the contributions of individual treatments. Very promising results have been seen with this approach. Table 23.3 summarizes representative trials in which chemotherapy has been utilized.

Table 23.3. *Combined-Modality Therapy in Carcinoma of the Esophagus: Results of Respective Trials*

Chemotherapy	Radiation Therapy (cGy)	No. of Patients	Median Survival (mo)
Cisplatin + bleomycin + vindesine	5,500 (postop)	34	16.2
Cisplatin + bleomycin	3,000 (postop)	34	10
Cisplatin + 5-fluorouracil	5,000 or more (postop)	20	16+
Cisplatin + 5-fluorouracil	3,000 (concurrent)	21	18
Mitomycin C + cisplatin	5,000 (concurrent)	35	<12
Mitomycin C + cisplatin	3,000 (concurrent)	30	11
Cisplatin + 5-fluorouracil	3,000 (concurrent)	21	18
Cisplatin + 5-fluorouracil	3,000 (concurrent)	110	12

There have been two different methods of incorporating chemotherapy in combined programs, namely, chemotherapy prior to surgery, and chemotherapy along with radiation therapy, followed by surgery in some studies.

Chemotherapy Plus Surgery

As mentioned above, only 6 of the 43 patients who received just one course of cisplatin and bleomycin in the Coonley et al. series (1984) achieved a partial remission. Thirty-four of these patients actually received surgery; their median survival was 10 months.

Kelsen et al.'s 1983 second-generation study mentioned above included the addition of vindesine to cisplatin and bleomycin. Forty-five patients with locally advanced disease received two courses of chemotherapy as preparation for surgery (Kelsen et al. 1983); 28 of these achieved a partial response with chemotherapy. Normalization of the esophagogram was noted in eight patients; however, none achieved endoscopic or pathological complete remission. Surgery was performed in 34 of the 45. The median survival in these 34 patients was 16.2 months. The median survival of 45 patients with locally advanced disease appears to be shorter than 16.2 months.

Addition of Radiation Therapy

In a 1985 study by Keane et al., 36 patients with locally advanced squamous cell carcinoma of the esophagus were treated with 5-fluorouracil and mitomycin C concurrently with radiation therapy. Twenty-one patients received split-course radiation and 15 received full-course radiation, at 4,500 to 5,000 cGy. The survival was 47% at one year and only 28% at two years. A survival advantage was seen in patients who received single-fraction radiation therapy. None of the patients in this study received surgery.

5-Fluorouracil (at 1,000 mg/m^2 infusion on days 1–4 and 29–32) and cisplatin (at 100 mg/m^2 on days 1 and 29) were combined with radiation therapy (3,000 cGy) in a pilot study of 21 patients (Leichman et al. 1984b). Nineteen patients underwent surgical resection; 5 died as a result of surgery. Five patients achieved a pathologically complete remission, and two additional patients had tumor only in the lymph nodes. The median survival of the whole group was 18 months; the patients who had pathologically complete remission survived longer.

A follow-up study utilizing the same therapy is being conducted by the Southwest Oncology Group and Radiation Therapy Oncology Group. Early results have been reported on 110 patients (Leichman et al. 1984). Twenty-four patients were not eligible for surgery on account of medical illness. Resection was not possible in 11 of 86 patients because of advanced disease. Nineteen (22%) of the 86 patients who underwent surgery were free of tumor. The median survival of the whole group, however, is 12 months.

Thirty patients with potentially resectable carcinoma of the esophagus were treated with mitomycin C and 5-fluorouracil and concurrent radiation therapy (3,000 cGy), followed by surgery in some patients and with some receiving postoperative radiation therapy for residual disease (Franklin et al. 1983). Resection was possible in 18, and only 6 of these achieved a pathologically complete remission. The median survival of the 18 surgical patients was 76 weeks; however, the median survival of all 30 patients was only 49 weeks. An additional 25 patients who had localized disease but who were not eligible for surgery had a median survival of only 16 weeks.

Another important study by the Wayne State University investigators was that of 42 patients with locally advanced squamous carcinoma who received preoperative chemotherapy with 5-fluorouracil and either mitomycin C or cisplatin. Thirty-five patients underwent surgery; 13 (37%) of these achieved a pathologically complete remission and an additional 6 (17%) had only microscopic disease (Steiger et al. 1981). The one-year survival of the surgical group was 52%. The median survival of 42 patients was much lower than 12 months. In studies of this type, in which chemotherapy is administered concurrently with radiation therapy, the pathologically complete remission rate has been high but the median survival has not been greatly improved.

Treatments incorporating multiple modalities have come a long way. A great deal of cooperation and unified understanding of the disease have marked the success of these trials. Many such trials are under way and the results are awaited.

DISCUSSION

Patients with carcinoma of the esophagus typically present with locally advanced disease; however, 80% of the patients have occult metastatic disease at presentation. The median survival of patients treated with palliative modalities is six months.

Only a few chemotherapeutic agents have been fully investigated, and there is an urgent need to evaluate investigational agents in this disease. Combinations of drugs have resulted in higher response rates than single-agent protocols. However, the median duration of response has been low (< eight months) in most trials of combination chemotherapy, and the response rate has been generally less than 50%. Thus, this approach has not affected median survival overall. There is an obvious need to develop combinations that yield higher response rates and longer response durations. Cisplatin has emerged as the most important agent in these combinations, but its chronic and dose-limiting toxicity (i.e., neurotoxicity) has restricted its use for prolonged periods. There is also a need to investigate cisplatin analogues in combination for squamous cell carcinoma of the esophagus.

Combined-modality therapy in esophageal cancer has demonstrated that (1) the local disease can be controlled successfully in a great majority of patients; (2) pathologically complete remission of the primary is rare with chemotherapy alone but can be as high as 37% with the addition of radiation therapy to chemotherapy, as noted in a small series (Steiger et al. 1981); and (3) in general, surgical mortality is not increased by the use of preoperative therapies. To a great extent, metastatic disease has been ignored in present designs of combined-modality therapy: a careful examination of the rationale of all published combined-modality studies reveals an emphasis only on the treatment of local disease. It follows that, even in situations in

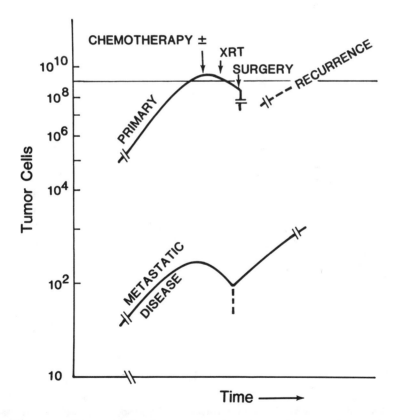

Fig. 23.2. A graphic model of the current design of combined-modality therapy in esophageal carcinoma. Emphasis is on local-regional disease only.

which local disease can be successfully eradicated, metastatic disease could ultimately overwhelm the patient and claim life. This observation is further illustrated
by the median survival of patients entered in combined-modality protocols, which
has ranged from 8 to 16 months. Figure 23.2 is a representative model of the current
design of combined-modality therapy in this disease.

If the goal in squamous cell carcinoma of the esophagus is to overcome or delay
metastatic disease, then this cancer should, perhaps, be treated like breast carcinoma in that, following the treatment of primary disease, systemic therapy for the
presumed microscopic metastatic disease would be continued for a defined length of
time. Such a schema is illustrated in figure 23.3.

The challenge lies in developing combination chemotherapy regimens that (1)
could be safely utilized in combined-modality therapy, (2) would yield high response rates, (3) would yield a high incidence of clinically and pathologically complete responses, and (4) could be given for prolonged periods without severe toxicity. Until such time, the contribution of chemotherapy in this disease will remain

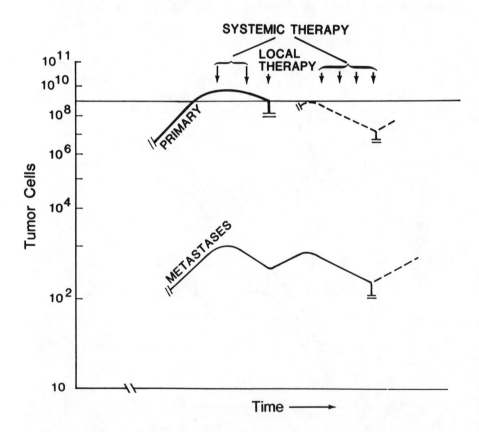

Fig. 23.3. Schema for improved therapy in carcinoma of the esophagus, with systemic treatment for presumed microscopic metastatic disease given after primary treatment.

limited. Another significant question is whether or not chemotherapy can prolong the survival of patients. Only future trials capable of recruiting a large number of patients could answer this question.

Squamous cell carcinoma of the esophagus has become an interesting disease for clinical trials since it is now considered quite sensitive to chemotherapy, a notion that has only recently opened up many avenues of dealing with this cancer and that allows optimism for future control of the disease.

REFERENCES

Bezwoda WR, Derman DP, Weaving A, et al. 1984. Treatment of esophageal cancer with vindesine: An open trial. *Cancer Treat Rep* 68:783–785.

Coonley CJ, Bains M, Hilaris B, et al. 1984. Cisplatin and bleomycin in the treatment of esophageal carcinoma: A final report. *Cancer* 54:2351–2355.

Dinwoodie WR, Bartolucci AA, Lyman GH, et al. 1986. Phase II evaluation of cisplatin, bleomycin, and vindesine in advanced squamous cell circinoma of the esophagus: A Southeastern Cancer Study Group trial. *Cancer Treat Rep* 70:267–270.

Engstrom PF, Lavin PT, Klaassen DJ. 1983. Phase II evaluation of mitomycin and cisplatin in advanced esophageal carcinoma. *Cancer Treat Rep* 67:713–715.

Franklin R, Steiger Z, Vaishampayan G, et al. 1983. Combined modality therapy for esophageal squamous carcinoma. *Cancer* 51:1062–1071.

Gisselbrecht C, Calvo F, Mignot L, et al. 1983. Fluorouracil (F), Adriamycin (A), and cisplatin (P) (FAP): Combination chemotherapy of advanced esophageal carcinoma. *Cancer* 52:974–977.

Keane TJ, Harwood AR, Elhakim T, et al. 1985. Radical radiation therapy with 5-fluorouracil infusion and mitomycin C for oesophageal squamous carcinoma. *Radiother Oncol* 4:205–210.

Kelsen D, Chapman R, Bains M, et al. 1982. Phase II study of methyl-GAG in the treatment of esophageal carcinoma. *Cancer Treat Rep* 66:1427–1429.

Kelsen D, Hilaris B, Coonley C, et al. 1983. Cisplatin, vindesine, and bleomycin chemotherapy of local-regional and advanced esophageal carcinoma. *Am J Med* 75:645–652.

Kelsen DP, Fein R, Coonley C, et al. 1986. Cisplatin, vindesine, and mitoguazone in the treatment of esophageal cancer. *Cancer Treat Rep* 70:255–259.

Leichman L, Steiger Z, Seydel HG, et al. 1984a. Combined preoperative chemotherapy and radiation therapy for cancer of the esophagus: The Wayne State University, Southwest Oncology Group and Radiation Therapy Oncology Group experience. *Semin Oncol* 11:178–185.

Leichman L, Steiger Z, Seydel HG, et al. 1984b. Preoperative chemotherapy and radiation therapy for patients with cancer of the esophagus: A potentially curative approach. *J Clin Oncol* 2:75–79.

Marsh JC. 1986. Management of cancer of the esophagus. *Current Concepts in Oncology* 8:15–22.

Panettiere FJ, Leichman LP, Tilchen EJ, et al. 1984. Chemotherapy for advanced epidermoid carcinoma of the esophagus with single-agent cisplatin: Final report on a Southwest Oncology Group study. *Cancer Treat Rep* 68:1023–1024.

Silverberg E. Lubera J (eds). 1987. Cancer statistics. *CA* 36:9–25.

Steiger Z, Franklin R, Wilson RF, et al. 1981. Complete eradication of squamous cell carcinoma of the esophagus with combined chemotherapy and radiotherapy. *Am Surg* 47:95–98.

Annual Clinical Conference on Cancer, Vol. 30
Gastrointestinal Cancer: Current Approaches to Diagnosis and Treatment
© 1988 by The University of Texas System Cancer Center

24. Laser Therapy for Esophageal Cancer

Jack S. Faintuch

LASER is an acronym for light amplification by stimulated emission of radiation. In essence, a laser is merely a generator of a unique form of light, one not found in nature, known as coherent radiation.

The heart of any laser is the medium that forms the laser beam. This medium can be a gas, as found in a carbon dioxide (CO_2) or argon laser; a liquid, as in a dye laser; or a solid material, as in an Nd:YAG (neodymium:yttrium aluminum garnet) laser. Virtually anything can be used as a medium and made to lase.

The various media must be "excited" to form a laser beam (fig. 24.1). If the lasing medium is a gas, it can be excited with an electrical discharge. If it is a solid, it requires a different energy source; in most cases the source is an intense lamp, which is energized in turn by an electrical power supply. The lamp transfers energy to the laser medium, part of which is absorbed by an active lasing element in that medium, i.e., neodymium in the case of Nd:YAG lasers. The active element then emits this energy spontaneously in the form of light. By placing mirrors outside the laser medium, one at each end, some of this spontaneous light is trapped and reflected back through the medium. When the light is reflected back through the laser medium it stimulates more of the excited atoms to release their excess energy, thereby increasing the intensity of the light. When one of the mirrors is a partial reflector, some of the light is transmitted through it and becomes the laser beam (Enderby 1983).

Laser light has three important properties: coherence (the light waves are all in phase in time and space); collimation (the light waves are propagated in a nearly parallel direction); and monochromaticity (the waves are all of the same wavelength). These unique properties make it possible to focus laser beams into very small spots in which the power density (power per unit area) can exceed a million watts per square centimeter. When a laser beam strikes the surface of a tissue mass, the light is either reflected, scattered, transmitted, or absorbed. Only the absorbed light can produce a biologic effect. The majority of the absorbed light is converted to thermal power. As the heat is absorbed, predictable tissue reactions occur. The first effect seen is thermal contraction in the immediate vicinity of the target area. As more heat is dissipated, local necrosis is produced, and if enough heat is delivered, the tissue is vaporized. The fate of the tissue depends on the extent of heating. At temperatures of 45°C, cell death, edema, and endothelial damage occur; as the temperature increases to 60°C, protein coagulates. At 80°C, collagen contracts and vasoconstriction occurs, and at 100°C, tissue water boils (Cummins 1983). The

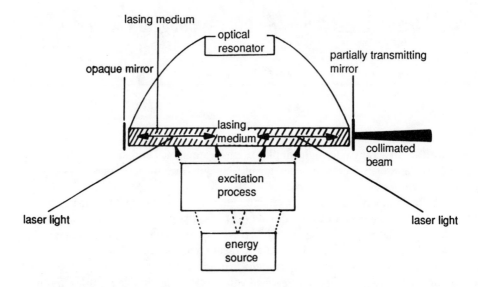

Fig. 24.1. Solid laser medium excited by an optical source.

tissue immediately under the laser beam is vaporized and that in adjacent areas below and laterally is necrosed, causing subsequent scarring or sloughing. Beyond this
area, only local warming and edema occur (Bown 1983). The predictability of the
nature and extent of these changes allows us to employ this modality in treating
esophageal carcinoma (Bown 1980).

PALLIATIVE THERAPY OF ESOPHAGEAL CARCINOMA

At the time of diagnosis most cases of cancer of the esophagus are advanced, and
the likelihood of cure is minimal (Kelsen 1982; Boyce 1984). A recent review by
Earlam and Cunha-Melo (1980a) of 83,383 cases of esophageal carcinoma confirms
the poor survival rates associated with this disease. In their critical review of surgery for esophageal cancer, these two authors stated that:

> out of any 100 patients, including all in the community who actually go to visit
> a doctor, 58 will be explored, 39 resected, 26 leave the hospital with tumor
> excised, 18 survive for 1 year, 9 for 2 years, and 4 for 5 years [fig. 24.2]. If
> there is any surgeon accepting all patients in the population he serves who can
> improve on these figures, he has not yet written an article with his results. The
> first question to be asked is whether these figures can be accepted as correct
> by surgeons. If they are taken as true, the second question follows: would the
> patient, being properly informed, consent to surgical exploration with a 29 per-
> cent operative mortality and an 18 percent chance of surviving 1 year or would

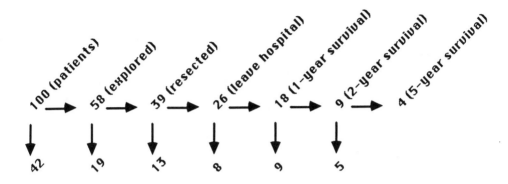

Fig. 24.2. Surgical results in esophageal carcinoma. *Source:* Earlam and Cunha-Melo 1980a, adapted.

he ask whether there was any other available treatment (Earlam and Cunha-Melo 1980a).

These statistics make it apparent that the majority of patients with esophageal cancer are not good surgical candidates. The question that must be answered, then, is which palliative therapy provides the most effective symptomatic relief, affording the patient the best quality of life.

Surgical and nonsurgical approaches—surgery, radiotherapy, chemotherapy, peroral dilatation, peroral prosthesis placement, endoscopic laser therapy, and gastrostomy/jejunostomy—can be applied as palliative forms of therapy. Surgical bypass with or without removal of the primary tumor relieves dysphagia in greater than 90% of treated patients, but unfortunately it requires prolonged hospitalization and is associated with high operative morbidity and mortality (Conlan et al. 1983; Hoffman et al. 1981). Radiation therapy can be used for palliation although the results are not quite as good as those with surgery: approximately 50% of patients have reported symptomatic relief. Unfortunately, a prolonged period of time is required to achieve palliation (1–3 weeks), and response is of limited duration (2–6 months) (Kelsen 1982; Earlam and Cunha-Melo 1980b). Chemotherapy alone or combined with radiotherapy may also be used for palliation. The effectiveness of chemotherapy for palliation remains to be determined, and unfortunately its morbidity often extends over a long time.

Another palliative option is peroral esophageal dilatation, a safe, simple, and effective method of treating esophageal obstruction (Boyce 1984). Peroral esophageal prosthesis placement is successful in approximately 90% of patients, but its complication rates are significant (10%–25%) (Boyce 1984; Tytgat et al. 1986). All of these modalities have significant drawbacks, making them less than ideal.

Laser therapy, using the Nd:YAG laser, has in many instances eliminated the need for less acceptable palliative measures aimed at decreasing dysphagia and improving the nutritional status of the patient (Fleischer and Kessler 1983; Mellow and Pinkas 1984; Pietrafitta and Dwyer 1986).

INDICATIONS

Endoscopic laser therapy is a palliative therapeutic modality that should be limited to patients considered surgically unresectable. Patients with residual or recurrent disease after surgery, radiotherapy, or chemotherapy are candidates for laser therapy.

The primary indication for laser therapy in esophageal carcinoma is to relieve dysphagia, malnutrition, or chest pain. It is contraindicated in the presence of an esophagomediastinal or esophagobronchial fistula. When submucosal disease without an exophytic component is extensive, laser therapy should not be attempted unless the precise extent of the tumor has been documented previously by computerized tomography or endoscopic ultrasound (Ell et al. 1986).

TECHNIQUE

The technique of laser recanalization to clear obstructing esophageal carcinoma is still evolving. A high-power laser is used, in essence, to burn through the obstructing tumor. We use the Medilase-II, a continuous-wave neodymium:YAG laser manufactured by MBB, Munich, Germany. The Nd:YAG laser produces an infrared beam of light at a wavelength of 1064 nm. This is transmitted via a glass or quartz fiber that is fixed in a 2-mm Teflon catheter. The system can be passed through an endoscope biopsy channel with a diameter of 2.8 mm or greater. The Teflon supports the fiber and provides a means of delivering a stream of CO_2 across the tip of the light guide that cools and cleans it.

The use of coaxial gas necessitates some type of removal system to prevent overdistention of the esophagus and stomach. This can be accomplished with a nasogastric tube passed alongside the endoscope or with continuous suctioning through a single-channel or double-channel endoscope. The procedure is carried out in the therapeutic endoscopy or laser suite, with the patient under general intravenous sedation plus topical pharyngeal anesthesia.

Antegrade

The first published reports on laser therapy for esophageal carcinoma recommended that the energy be applied from the proximal margin of the tumor and then distally throughout one or several sessions, the so-called antegrade technique (fig. 24.3) (Bown et al. 1982; Fleischer and Kessler 1983). Once the tumor has been identified,

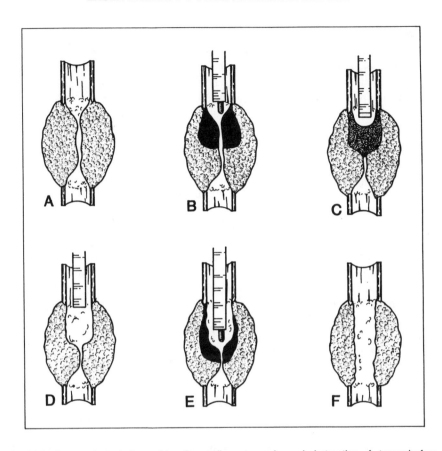

Fig. 24.3. Antegrade technique of treating malignant esophageal obstruction. *A,* tumor before treatment; *B,* proximal 1 to 2 cm of tumor coagulated; *C,* 48 hrs later, tumor has necrosed and liquified, leaving 1 to 2 cm of lumen open; *D,* necrotic material is aspirated before further therapy; *E,* next 1 to 2 cm of tumor coagulated; *F,* lumen reestablished at completion of therapy. *Source:* Pietrafitta and Dwyer 1986, adapted with permission.

the endoscope is held in position with the fiber delivery system 5 to 10 mm from the tumor. Usual energy settings range from 60 to 100 watts. Using one- to two-second pulses, the operator vaporizes the tumor from its medial edge toward the esophageal wall. The total amount of tumor that can be treated in one session depends on the extent of the tumor and the patient tolerance. When more than one session is required to complete the primary course of therapy, two to three days should elapse between treatments to maximize tumor slough and late thermal necrosis resulting from the first treatment. At the second session, the previously lasered areas appear yellow-white and necrotic; as much of this necrotic material as possible should be removed before beginning the second treatment. Treatments are repeated until the esophagus is recanalized, at which time all obviously malignant areas should have been treated.

Several problems are associated with this approach. Depending on the degree of stenosis, the natural course of the esophagus cannot always be determined, making safe lasering difficult. In addition, the tissue that is not actually vaporized may become edematous and obstruct the lumen. The result can be an increase of dysphagia and decreased visualization of the lumen, leading to a greater chance of complications—in particular, perforation—during treatment (Fleischer and Sivak 1984).

Retrograde

The retrograde technique combines laser therapy of the esophagus with prior bougienage (fig. 24.4). A guide wire is passed through the stenotic mass under direct vision and its position is confirmed by fluoroscopy. Esophageal dilation is then performed to achieve a lumen diameter of at least 12 to 13 mm. The endoscope is then passed to the distal margin of the tumor, and the tumor is vaporized as previously described (Reimann et al. 1985; Pietrafitta and Dwyer 1986; Sabben, Lambert, and Lenz 1983). With this technique, the entire tumor can be treated in a single session, and visualization of the lumen is good throughout the procedure. A relative disadvantage of this method is that it requires more treatment steps. Controversy exists about dilation: some investigators are hesitant to dilate too vigorously in a single session fearing that it may perforate or crack the tumor rather than stretch the lesion (Boyce 1984).

Contact Approach

A third available technique uses a contact, rather than the standard noncontact, approach. Recently, manufacturers have produced sapphire tips (Surgical Laser Technologies, Cincinnati, Ohio) or titanium probes (Trimedyne, Santa Ana, California) that can deliver the laser energy to the tumor. Instead of holding the fiber above the tissue, the operator keeps the tip in direct contact with the lesion (fig. 24.5). These tips allow controlled tumor vaporization at lower power settings and do not require coaxial CO_2. They are most valuable in treating an extremely tight stenosis where precise destruction of the tumor is mandated. Once the tip has passed through the tumor, more aggressive laser therapy using the noncontact method is appropriate. The relative advantages and disadvantages of the contact and noncontact methods of Nd:YAG laser therapy are illustrated in table 24.1.

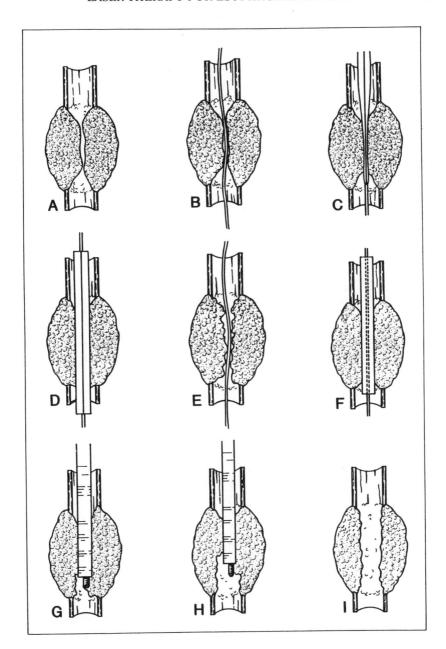

Fig. 24.4. Retrograde technique of treating malignant esophageal obstruction. *A,* tumor before treatment; *B,* Savary-Guillard wire is passed through tumor and into stomach; *C,* first dilator is passed through tumor; *D,* tumor is dilated up to 15 mm; *E,* wire is left in place after dilatation is complete; *F,* endoscope is passed over guide wire into stomach; *G,* laser waveguide is in place, and tumor destruction begins at distal tumor margin; *H,* 50% of treatment completed; *I,* lumen is reestablished at completion of therapy.

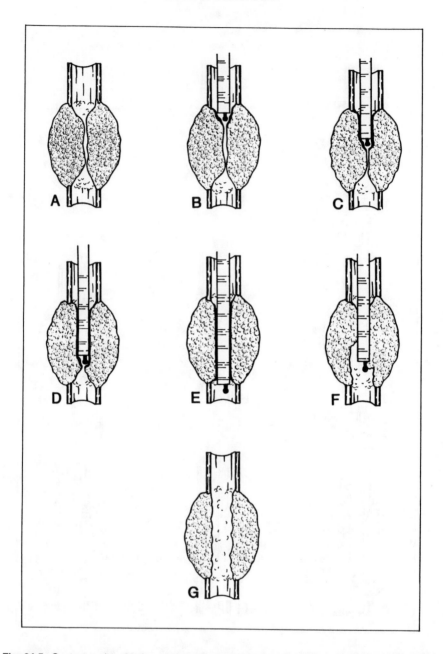

Fig. 24.5. Contact-probe ablation of malignant esophageal obstruction. *A,* tumor before treatment; *B,* proximal 1 to 3 cm is coagulated with contact probe; *C, D, E, F,* continued coagulation of narrow rim of tumor adjacent to lumen until distal margin is reached; *G,* narrow coagulated area traverses the stenotic tumor.

Table 24.1. *Relative Advantages and Disadvantages of the Contact and Noncontact Methods of Nd-YAG Laser Therapy in Clinical Practice*

Feature of the Treatment	Contact Method	Noncontact Method
Tissue contact necessary	Yes	No
Therapy under direct vision	No	Yes
Technique used	Punctiform	Paintbrush
Distension of the bowel	No	Yes
Pain	No	Yes
Laser edema	Less	More
Smoke	Less	More
Light-guide ignition	No	Yes
Light-guide adhesion	Yes	No
Large tumor mass	Less effective	More effective
Exophytic tumor	Less effective	More effective
Tumor destruction		
From distal to proximal	Less effective	More effective
From proximal to distal	More effective	Less effective
Total stenosis:		
tumor overgrowth of the tube	More effective	Less effective

Source: Adapted from Ell, Hochberger, and Lux 1986.

In my opinion, laser therapy should be limited to those lesions with a predominant mucosal or exophytic component. When possible, the retrograde approach should be used, as it is much more controlled and safer. When the esophagus is totally or almost totally obstructed, the contact probes can be invaluable in recannulating the lumen prior to bougienage or further noncontact laser therapy.

RESULTS

Investigators from several countries have reported the results of endoscopic laser treatment of advanced esophageal cancer (Fleischer and Sivak 1985; Mellow and Pinkas 1984; Krasner and Beard 1984; Buset et al. 1983; Swain et al. 1984; Pietrafitta and Dwyer 1986). All report good immediate relief of dysphagia in the majority of cases. Individual series include from 6 to 76 patients and have 80% to 100% success rates. A recent international survey evaluated the results of 1,359 patients submitted to laser therapy for malignant obstruction of the upper gastrointestinal tract (Ell et al. 1986). In the final analysis, only the data from investigators who had treated more than 15 patients were used in order to minimize the influence of inexperience on the results; therefore, the final total was 1,184 patients from 20 hospitals. The location and extent of the cancers can be seen in table 24.2. The majority of investigators combined laser therapy and bougienage. The average amount of energy used was 11,000 joules (range 7,000–24,000) applied over three sessions (table 24.3). The average success rate for the initial treatment was greater than 80%, and the total complication rate was 4.1% (table 24.4).

In our early experience, we have treated eight patients (table 24.5). The primary

Table 24.2. *International Inquiry: Patients, Prior Treatment, and Pretherapy Tumor Characteristics (20 Hospitals with > 15 Treated Patients)*

Characteristic	Patients Treated	
	No.	%
Treated patients (total)	1184	100
Tumor location		
Esophagus	816	68.9
Proximal	174	14.7
Middle	348	29.4
Distal	294	24.8
Stomach	265	22.3
Anastomosis	100	8.4
Duodenum/jejunum	3	0.3
Degree of stenosis:		
endoscopically impassable (lumen < 9mm)	660	55.7
Length of stenosis > 4 cm	686	57.9
Pretreatment		
Radiotherapy	152	12.8
Chemotherapy	50	4.2

Source: Adapted from Ell et al. 1986.

Table 24.3. *International Inquiry: Premedication and Technical Data on Laser Therapy (20 Hospitals with > 15 Treated Patients)*

Treatment	No. of Hospitals
Premedication	
Tranquilizers + analgesics	10
Tranquilizers	5
Analgesics	1
Hypnotics	1
Tranquilizers + analgesics/anesthesia	3
Laser sessions (initial treatment)	
on average 11,000 (7,000–24,000) joules	
Technique employed	
Combined laser therapy (laser + bougienage)	
and laser therapy alone	16
Laser therapy alone	4

Source: Adapted from Ell et al. 1986.

course of treatment was completed in an average of two treatment sessions (range 1–3). Total energy used ranged from 5,124 to 37,979 joules (average, 11,775). In all patients treated, a patent esophageal lumen was reestablished, and all resumed eating solid foods. Two patients required repeated procedures during the course of their disease. The average time to recurrence of symptoms that necessitated retreat-

Table 24.4. *International Inquiry: Results of Palliative Laser Therapy (20 Hospitals with > 15 Treated Patients; Total Number of Patients Treated: 1,184)*

	Patients	
Result	No.	%
Initial treatment successful (solid food can be taken)	983	83.0
Complications (total)	49	4.1
Perforation	25	2.1
Fistulas	9	0.8
Hemorrhage	8	0.7
Sepsis	7	0.6
Complications resulting in death	12	1.0

Source: Adapted from Ell et al. 1986.

Table 24.5. *Laser Therapy for Malignant Esophageal Obstruction: (UT M. D. Anderson Hospital Experience)*

Patient	Histology	No. of Treatments	Technique	Total Energy (joules)	Outcome
1	Adenosquamous	2	Noncontact	37,979	Excellent
		1	Noncontact	12,559	Excellent
2	Adenocarcinoma	2	Noncontact	8,653	Good
		2	Noncontact	12,302	Good
		1	Noncontact	6,976	Good
3	Squamous	1	Noncontact	5,035	Good
4	Squamous	2	Noncontact	13,900	Excellent
5	Squamous	2	Noncontact	7,918	Good
6	Squamous	2	Noncontact	10,963	Excellent
7	Squamous	2	Noncontact	5,124	Good
8	Adenocarcinoma	3	Contact	8,125	Good

ment was 10 weeks (8–16 weeks). No complications have occurred among our patients.

CONCLUSION

Current data suggest that endoscopic laser therapy is an effective and safe means of achieving a good quality of palliation in patients with esophageal carcinoma. So far, few data are available regarding the effect, if any, of this treatment modality on survival. Only one report has shown a survival benefit for patients with esophageal carcinoma treated with laser therapy (Mellow and Pinkas 1984). This report was based on a nonrandomized study that used a historical control group from the same hospital. As yet, no one has compared endoscopic laser therapy with any other palliative treatment for esophageal carcinoma.

In an effort to clarify the role of this therapeutic modality, we have initiated a randomized clinical trial comparing endoscopic laser therapy and surgical bypass to relieve dysphagia in patients with unresectable carcinoma of the esophagus. Through this study we hope to gain meaningful information regarding the quality of palliation, the morbidity, mortality, and survival rates, and the cost effectiveness of these two treatments.

REFERENCES

Bown SG. 1983. Phototherapy of tumours. *World J Surg* 7:700–709.

Bown SG, Salmon PR, Storey DW, et al. 1980. Nd:YAG laser photocoagulation in the dog stomach. *Gut* 21:818–825.

Bown SG, Swain CP, Edwards DA, et al. 1982. Palliative relief of malignant upper gastrointestinal obstruction by endoscopic laser therapy (abstract). *Gut* 23:918.

Boyce HW Jr. 1984. Palliation of advanced esophageal cancer. *Semin Oncol* 11:186–195.

Buset M, Dunham F, Baize M, et al. 1983. Nd:YAG laser: A new palliative alternative in the management of esophageal cancer. *Endoscopy* 15:353–356.

Conlan AA, Nicolaou N, Hammond CA, et al. 1983. Retrosternal gastric bypass for inoperable esophageal cancer. A report of 21 patients. *Ann Thorac Surg* 36:396–401.

Cummins L. 1983. Laser tissue interaction. In *Therapeutic Laser Endoscopy in Gastrointestinal Disease*, D Fleischer, D Jensen, P Bright-Asare, eds., pp. 9–28. Boston: Martinus Nijhoff.

Earlam R, Cunha-Melo JR. 1980a. Oesophageal squamous cell carcinoma. I. A critical review of surgery. *Br J Surg* 67:381–390.

Earlam R, Cunha-Melo JR. 1980b. Oesophageal squamous cell carcinoma. II. A critical review of radiotherapy. *Br J Surg* 67:457–467.

Ell C, Hochberger J, Lux G. 1986. Clinical experience of non-contact and contact Nd:YAG laser therapy in inoperable tumour stenoses of the oesophagus and stomach. *Laser Med Sci* 1:143–146.

Ell C, Riemann JF, Lux G, et al. 1986. Palliative laser treatment of malignant stenoses in the upper gastrointestinal tract. *Endoscopy* 18:21–26.

Enderby CE. 1983. Medical laser fundamentals. In *Therapeutic Laser Endoscopy in Gastrointestinal Disease*, D Fleischer, D Jensen, P Bright-Asare, eds., pp. 1–8. Boston: Martinus Nijhoff.

Fleischer D, Kessler F. 1983. Endoscopic Nd:YAG laser therapy for carcinoma of the esophagus: A new form of palliative treatment. *Gastroenterology* 85:600–606.

Fleischer D, Sivak MV. 1984. Endoscopic Nd:YAG laser therapy as palliative treatment for advanced adenocarcinoma of the gastric cardia. *Gastroenterology* 87:815–820.

Fleischer D, Sivak MV. 1985. Endoscopic Nd:YAG laser therapy as a palliation for esophagogastric cancer. *Gastroenterology* 89:827–831.

Hoffman TH, Kelly JR, Grover FL, et al. 1981. Carcinoma of the esophagus. *J Thorac Cardiovasc Surg* 81:44–49.

Kelsen D. 1982. Treatment of advanced esophageal cancer. *Cancer* 50:2576–2581.

Krasner N, Beard J. 1984. Laser irradiation of tumours of the oesophagus and gastric cardia. *Br Med J* 288:829.

Mellow MM, Pinkas H. 1984. Endoscopic therapy for esophageal carcinoma with Nd:YAG laser: Prospective evaluation of efficacy, complications and survival. *Gastrointest Endosc* 30:334–339.

Pietrafitta JJ, Dwyer RM. 1986. Endoscopic laser therapy of malignant esophageal obstruction. *Arch Surg* 121:395–400.

Riemann JF, Ell C, Lux C, et al. 1985. Combined therapy of malignant stenoses of the upper gastrointestinal tract by means of laser beam and bougienage. *Endoscopy* 17:43–48.

Sabben G, Lambert R, Lenz P. 1983. Laser therapy with quartz fibers in tissue contact (abstract). *Gastrointest Endosc* 29:183.

Swain CP, Bown SG, Edwards DAW, et al. 1984. Laser recanalization of obstructing foregut cancer. *Br J Surg* 71:112–115.

Tytgat GN, den Hartog Jager FCA, Bartelsman JFWM. 1986. Endoscopic prosthesis for advanced esophageal cancer. *Endoscopy* 18:32–39.

PANCREATIC, ENDOCRINE, AND HEPATOBILIARY CANCER

Annual Clinical Conference on Cancer, Vol. 30
Gastrointestinal Cancer: Current Approaches to Diagnosis and Treatment
© 1988 by The University of Texas System Cancer Center

25. Overview: Biology and Diagnosis of Pancreatic Cancer

Eugene P. DiMagno

The incidence and mortality of adenocarcinoma of the pancreatic duct are gradually increasing. In the decades from 1950 to 1970, the incidence increased from 6/100,000 to 10/100,000 population. Since 1970, this incidence has continued to increase, and now it is 11–12/100,000. Unfortunately, the overall five-year survival rate (2%) and the five-year survival rate of patients with resectable tumors (10%) have not improved (Gordis and Gold 1986). Interestingly, survival is not related to the histological grade or the presence of metastatic lesions (Edis, Kiernan, and Taylor 1980). In our experience, patients who have tumors that are Broder's histological grades III and IV live as long as patients with tumors of grades I and II, and the overall survival rate is not affected by the presence of metastases in regional lymph nodes. No patients with unresectable tumors who have been treated with biliary bypass surgery have survived more than four years, and only 10% have survived as long as two years (van Heerden, Heath, and Alden 1980).

Virtually all patients with pancreatic ductal adenocarcinoma have advanced disease at the time of diagnosis. Thus, as physicians, our major task is to treat the symptoms of pancreatic cancer. We continue, however, to make advances in the diagnosis of pancreatic cancer with the hope that if we can identify early pancreatic cancer, survival may be improved by modern treatment. My objectives in this chapter will be to discuss the diagnosis of pancreatic cancer and to address the pathophysiology and symptomatic treatment of weight loss and malabsorption.

DIAGNOSIS OF PANCREATIC CANCER

Symptoms

The symptoms of pancreatic cancer are nonspecific. A variety of nonpancreatic diseases as well as pancreatitis may cause symptoms identical to symptoms experienced by patients with pancreatic cancer. In a prospective study comparing diagnostic tests for pancreatic cancer (DiMagno et al. 1977b), we admitted patients if they were more than 35 years old and had abdominal pain, weight loss, or jaundice but otherwise normal findings on physical examination and routine laboratory tests, cholecystography (which they underwent if not jaundiced), and barium gastrointestinal roentgenography. Therefore, only patients who had symptoms unexplained by gastrointestinal test results but suggestive of pancreatic cancer were considered for acceptance. After testing, the final diagnosis was established by laparotomy in 68 patients and by liver biopsy in 2. Of the 70 patients, 30 had patcreatic cancer; 7 had pancreatitis; 9 had nonpancreatic, intraabdominal neoplasms (3 lymphomas, 4 carcinomas of the small intestine, 1 ovarian cancer, and 1 uterine cancer with retroperitoneal metastasis); 8 had miscellaneous nonpancreatic, nonneoplastic disease (1 celiac artery aneurysm, 1 granuloma of the abdominal wall, 1 alcoholic hepatitis, 1 multiple small bowel ulcer, 2 cholecystitis, 1 abdominal sarcoidosis, and 1 active duodenal ulcer); and 16 had negative results at laparotomy. Thus only 40% of patients who present with symptoms very suggestive of pancreatic carcinoma will turn out to have pancreatic cancer, and sensitive and specific tests for pancreatic cancer are needed to make the diagnosis.

SENSITIVITY, SPECIFICITY, AND PREDICTIVE VALUE OF CURRENT DIAGNOSTIC TESTS

Routine Clinical Tests

Although some routine laboratory tests show statistically significant differences between laboratory values of patients with pancreatic cancer and those of patients with pancreatitis, other cancers, and benign gastrointestinal disorders, there is a significant overlap, which limits the values' usefulness (Go, Taylor, and DiMagno 1981; table 25.1). Patients with pancreatic disease have higher values for serum lipase, amylase, and glucose than do other patients; however, these tests do not distinguish between pancreatic cancer and pancreatitis. Alkaline phosphatase, aspartate aminotransferase (AST), and bilirubin levels are elevated in patients with pancreatic cancer, but these tests lack the specificity to exclude benign hepatic disorders. Nevertheless, I recommend that patients suspected of having pancreatic cancer undergo a battery of tests. These tests include a hematology group, a chemistry group, total serum amylase level, urinary amylase level, and x-ray films, including an abdominal film (to determine if any calcification is present) and a chest film. I include the total serum amylase level among these tests because this test is routinely available. If lipase or pancreatic isoamylase tests are available, they may be preferable. Urinary amylase is measured because this level is elevated for long periods of time during exacerbation of acute pancreatitis, which may complicate pancreatic cancer.

If the level of enzymes is elevated, my suspicion of pancreatic disease increases, but further special tests are needed to make the diagnosis. Nonspecific signs such as bony lesions, pleural effusion, or ascites can be seen on chest and abdominal x-ray films and indicate pancreatitis or pancreatic cancer. However, if pancreatic calcifications are present on the abdominal films, a diagnosis of chronic pancreatitis can be made with 90% confidence and no further tests. Finding obvious pulmonary or bony metastases is diagnostic of metastatic cancer, but it poses a philosophical problem. In this situation, some physicians may opt to go no further, but some who believe even metastatic diseases should be treated aggressively would get special tests to find the primary tumor.

Table 25.1. Serological Tests in Patients Suspected of Having Pancreatic Cancer

Laboratory Tests	Pancreatic Cancer (N = 28)	Pancreatitis (N = 9)	Other Benign Disease (N = 28)
Glucose (mg/dl)	122.5 ± 6.9	103.8 ± 8.2	100.0 ± 2.9
Calcium (mg/dl)	9.6 ± 0.1	9.5 ± 0.1	9.4 ± 0.1
Phosphorus (mg/dl)	3.5 ± 0.1	3.6 ± 0.2	3.2 ± 0.1
Prothrombin time (sec)	12.2 ± 0.3	11.9 ± 0.2	11.4 ± 0.3
Direct bilirubin (mg/dl)	2.4 ± 0.6	0 ± 0	0.6 ± 0.5
Indirect bilirubin (mg/dl)	1.9 ± 0.4	0.5 ± 0.1	1.3 ± 0.7
Alkaline phosphatase (U/liter)	565.2 ± 71.8	239.0 ± 76.2	237.8 ± 14.1
Serum glutamic oxaloacetic transaminase (U/liter)	47.6 ± 6.1	19.1 ± 3.8	20.9 ± 4.7
Lipase (U/liter)	95.8 ± 21.7	245.8 ± 55.2	50.3 ± 12.1
Amylase (U/liter)	337.3 ± 152.4	609.6 ± 113.4	237.8 ± 14.1

Source: Adapted from Go, Taylor, and DiMagno 1981.

Immunological Tests

Because of the lack of sensitivity and specificity of the routine laboratory investigations, there has been and continues to be an intense effort by many investigators to find a sensitive and specific serological marker for pancreatic cancer. However, it is indeed quite disappointing that none of the available tumor markers evaluated has neither the sensitivity nor the specificity to be used routinely in cancer screening or diagnosis (table 25.2). In our hands, tests of hormones such as total thyroxin, insulin, gastrin, parathyroid hormone, calcitonin, immunoglobulins (IgA, IgG, IgM), and carcinoembryonic antigen (CEA) are not sufficiently sensitive or specific (table 25.3). The serum CEA level is elevated in patients with nonpancreatic and pancreatic cancer but not in patients with benign pancreatic disease. Others have found similar results. Elevated CEA levels are present in up to 85% of patients with cancer of the pancreas; unfortunately, 65% of patients with other cancers and 46% of patients with benign diseases also have had elevated CEA levels (Holyoke et al. 1979; Klavins 1981; Moossa and Levin 1981; Zamcheck and Martin 1981).

Other tumor markers such as α-fetoprotein and pancreatic oncofetal antigen have been evaluated by a number of investigators, who found that they are not useful markers for pancreatic cancer. Pancreatic oncofetal protein, non-cross-reacting antigen, α_2 glycoprotein, β_2 microglobulin, and CA 19-9 and DU-Pan-2 monoclonal antibodies have been or are being evaluated. Similarly, many enzymes (table 25.2) have been investigated, but none have proved to be clinically useful in the diagnosis of pancreatic cancer.

Some of the tumor markers have some promise but require further testing. The leukocyte adherence inhibition test, based on the presence of specific tumor anti-

Table 25.2. *Tumor Markers in Pancreatic Cancer*

Oncofetal Antigens	Enzymes
Carcinoembryonic antigen	Trypsin
α_1-fetoprotein	Trypsinogen
Pancreatic oncofetal antigen	Chymotrypsin
Basic fetoprotein	Amylase
α-CAP 1	Pancreatic ribonuclease
	Galactosyltransferase II
Proteins	
Lactoferrin	Monoclonal antibodies
Ferrin	CA 19-9
B$_2$ microglobulin	DU-Pan-2
Immunosuppressive acidic protein	
	Glycoproteins
Peptide hormones	Non-cross-reacting antigen
B human chorionic gonadotropin	EDC 1
Parathormone	B$_2$ glycoprotein
Calcitonin	Tennagen
C peptide	
Gastrin	Others
Glucagon	Fucose
Insulin	Leukocyte adherence inhibition assay

Source: Adapted from Faintuch and Levin 1986.

Table 25.3. Additional Serological Tests in Patients Suspected of Having Pancreatic Cancer

Laboratory Tests	Pancreatic Cancer (N = 48)	Pancreatitis (N = 9)	Other Cancers (N = 10)	Other Benign Disease (N = 28)
Total thyroxine (μg/dl)	6.7 ± 0.4	7.8 ± 0.9	6.5 ± 0.5	6.2 ± 0.4
Insulin (U/ml)	16.8 ± 4.0	8.7 ± 2.1	6.8 ± 2.1	13.4 ± 2.3
Gastrin (pg/ml)	109.6 ± 15.3	150.2 ± 26.3	208.1 ± 55.4	121.2 ± 21.6
Parathyroid hormone (μl eq/ml)	25.3 ± 1.3	20.3 ± 4.0	29.7 ± 4.5	24.3 ± 1.4
Calcitonin (pg/ml)	78.0 ± 16.6	51.0 ± 11.4	67.0 ± 11.9	46.0 ± 8.3
IgA (mg/ml)	2.1 ± 0.2	2.2 ± 0.1	2.3 ± 0.3	2.4 ± 0.2
IgG (mg/ml)	9.5 ± 0.4	10.0 ± 1.2	9.9 ± 0.5	10.3 ± 0.6
IgM (mg/ml)	1.2 ± 0.1*	1.4 ± 0.3	0.8 ± 0.1	1.8 ± 0.2
Carcinoembryonic antigen (ng/ml)	12.4 ± 3.8*	5.2 ± 3.8	18.3 ± 7.0	2.3 ± 0.4

Source: Adapted from Go Taylor and DiMagno 1981.

Note: Values represent mean plus or minus standard error of the mean.

*$p < .05$.

gens in the serum of cancer patients that inhibit normal adherence of sensitized leukocytes on a glass surface, predicts the presence of cancer accurately in 80% of patients. The specificity for pancreatic cancer is currently under investigation. Galactosyltransferase has a sensitivity of 67% in detecting pancreatic cancer (Podolsky et al. 1981). When this test is combined with ultrasonography, endoscopic retrograde pancreatography, or computed tomography (CT), the sensitivities of the combined tests are 80% to 100%. Thus, this marker has some promise but needs to be investigated further.

A number of groups, including ours, have prospectively evaluated mouse hybridoma-generated monoclonal antibodies. In a study of more than 5,000 patients in our gastrointestinal clinic (Ritts et al. 1984), this marker appeared to have some promise in the diagnosis of early resectable lesions: results were positive in 100% of early resectable lesions but positive in only 53% of specimens from patients with advanced pancreatic cancer. It also detects, however, other neoplasms of the gastrointestinal tract, such as gastric cancer, and has a false-positive rate of 11% in patients with pancreatitis and 2% in normal subjects. We found the CA 19 and the CA 125 antibodies had approximately the same sensitivity (about 75%), which is somewhat better than CEA, which ranges from 25% to 62% (Ritts et al. 1984).

Imaging Tests

The cornerstone for the diagnosis of pancreatic cancer is pancreatic imaging. Ultrasonography, CT, and endoscopic pancreatography and ultrasonographic or computed tomographic transcutaneous pancreatic biopsy are the tests most commonly used today. Radioselenium pancreatic scanning, thermography, and arteriography are no longer widely used because they are nonspecific, insensitive, and too expensive, respectively.

Ultrasonography and Computerized Tomography

The sensitivity and specificity for ultrasonography and CT are similar for detecting a pancreatic mass or cancer. In chronic pancreatitis, it has been shown rather consistently that CT is 10% to 20% more sensitive than ultrasonography, whereas the sensitivity of those two techniques for detecting pancreatic cancer is similar and approximates 80% (Fitzgerald et al. 1978; DiMagno et al. 1977b; Moossa and Levin 1979). In my view, because ultrasonography is less expensive and does not expose the patient to ionizing radiation, it should be used as the first special imaging test to diagnose chronic pancreatic disease, even though it may be a bit less sensitive. When ultrasonography fails for technical reasons ($\simeq 10\%$) or if the diagnosis is uncertain ($\simeq 20\%$), CT scanning should be the next step.

Endoscopic Retrograde Pancreatography

Endoscopic retrograde pancreatography (ERP) has a sensitivity and specificity of 90% (DiMagno et al. 1977b; Moossa and Levin 1979) for the diagnosis of pancreatic cancer. The usual ERP abnormalities in pancreatic cancer are pancreatic duct obstruction and encasement of the pancreatic duct. If the tumor is in the head of the pancreas, contiguous involvement of both the pancreatic and bile ducts—the "double duct" sign—is found. In pancreatic cancer the common duct obstruction is abrupt. Although in chronic pancreatitis, parenchymal fibrosis may cause obstruction of the distal common bile duct, the narrowing is tapered. A tumor located in the parenchyma of the pancreas may be seen by forcing contrast media into the entire collection system (acinarization), but this technique may cause acute pancreatitis. It is rare that filling of a tumor cavity occurs during ERP, but it is a sign of pancreatic cancer.

Ultrasonography- or CT-Guided Percutaneous Pancreatic Biopsy

Ultrasonography- or CT-guided percutaneous pancreatic biopsy is becoming increasingly popular for obtaining a tissue diagnosis in patients with pancreatic cancer. It is performed in patients who have cancer of the body or tail of the pancreas (there are no five-year survivors who have cancer of the pancreas in these locations) or in patients who have unresectable lesions. However, it is not indicated in patients who have resectable lesions (no metastases detected and no extension of the tumor beyond the confines of the pancreas).

The procedure requires localization of the tumor by either ultrasonography or CT. A focused linear array real-time ultrasound technique or CT scanning allows visualization of the tip of the aspiration needle so that it can be positioned within the tumor mass. Performed in this manner, the technique is 90% sensitive for diagnosis of pancreatic cancer (Ferrucci and Wittenberg 1978; Yeh 1981).

Newer Imaging Tests

Evaluation of newer imaging tests—endoscopic ultrasonography (DiMagno et al. 1982) and magnetic resonance imaging—for the diagnosis of pancreatic cancer is under way. However, these techniques do not appear to be any more sensitive or specific than the usual imaging tests.

Pancreatic Function Tests

In the past, pancreatic function tests that require gastrointestinal intubation to obtain exocrine pancreatic secretion have played a prominent role in the diagnosis of pancreatic cancer. In these tests, secretin, cholecystokinin, or a combination of these hormones is used to stimulate the pancreas after the patient is intubated. We have always quantified the recovery of volume, bicarbonate, and enzymes by perfusing nonabsorbable markers. In experienced hands, these tests have a sensitivity and specificity between 80% and 90% (DiMagno et al. 1977b). We have found low outputs of pancreatic enzymes in 90% of the patients with cancer of the pancreatic head and 70% of patients with cancer of the body and the tail of the pancreas (DiMagno et al. 1977a). A few patients with malabsorption from causes other than chronic pancreatitis (for example, mucosal small bowel disease) or who have another gastrointestinal cancer may have an abnormal test result. However, because of the invasiveness of these tests and the emergence of sensitive and specific imaging tests, the use of invasive pancreatic function tests to detect pancreatic cancer has declined sharply.

Unfortunately, noninvasive tests of pancreatic function, although they are simpler and cheaper than invasive tests, are too insensitive or nonspecific for use in the diagnosis of pancreatic cancer and their results are not reliably reproducible (DiMagno 1982). Noninvasive tests are of three types according to measurement of (1) undigested food in stool or diminished products of digestion in breath; (2) products of synthetic compounds that are hydrolyzed by intraluminal pancreatic enzymes, absorbed by the gut, and found in blood and urine; and (3) hormones that are decreased in the fasting or stimulated (postprandial or after intravenous hormone infusion) states, or both.

ALGORITHM FOR THE DIAGNOSIS OF PANCREATIC CANCER

In prospective studies, we have shown that pancreatic disease could be identified with 90% sensitivity and specificity by a combination of ultrasonography, ERP, and a pancreatic function test that requires gastrointestinal intubation and cholecystokinin stimulation. Formerly, we recommended that ultrasonography be done first; if the results were negative, a pancreatic function test was performed next. If either of these procedures yielded a positive test result, we suggested that ERP be done to differentiate between cancer and pancreatitis. In our studies, this sequence of testing identified 89% of patients with pancreatic disease and all patients without pancreatic disease (DiMagno et al. 1977b).

We now recommend (fig. 25.1) that ultrasonography be done first. If the results are negative or indeterminate, a CT scan (if possible) should be done next, followed by ERP. The pancreatic function test is only rarely needed. This sequence of tests should identify pancreatic disease and make the differentiation between pancreatitis and cancer in 90% of patients. We choose to do ultrasonography first and reserve CT scanning and ERP as second and third tests because ultrasonography, in contrast to the other tests, does not require ionizing radiation, is more widely available, is not invasive, and has the same sensitivity and specificity as CT scanning.

BIOLOGY AND TREATMENT OF WEIGHT LOSS

Weight loss in pancreatic cancer because of caloric deprivation may occur because of malabsorption, decreased oral intake of calories, or abnormally rapid utilization of ingested calories. When we investigated the relationship among weight loss, decreased calorie intake, and malabsorption, we found that 75% of patients with pancreatic cancer had malabsorption (Perez et al. 1983). When we investigated the relationship between the location of ductal cancer by ERP and exocrine function in patients with pancreatic cancer, we found that the rate of maximal enzyme secretion was related to the length of ductal opacification by ERP (DiMagno, Malagelada, and Go 1979). Obstruction of the pancreatic duct in the body or the tail of the gland was associated with normal enzyme secretion. But when the obstruction occurred close to the entry of the pancreatic duct into the duodenum, pancreatic enzyme secretion fell markedly. Therefore, patients with carcinomas of the head of the pancreas (75% of patients with pancreatic cancer) have diminished enzyme secretion, whereas those whose tumors are located in the body or tail may have normal enzyme

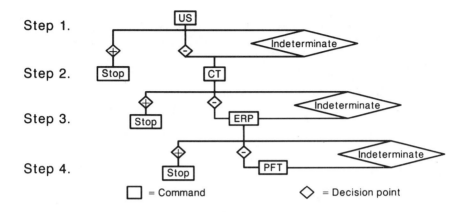

Fig. 25.1. Algorithm for diagnosis of pancreatic cancer if ultrasonography (*US*), computed tomography (*CT*), endoscopic retrograde pancreatography (*ERP*), and pancreatic function test (*PFT*) are available.

secretion. In physiological terms, this means that the acinar tissue in the head of the pancreas is capable of maximal enzyme secretion.

We have investigated the relationship between malabsorption, decreased caloric consumption, and weight loss in 12 patients with pancreatic cancer (Perez et al. 1983). Eleven of the 12 patients had weight loss, 9 had malabsorption, and 7 had decreased caloric consumption. In these patients, the coefficients of protein and fat absorption were correlated with the percentage of body weight loss. However, the percent body weight loss did not correlate with the coefficient of caloric consumption. Therefore, at least in these patients, malabsorption, rather than decreased caloric intake, was the major reason for weight loss.

Because of these findings, we believe it is prudent to treat patients with pancreatic cancer and weight loss with pancreatic enzyme replacements. In our experience (Perez et al. 1983), every patient with significant fat and protein malabsorption improved his coefficient of fat and protein absorption by ingesting eight pancreatin tablets with meals (two at the beginning and end of the meal and four during the meal), except one patient who had a biliary cutaneous fistula, which was probably a major contributing factor to fat malabsorption. Thus, these patients should be treated with pancreatic enzymes, which may decrease weight loss.

REFERENCES

DiMagno EP. 1982. Diagnosis of chronic pancreatitis: Are noninvasive tests of exocrine pancreatic function sensitive and specific? *Gastroenterology* 83:143–146.

DiMagno EP, Malagelada JR, Go VLW. 1979. The relationships between pancreatic ductal obstruction and pancreatic secretion in man. *Mayo Clin Proc* 54:157–162.

DiMagno EP, Malagelada JR, Moertel CG, et al. 1977a. Prospective evaluation of the pancreatic secretion of immunoreactive carcinoembryonic antigen, enzyme, and bicarbonate in patients suspected of having pancreatic cancer. *Gastroenterology* 73:457–461.

DiMagno EP, Malagelada JR, Taylor WP, et al. 1977b. A prospective comparison of current diagnostic tests in pancreatic cancer. *N Engl J Med* 297:737–742.

DiMagno EP, Regan PT, Clain JE, et al. 1982. Human endoscopic ultrasonography. *Gastroenterology* 83:824–829.

Edis AJ, Kiernan PD, Taylor WF. 1980. Attempted curative resection of ductal carcinoma of the pancreas: Review of Mayo Clinic experience, 1951–1975. *Mayo Clin Proc* 55: 531–536.

Faintuch J, Levin B. 1986. Clinical presentation and diagnosis of exocrine tumors of the pancreas. In *The Exocrine Pancreas: Biology, Pathobiology and Diseases*, VLW Go et al., eds., pp. 675–687. New York: Raven Press.

Ferrucci JF Jr, Wittenberg J. 1978. CT biopsy of abdominal tumors: Aids for lesion localization. *Radiology* 129:739–744.

Fitzgerald PJ, Fortner JG, Watson RC, et al. 1978. The value of diagnostic aids in detecting pancreas cancer. *Cancer* 41:868–879.

Go VL, Taylor WF, DiMagno EP. 1981. Efforts at early diagnosis of pancreatic cancer: The Mayo Clinic experience. *Cancer* 3:1698–1703.

Gordis L, Gold EB. 1986. Epidemiology and etiology of pancreatic cancer. In *The Exocrine Pancreas: Biology, Pathobiology and Diseases*, VLW Go et al., eds., pp. 621–636. New York: Raven Press.

Holyoke ED, Douglass HO, Goldrosen MH, et al. 1979. Tumor markers in pancreatic cancer. *Semin Oncol* 6:3.

Klavins JV. 1981. Tumor markers of pancreatic carcinoma. *Cancer* 47:1597–1601.

Moossa AR, Levin B. 1979. Collaborative studies in the diagnosis of pancreatic cancer. *Semin Oncol* 6:298–308.

Moossa AR, Levin B. 1981. The diagnosis of "early" pancreatic cancer: The University of Chicago experience. *Cancer* 47:1688–1697.

Perez MM, Newcomer AD, Moertel CG, et al. 1983. Assessment of weight loss, food intake, fat metabolism, malabsorption, and treatment of pancreatic insufficiency in pancreatic cancer. *Cancer* 52:346–352.

Podolsky DK, McPhee MS, Alpert E, et al. 1981. Galactosyltransferase isoenzyme II in the detection of pancreatic cancer: Comparison with radiologic, endoscopic, and serologic tests. *N Engl J Med* 304:1313–1318.

Ritts R R Jr, Jacobsen D, Ilstrup D, et al. 1984. A prospective evaluation of MoAb CA 19-9 to detect GI cancer in a high risk clinic population. *Cancer Detect Prev* 7:525.

Ritts R R Jr, Klug T, Jacobsen D, et al. 1984. Multiple tumor marker tests enhance sensitivity of pancreatic carcinoma detection. *Cancer Detect Prev* 7:459.

van Heerden JA, Heath PM, Alden CR. 1980. Biliary bypass for ductal adenocarcinoma of the pancreas: Mayo Clinic experience, 1970–1975. *Mayo Clin Proc* 55:537–540.

Yeh H. 1981. Percutaneous fine needle aspiration biopsy of intraabdominal lesions with ultrasound guidance. *Am J Gastroenterol* 75:148–152.

Zamcheck N, Martin EW. 1981. Factors controlling the circulating CEA levels in pancreatic cancer. *Cancer* 47:1620–1627.

Annual Clinical Conference on Cancer, Vol. 30
Gastrointestinal Cancer: Current Approaches to Diagnosis and Treatment
© 1988 by The University of Texas System Cancer Center

26. Percutaneous Biliary Drainage

C. Humberto Carrasco

Although Burkhardt and Muller described percutaneous cholecystography in 1921 and Huard and Do-Xuan-Hop performed percutaneous transhepatic cholangiography in 1937, these diagnostic techniques remained largely ignored for almost four decades. Early investigators, however, realized that percutaneous cholangiography was useful in the differential diagnosis of jaundice. They also recognized that peritoneal bile leakage, the main problem of this diagnostic modality, could be prevented by leaving a drainage catheter within the bile ducts until definitive surgical procedures could be performed (Atkinson, Happey, and Smiddy 1960; Shaldon, Barber, and Young 1962; Dodd, Greening, and Wallace 1965). Subsequently, biliary catheters were maintained for continuous drainage in patients who were poor operative candidates (Kaude, Weidenmeir, and Agee 1969; Molnar and Stockum 1974). Thus, percutaneous transhepatic biliary drainage was developed as an extension of percutaneous needle cholangiography.

The development of noninvasive imaging techniques like ultrasonography, computerized tomography (CT), and nuclear scintigraphy have aided in the often difficult diagnostic differentiation of obstructive jaundice from that caused by parenchymal disease by confirming or excluding the presence of biliary duct dilatation. These techniques often fail to demonstrate the site of the obstruction, whereas percutaneous cholangiography will confirm the presence of ductal obstruction and reveal its site, thus suggesting its possible etiology.

Malignant biliary obstruction may be secondary to carcinomas arising in the pancreas, bile ducts, and liver; to metastases from primary neoplasms of the gastrointestinal tract, lungs, and breast; and to lymphoma or melanoma. Patients with malignant biliary obstruction have a poor prognosis with few prospects for cure because current therapeutic and palliative modalities have had little effect on the course of the disease.

Although prolonged survivals may be achieved in some patients with resectable primary neoplasms causing biliary obstruction, obstructive jaundice caused by metastatic disease from most primary neoplasms is usually a terminal event. The lifespan of these patients may be shortened even more by recurrent cholangitis, progressive hepatic decompensation, and nutritional deficiencies caused by the interruption of bile flow. Pruritus is often an incapacitating symptom that is unresponsive to the usual medical therapy. Percutaneous biliary decompression will relieve jaundice, its symptoms, and the metabolic alterations associated with it in patients with malignant obstruction, most of whom are poor candidates for surgical bilioenteric bypass.

Three types of biliary drainage are performed percutaneously: external, combined internal-external, and internal employing indwelling stents. External biliary drainage, achieved by placing a catheter proximal to the site of the biliary obstruction, does not allow flow of bile into the duodenum and intestines, resulting in fluid and electrolyte losses, malabsorption, and malnutrition. Oral ingestion of the drained bile has been suggested to prevent its loss, but patients do not tolerate this for long. Bile flow into the duodenum may be reestablished by passing a catheter through the lumen of the obstructed segment, which is combined internal-external drainage, or by placing an indwelling stent at the level of the obstruction.

INDICATIONS AND CONTRAINDICATIONS

Patients with biliary obstruction secondary to resectable malignancies may benefit from preoperative biliary decompression. The morbidity and mortality rates associated with pancreatoduodenectomy in patients with total serum bilirubin greater than 10 mg/dl have been reported to be higher than in those with lesser degrees of jaundice. It has been recommended, therefore, that the operative procedure be performed in two stages: (1) a preliminary bilioenteric bypass to improve hepatic function, bleeding parameters, and overall metabolic condition, and (2) second-stage pancreatoduodenectomy (Braash and Gray 1977; Brooks and Culebras 1976; Maki et al. 1966). Operative mortality rates of 10% to 33% have been reported, however, for various types of surgical decompressive procedures (Brooks and Culebras 1976; Feduska, Dent, and Lindenauer 1971; Buckwalter, Lawton, and Adrick 1965; Nakase et al. 1977; Hertzberg 1974) for which the complications may be as high as 59% in patients with metastatic disease (Feduska, Dent, and Lindenauer 1971). Preoperative percutaneous biliary drainage has been found by some investigators (Nakayama, Ikeda, and Okuda 1978; Dawson 1965) to decrease the incidence of postoperative complications, whereas others (Norlander, Kalin, and Sundblad 1982; Hatfield et al. 1982) have not found any benefit in the preoperative reduction of the serum bilirubin.

The percutaneous drainage modality is an important adjunct to palliative treatment in patients with unresectable carcinomas because it also allows the administration of chemotherapeutic agents that require low serum bilirubin levels. In addition, percutaneous biliary drainage is used in treating acute suppurative cholangitis (Nakayama, Ikeda, and Okuda 1978; Kadir et al. 1982; Ferrucci, Mueller, and Harbin 1980), in cases of failed bilioenteric bypass, and for diversion of bile flow in treating bile leaks and fistulas where it may be used in conjunction with percutaneous drainage of the extraductal bile collections (Kaufman et al. 1985). Percutaneous access to the biliary system also allows the performance of biopsies of intraductal lesions. Biopsies of extraductal lesions are performed percutaneously with a fine needle aimed at the site of the obstruction.

Percutaneous biliary drainage is contraindicated in the presence of multiple sites of intrahepatic biliary obstruction, which is usually caused by hepatic metastases. Catheter drainage for patients in this situation is impractical because multiple catheters would be required for adequate drainage. These patients are usually in the terminal stages of their disease; thus, biliary drainage is not likely to offer significant palliation. Moreover, drainage of an isolated segment results in bacterial contamination, which may lead to intractable infection of the undrained segments. Abnormal coagulation parameters constitute a relative contraindication and should be corrected whenever possible.

PREPROCEDURAL CONSIDERATIONS

The clinically suspected bile duct obstruction should be confirmed by a noninvasive imaging study, such as ultrasound, CT, or radionuclide scintigraphy, which may also suggest its etiology. Preprocedural administration of appropriate antibiotics is required in patients suspected of having cholangitis. The patient must have a thorough understanding of the procedure and should be informed of the possibility of experiencing severe pain during and after insertion of the drainage catheter. Intravenous sedatives and analgesics should be titrated according to each patient's needs; nitrous oxide, when available, provides adequate analgesia.

TECHNIQUE

The most commonly used method for percutaneous biliary drainage is the modified Seldinger technique, which may be divided into two stages: fine-needle percutaneous cholangiography, and definitive puncture for insertion of the drainage catheter.

The puncture site should be located in the mid or anterior axillary line below the tenth rib to avoid violating the pleural space. For drainage through the left hepatic duct, the puncture site is located below the sternal xiphoid, which avoids the pleural space.

Fine-needle percutaneous cholangiography under fluoroscopic guidance is done initially for visualization of the obstructed bile ducts. A 22- or a 23-gauge needle is inserted through the hepatic parenchyma into an intrahepatic bile duct, and contrast medium is injected until a duct adequate for the definitive puncture is opacified. If a bile duct is not punctured on the first attempt, the fine needle is reinserted at a slightly different angle. Usually, no more than two or three passes are necessary to puncture a dilated biliary system, but up to 10 or more attempts may be required for entering nondilated intrahepatic ducts. Although the number of passes performed has no direct bearing on morbidity, if a duct is not entered after six passes, ductal dilatation and, therefore, biliary obstruction is unlikely (Harbin, Mueller, and Ferrucci 1980). The success rate of ductal opacification in the presence of dilated intrahepatic ducts has been reported to be 99%; however, in patients with nondilated ducts, it is only 74% (Mueller et al. 1981).

Inserting the Drainage Catheter

After cholangiography, the fine needle is left in place to prevent bile leakage and allow injection of more contrast medium if necessary. A horizontal duct in the right lobe of the liver is selected for the definitive puncture and catheterization. The selected duct is punctured with an 18-gauge sheathed needle through which a guide wire is inserted. Subsequently, the tract is progressively dilated and the drainage catheter inserted.

Simplified single-puncture insertions have been devised in an attempt to decrease risks of hemorrhage and bile leakage. Hawkins (1979) designed a 45-cm-long 22-gauge needle over which a sheath is introduced if the initial puncture is satisfactory; however, the needle's long length and flexibility have made its use cumbersome (Ferrucci, Mueller, and Harbin 1980). Cope (1982) devised a method for making the initial puncture with a 21-gauge needle, then inserting a 0.018-inch guide wire through the needle into the bile ducts, and exchanging the needle for a dilator that could accommodate a 0.038-inch guide wire for final placement of the drainage catheter. However, this procedure may be prolonged because of suboptimal fluoroscopic visualization of the initial guide wire.

Internal-External Drainage

The initial procedure should be limited to external drainage, which will minimize manipulations to decrease the risk of sepsis. If bile flow is to be directed into the duodenum, the obstruction is traversed two or three days later by a 10- to 12-F drainage catheter with sideholes appropriately placed above and below the level of the obstruction. Using catheters of adequate size is important because inadequate drainage leads to bile stasis predisposing the patient to cholangitis (Mueller, van Sonnenberg, and Ferrucci 1982).

After the internal-external catheter has been in place for one or two days, its hub is capped to initiate internal drainage and the patient is observed for signs of cholangitis. If the patient experiences pain, fever, or chills, the catheter is uncapped and also allowed to drain externally. Cholangitis usually signals inadequate bile drainage and stasis, which may be related to abnormal choledochoduodenal pressure gradients. In patients who have had gastroenterostomies, passage of a long catheter through the obstruction for bile drainage into the efferent loop may improve drainage. If the drainage catheter cannot be internalized and fluid and electrolyte losses are excessive, jejunal intubation through an endoscopic (Ponsky and Aszodi 1982) or percutaneous gastrostomy may be used as an external bypass.

DRAINAGE IN OBSTRUCTIVE CHOLANGITIS

Acute obstructive cholangitis with fever, chills, pain, and jaundice may be caused by total or partial obstruction of the common bile duct or one of its branches. The morbidity and mortality rates of surgical decompression in acute obstructive cholangitis are reported to be as high as 50% to 75% (Dow and Lindenauer 1969; Ostermiller et al. 1965; Boey and Way 1980); failure to decompress the biliary system may, however, cause suppurative cholangitis, hepatic abscesses, septicemia, and shock leading to death. The use of percutaneous biliary drainage has reduced the mortality rates associated with this condition; in a series of 18 patients, nine of whom had the suppurative form of cholangitis, the mortality rate was 17% (Kadir, Baassiri, and Barth 1982).

Although, in an obstructed biliary system, antibiotic drugs do not reach the concentrations needed to alter the system's bacterial content, they must be administered to control the bacteremia that occurs during the drainage procedure. Bile antibiotic levels increase when biliary drainage is reestablished. The predrainage cholangiogram should be done with a small amount of contrast medium to avoid excessive intraductal pressures that produce cholangiovenous or cholangiolymphatic backflow (Huang, Bass, and Williams 1969; Jacobsson, Kjellander, and Rosengren 1962), which may cause bacteremia. For the same reason, manipulations should be minimized.

POSTPROCEDURAL CARE

During the first few days after the procedure, patients' water and electrolyte losses are closely monitored and replaced by intravenous solutions, and infections are treated with appropriate antibiotics.

Combined internal-external drainage catheters that have been capped are flushed with 10 ml of physiological solution once every other day to maintain longer patency. We do not routinely flush external drainage catheters. Since these catheters eventually become obstructed, one recommendation is to exchange them every three months (Ring et al. 1979), although we and others (Ferrucci, Mueller, and Harbin 1980) prefer to exchange them only when they become dysfunctional. The function and patency of an internally draining catheter are reliably evaluated by routine measurement of intraductal pressures through the drainage catheter. Catheters are exchanged only when the intraductal pressures exceed 20 cm of water (Beinart et al. 1982).

Patients and family members are taught that periodic cleansing and dressing changes reduce skin damage around the catheter insertion site. Patients are allowed to shower but not to immerse themselves in water.

RESULTS

The serum bilirubin level usually declines rapidly after the drainage procedure. In 25 patients with biliary obstruction but no hepatic metastases, Hansson et al. (1979) reported a mean serum bilirubin decrease from 17 mg/dl to 5 mg/dl after two weeks of drainage and mean bile output of 610 mg/24 hours. In 13 patients with obstruction and hepatic metastases, the mean serum bilirubin of 17 mg/ml decreased to 9 mg/ml after two weeks of drainage, and the mean volume of bile drained was 360 ml/24 hours. Berquist et al. (1980) reported resolution of pruritus and jaundice in 88% of their 50 patients who underwent percutaneous biliary drainage. Patients undergoing drainage because of sepsis usually become afebrile within 24 hours.

In 131 of our patients with cancer, the overall median survival from the time of percutaneous drainage was only 57 days. This short survival reflects the terminal nature of biliary obstruction in patients with metastatic disease who frequently undergo the procedure before starting chemotherapy regimens that require low serum bilirubin. Patients who underwent subsequent surgical biliary bypass had a somewhat better median survival (172 days) than did those for whom percutaneous drainage was definitive (46 days). This reflects the better clinical status of the surgical candidates, most of whom had carcinoma of the pancreas, a disease in which jaundice often occurs relatively early (Carrasco, Zornoza, and Bechtel 1984).

COMPLICATIONS

The acute complications of biliary drainage are related to the procedure, whereas delayed complications are related to chronic catheter drainage. The incidence of acute complications is low; a review of 200 patients who underwent percutaneous biliary drainage showed that sepsis occurred in seven, clinically apparent hemorrhage occurred in six, and three patients died, including two of the six who had hemorrhaged. Fever and hemobilia occurred in 21 and 18 patients, respectively (Mueller, van Sonnenberg, and Ferrucci 1982).

Cholangitis is the most frequent complication in patients with chronic drainage (Hansson et al. 1979). In our series of 161 cancer patients who underwent the procedure, cholangitis was documented in 47%, often during periods of myelosuppression. The most frequently cultured organisms in bile were enterococci, *Klebsiella, Escherichia coli, Pseudomonas,* and *Candida.*

Although bacterial colonization of the biliary tree occurs soon after the drainage catheter is placed, it alone does not produce symptoms. An inadequate bile flow caused by a small catheter lumen, catheter occlusion, or increased intraduodenal pressures leads to bile stasis, bacterial overgrowth, and clinical cholangitis. Epithelial damage during catheter insertion may also predispose to bacterial invasion.

Partial catheter dislodgement may predispose patients to cholangitis because of inadequate drainage, or to bleeding, when the catheter sideholes abut a vessel. Partial displacement can usually be easily corrected. Complete dislodgement of the catheter, however, in patients who do not have a well-established biliocutaneous tract, may cause significant complications because reestablishing percutaneous drainage may be impossible in a nondilated biliary tree that is decompressed into the peritoneal cavity. The catheter became dislodged in 18% of our patients and it became occluded in 14% (Carrasco, Zornoza, and Bechtel 1984).

Occlusion would probably occur in most patients if catheter drainage were maintained for long periods. It is usually caused by encrustations and manifested by sepsis, hyperbilirubinemia, and external bile drainage around the catheter. Obstructed catheters should be exchanged for new ones because success with unclogging is usually short-lived. Leakage of ascitic fluid around the catheter cannot be corrected mechanically.

Intrahepatic vascular lesions, including pseudoaneurysms and arterioportal fistulas, have been reported in 26% to 33% of the patients undergoing percutaneous transhepatic biliary drainage (Hoevels and Nilsson 1980; Okuda et al. 1978), but the majority remain asymptomatic and rarely experience severe bleeding. When these vascular lesions become symptomatic, they are best treated by transcatheter embolization (Mitchell et al. 1985; Kadir et al. 1980; Druy 1981). McLean et al. (1982) described massive hemobilia in three patients who had been irradiated in the area traversed by the percutaneous drainage catheter.

Pleural complications including empyema, hemothorax, pneumothorax, and bilious pleural effusion occur in 1% to 2.5% of patients (Nakayama, Ikeda, and Okuda 1978; Mueller, van Sonnenberg, and Ferrucci 1982; Berquist et al. 1980; Clark et al. 1981; Oleaga and Ring 1981). The incidence of these complications is low, considering that procedures performed by the lateral intercostal approach may easily violate the pleural space. Use of the left subxiphoid approach, which avoids pleural puncture, has been suggested for patients who are uncooperative or obese, for patients who have ascites, pleural effusion, or emphysema, or for those in whom only the left hepatic duct is obstructed (Nichols, Cooperberg, and Golding 1984).

We have observed a cholerrhagic state with bile output as high as 7 liters per day in 5% of our patients (Carrasco, Zornoza, and Bechtel 1984). This is an unusual complication that occurs within the first few days after the percutaneous drainage procedure. It is temporary and its pathophysiology is unknown but it brings severe fluid and electrolyte losses and may result in hypotension and symptomatic hyponatremia that require aggressive replacement therapy.

INDWELLING STENTS

The disadvantages of biliary drainage by percutaneous catheters—persistent pain at the catheter entry site, catheter dislodgement, leakage of bile around the catheter, and the negative psychological effects—are avoided with indwelling stents. These are short tubes of various designs introduced percutaneously through the tract of a biliary drainage catheter or endoscopically, after papillotomy.

An indwelling stent is inserted percutaneously at least two or three days after insertion of the drainage catheter, which allows for maturation of the tract and thus facilitates the procedure. The drainage catheter is removed over a guide wire, and the endoprosthesis is inserted into the obstructed segment.

Theoretically, the adequacy of catheter drainage depends on the physical properties of the catheter material, its luminal diameter, its length, and the total area of its inflow and outflow sideholes, as well as the pressure gradient and the type of fluid being drained (Kerlan et al. 1984). Although stents larger than 8- to 10-F are best for internal drainage, transhepatic insertion of them is painful and requires a well-established tract. A combined peroral-transhepatic method (Kerlan et al. 1984) and an endoscopic technique (Siegel and Daniel 1984) have been described for passage of a relatively large endoprosthesis. To improve drainage and possibly prolong patency without excessive hepatic trauma, we introduce two 8- to 10-F stents placed alongside each other.

After the indwelling stent is inserted, an external drainage catheter is left in place and allowed to drain for 24 to 48 hours to clear clots and other debris. Then the external drain is clamped for 24 hours for a trial of internal drainage. If the patient has no fever, chills, pain, or increasing serum bilirubin, the external catheter is removed. The risks of external biliary fistula or intraperitoneal bile leakage are probably decreased when the transhepatic tract is plugged with a piece of Gelfoam as the external drainage catheter is removed.

Migrating stents can be repositioned with preplaced sutures through the proximal end of the prosthesis (Miskowiak et al. 1982), with a threaded sling (Owman and Lunderquist 1983), and with balloon catheters (Honickman et al. 1982; Harries-Jones, Fataar, and Tuft 1982). In our use of stents with Mallecott tips at both ends, migration has not been a problem. In the case of stent occlusion by encrustations and tumor, which may eventually be inevitable, a new stent can be introduced percutaneously and placed alongside the obstructed one, or the occluded stent can be pushed into the duodenum to be excreted by the patient and a new one inserted in its place.

In patients with malignant biliary obstruction, the complications of indwelling stents seem to be lower than those of external-internal catheters. The early complication rate of 17% in a series of 113 patients who underwent stent placement was mainly related to unstable stent positioning in periportal obstructions, and the late complication rate of 31% was related to lumen occlusion and stent migration (Mueller et al. 1985). In another series of 99 patients undergoing drainage with indwelling stents, cholangitis occurred in only seven patients and was treated successfully with antibiotics; subphrenic and subhepatic abscesses occurred in three patients (Burcharth et al. 1981). Coons and Carey (1983) reported a 13% incidence of complications in 62 patients in whom biliary endoprostheses were inserted.

Median survival among 94 patients with malignant biliary obstruction who received indwelling stents was 62 days and ranged from 1 week to 2.5 years (Burcharth et al. 1981), a survival rate comparable to that of cancer patients with other types of biliary drainage (Carrasco, Zornoza, and Bechtel 1984).

PERCUTANEOUS CHOLECYSTOSTOMY

Decompressive cholecystostomy is performed with fluoroscopy or ultrasound for patients who have acute cholecystitis or common bile duct obstruction (Burkhardt and Muller 1982; Shaver, Hawkins, and Soong 1982; Teplick et al. 1982). Although a transhepatic approach to the gallbladder theoretically might decrease the risk of peritoneal bile leakage, puncture through its peritoneal surface has been reported without complications (Shaver, Hawkins, and Soong 1982; Teplick et al. 1982). In patients with common bile duct obstruction, however, puncture of the gallbladder's peritoneal surface without subsequent drainage may lead to significant intraperitoneal bile leakage.

DILATATION OF STRICTURES

Malignant strictures are not amenable to dilatation. Although benign biliary strictures are uncommon, they may cause many problems including progressive hepatic failure and sepsis, and operative repair of them is associated with a high rate of failure (Warren and Jefferson 1973). In one study of percutaneous balloon catheter dilatation of these strictures (Gallacher et al. 1985), patency rates after 36 months were higher than 67% for anastomotic strictures, 76% for iatrogenic strictures, and 42% for strictures associated with sclerosing cholangitis. The complications of the procedure were mostly minor and occurred in less than 7% of the patients.

CONCLUSION

Although percutaneous biliary drainage is an effective method of biliary decompression and usually palliates the symptoms associated with jaundice, it is not without potential for multiple problems. Complications that may be considered minor have a greater significance in the cancer patient whose organism is being deranged by a multitude of insults related to the disease and the therapeutic measures employed in attempts at palliation.

REFERENCES

Atkinson M, Happey MG, Smiddy FG. 1960. Percutaneous transhepatic cholangiography. *Gut* 1:357–365.

Beinart C, Sniderman KW, Tamura S, et al. 1982. Biliary pressure measurement: An aid in the management of patients on internal biliary drainage. *Invest Radiol* 17:356–361.

Berquist TH, May GR, Johnson CM, et al. 1981. Percutaneous biliary decompression: Internal and external drainage in 50 patients. *AJR* 136:901–906.

Boey JH, Way LW. 1980. Acute cholangitis. *Ann Surg* 191:264–270.

Braash JW, Gray BN. 1977. Considerations that lower pancreatoduodenectomy mortality. *Am J Surg* 129:480–483.

Brooks JR, Culebras JM. 1976. Cancer of the pancreas. Palliative operation, Whipple procedure or total pancreatectomy? *Am J Surg* 131:516–520.

Buckwalter JA, Lawton RL, Adrick RT. 1965. Bypass operations for neoplastic biliary tract obstruction. *Am J Surg* 109:100–106.

Burcharth F, Efsen F, Christiansen LA, et al. 1981. Nonsurgical internal biliary drainage by endoprosthesis. *Surg Gynecol Obstet* 153:857–860.

Burkhardt H, Muller WJ. 1921. Versuche uber die Punktion er Gallenblase und ihre Rontgendarstellung. *Deutsche Zeitschrift Fuer Chirurgie* 162:168–197.

Carrasco CH, Zornoza J, Bechtel WJ. 1984. Malignant biliary obstruction: Complications of percutaneous biliary drainage. *Radiology* 152:343–346.

Clark RA, Mitchell SE, Colley DP, et al. 1981. Percutaneous catheter biliary decompression. *AJR* 137:503–509.

Coons HG, Carey PH. 1983. Large-bore, long biliary endoprostheses (biliary stents) for improved drainage. *Radiology* 148:89–94.

Cope C. 1982. Conversion from small (0.018 inch) to large (0.038 inch) percutaneous drainage procedures. *AJR* 138:170–171.

Dawson JL. 1965. The incidence of post-operative renal failure in obstructive jaundice. *Br J Surg* 52:663–665.

Dodd GD, Greening RR, Wallace S. 1965. The radiologic diagnosis of cancer. In *Management of the Patient with Cancer,* TF Nealon Jr, ed., pp. 72–113. Philadelphia: W.B. Saunders.

Dow RW, Lindenauer SM. 1969. Acute obstructive suppurative cholangitis. *Ann Surg* 169:272–276.

Druy EM. 1981. Hepatic artery-biliary fistula following percutaneous transhepatic biliary drainage. *Radiology* 141:369–370.

Feduska NJ, Dent T, Lindenauer SM. 1971. Results of palliative operations for carcinoma of the pancreas. *Arch Surg* 103:330–334.

Ferrucci JT Jr, Mueller PR, Harbin WP. 1980. Percutaneous transhepatic biliary drainage: Technique, results, and applications. *Radiology* 135:1–13.

Gallacher DJ, Kadir S, Kaufman SL, et al. 1985. Nonoperative management of benign postoperative biliary strictures. *Radiology* 156:625–629.

Hansson JA, Hoevels J, Simert G, et al. 1979. Clinical aspects of nonsurgical percutaneous transhepatic bile drainage in obstructive lesions of the extrahepatic bile ducts. *Ann Surg* 189:58–61.

Harbin WP, Mueller PR, Ferrucci JT Jr. 1980. Transhepatic cholangiography: Complications and use patterns of the fine-needle technique. A multi-institutional survey. *Radiology* 135:15–22.

Harries-Jones EP, Fataar S, Tuft RJ. 1982. Repositioning of biliary endoprosthesis with Grüntzig balloon catheters. *AJR* 138:771–772.

Hatfield AR, Tobias R, Terblanche J, et al. 1982. Preoperative external biliary drainage in obstructive jaundice: A prospective controlled clinical trial. *Lancet* 2:896–899.

Hawkins IF Jr. 1979. A new fine needle for cholangiography with optional sheath for decompression. *Radiology* 131:252–253.

Hertzberg J. 1974. Pancreaticoduodenal resection and bypass operation in patients with carcinoma of the head of the pancreas, ampulla, and distal end of the common duct. *Acta Chir Scand* 140:523–527.

Hoevels J, Nilsson U. 1980. Intrahepatic vascular lesions following nonsurgical percutaneous transhepatic bile duct intubation. *Gastrointest Radiol* 5:127–135.

Honickman SP, Mueller PR, Ferrucci JT Jr, et al. Malpositioned biliary endoprosthesis: Retrieval using a vascular balloon catheter. *Radiology* 144:423–425.

Huang T, Bass JA, Williams RD. 1969. The significance of biliary pressure in cholangitis. *Arch Surg* 98:629–632.

Huard P, Do-Xuan-Hop. 1937. La ponction transhépatique des canaux biliaires. *Bull Soc Med Chir de l'Indochine* 15:1090–1100.

Jacobsson B, Kjellander J, Rosengren B. 1962. Cholangiovenous reflux: An experimental study. *Acta Chir Scand* 123:316–321.

Kadir S, Athanasoulis CA, Ring EJ, et al. 1980. Transcatheter embolization of intrahepatic arterial aneurysms. *Radiology* 134:335–339.

Kadir S, Baassiri A, Barth KH, et al. 1982. Percutaneous biliary drainage in the management of biliary sepsis. *AJR* 138:25–29.

Kaude JV, Weidenmier CH, Agee OF. 1969. Decompression of bile ducts with the percutaneous transhepatic technique. *Radiology* 93:69–71.

Kaufman SL, Kadir S, Mitchell SE, et al. 1985. Percutaneous transhepatic biliary drainage for bile leaks and fistulas. *AJR* 144:1055–1058.

Kerlan RK Jr, Ring EJ, Pogany AC, et al. Biliary endoprostheses: Insertion using a combined peroral-transhepatic method. *Radiology* 150:828–830.

Kerlan RK Jr, Stimac G, Pogany AC, et al. 1984. Bile flow through drainage catheters: An in vitro study. *AJR* 143:1085–1087.

McLean GK, Ring EJ, Freiman DB. 1982. Therapeutic alternatives in the treatment of intrahepatic biliary obstruction. *Radiology* 145:289–295.

Maki T, Sato T, Kakizaki G, et al. 1966. Pancreatoduodenectomy for periampullary carcinomas. *Arch Surg* 92:825–833.

Miskowiak J, Mygind T, Baden H, et al. 1982. Biliary endoprosthesis secured by a subcutaneous button to prevent dislocation. *AJR* 139:1019–1020.

Mitchell SE, Shuman LS, Kaufman SL, et al. 1985. Biliary catheter drainage complicated by hemobilia: Treatment by balloon embolotherapy. *Radiology* 157:645–652.

Molnar W, Stockum AE. 1974. Relief of obstructive jaundice through percutaneous transhepatic catheter: A new therapeutic method. *AJR* 122:356–367.

Mueller PR, Ferrucci JT Jr, Teplick SK, et al. 1985. Biliary stent endoprosthesis: Analysis of complications in 113 patients. *Radiology* 156:637–639.

Mueller PR, Harbin WP, Ferrucci JT Jr, et al. 1981. Fine needle transhepatic cholangiography: Reflections after 450 cases. *AJR* 136:85–90.

Mueller PR, van Sonnenberg E, Ferrucci JT. 1982. Percutaneous biliary drainage: Technical and catheter-related problems in 200 procedures. *AJR* 138:17–23.

Nakase A, Matsumoto Y, Uchida K, et al. 1977. Surgical treatment of cancer of the pancreas and the periampullary region. *Ann Surg* 185:52–57.

Nakayama T, Ikeda A, Okuda K. 1978. Percutaneous transhepatic drainage of the biliary tract. *Gastroenterology* 74:554–559.

Nichols DM, Cooperberg PL, Golding RH, et al. 1984. The safe intercostal approach? Pleural complications in abdominal interventional radiology. *AJR* 141:1013–1018.

Norlander A, Kalin B, Sundblad R. 1982. Effect of percutaneous transhepatic drainage upon liver function and postoperative mortality. *Surg Gynecol Obstet* 155:161–166.

Okuda K, Mucha H, Nakajima Y, et al. 1978. Frequency of intrahepatic arteriovenous fistula as a sequela to percutaneous needle puncture of the liver. *Gastroenterology* 74:1204–1207.

Oleaga JA, Ring EJ. 1981. Interventional biliary radiology. *Semin Roentgenol* 16:116–134.

Ostermiller W Jr, Thompson RJ Jr, Carter R, et al. 1965. Acute obstructive cholangitis. *Arch Surg* 90:392–395.

Owman T, Lunderquist A. 1983. Sling retraction for proximal placement of percutaneous transhepatic biliary endoprosthesis. *Radiology* 146:228–229.

Ponsky JL. Aszodi A. 1982. External biliary-gastric fistula: A simple method for recycling bile. *Am J Gastroenterol* 77:939–940.

Ring EJ, Husted JW, Oleaga JA, et al. 1979. A multihole catheter for maintaining long-term percutaneous antegrade biliary drainage. *Radiology* 132:752–754.

Shaldon S, Barber KM, Young WB. 1962. Percutaneous transhepatic cholangiography. *Gastroenterology* 42:371–379.

Shaver RW, Hawkins IF Jr, Soong J. 1982. Percutaneous cholecystostomy. *AJR* 138:1133–1136.

Siegel JH, Daniel SJ. 1984. Endoscopic and fluoroscopic transpapillary placement of a large caliber biliary endoprosthesis. *Am J Gastroenterol* 79:461–465.

Teplick SK, Wolferth CC Jr, Hayes MF Jr, et al. 1982. Percutaneous cholecystostomy in obstructive jaundice. *Gastrointest Radiol* 7:259–261.

Warren KW, Jefferson MF. 1973. Prevention and repair of strictures of the extrahepatic bile ducts. *Surg Clin North Am* 53:1169–1190.

Annual Clinical Conference on Cancer, Vol. 30
Gastrointestinal Cancer: Current Approaches to Diagnosis and Treatment
© 1988 by The University of Texas System Cancer Center

27. Endoscopic Palliation of Malignant Obstructive Jaundice: A New Wave

Robert E. Davis

Malignant neoplasms causing obstruction of the biliary system in most cases are found to be surgically unresectable for cure. This is determined by preoperative evaluation or at the time of exploratory surgery (Fedusca, Dent, and Lindenauer 1971; Gudjonsson 1981; Hermann and Vogt 1983; Huibregtse and Tytgat 1983; Arnesjo and Bakkevold 1984; Kuperman 1981; Ihse 1982). Most of these patients will be found to have adenocarcinoma of the pancreas (Sarr and Cameron 1984; Longmire 1984). Despite attempts to cure such patients through surgery, the reported five-year survival rate is only 5% (Gudjonsson 1981; Longmire 1984). Certain other types of malignancy involving the pancreas such as ampullary carcinoma, duodenal carcinoma, cystadenocarcinoma, islet cell tumors, and less frequent causes of malignant obstruction such as cholangiocarcinoma are associated with better survival rates (van Heerden 1984; Edmondson and Peters 1982). By use of improved preoperative screening procedures, including computerized tomography, ultrasound, and endoscopic retrograde cholangiopancreatography (ERCP), operative intervention is now focused on those lesions with a higher potential for cure; however, even T1N0M0 patients with adenocarcinoma of the pancreas have been reported to survive only an average of eight months (Kummerle and Ruckert 1984).

In those patients with unresectable tumors, relief of the biliary obstruction will lead to a better quality of life by alleviating pruritus, malabsorption, and liver dysfunction and by reducing possible life-threatening sequelae including cholangitis and related malabsorptive bleeding disorders (Sarr and Cameron 1984). Palliative bypass of the obstructed segment in the biliary system can be accomplished by surgical, percutaneous transhepatic, or endoscopic methods.

Nonoperative endoscopic placement of a biliary endoprosthesis has become the preferred therapy for incurable obstructive jaundice as either a primary therapy or for preoperative disease stabilization (Huibregtse and Tytgat 1983; Cotton 1984; van Heerden 1984; Tytgat et al. 1986; Huibregtse et al. 1986). Surgical bypass procedures require longer hospitalization and may have a higher mortality than other decompressive methods but are recommended initially in cases involving duodenal obstruction (Huibregtse and Tytgat 1983; Sarr and Cameron 1984; Cotton 1984; Huibregtse et al. 1986). Percutaneous drainage or insertion of an endoprosthesis is beneficial but may create more trauma for the patient because of the associated risks of bleeding, pneumothorax, and bile peritonitis (Cotton 1984; Hagenmuller 1984; Tytgat et al. 1986). Percutaneous approaches are now recommended as follow-up to a failed endoscopic attempt but are considered most effective when combined with endoscopy.

HISTORY OF ENDOSCOPIC PROCEDURES OF THE BILIARY SYSTEM

The evolution toward endoscopic prosthetic therapy for biliary obstruction began in the late 1960s with successful endoscopic cannulation of the biliary system (Oi 1970). Endoscopic papillotomy was first used in 1974 in Germany and Japan for biliary calculi extraction. As endoscopists became more experienced, they began in 1980 to use the access to the common bile duct for placement of wire guides, catheters, and stents. Endoscopic sphincterotomy is now a commonplace procedure. Multiple technical advancements in sphincterotomies, including precut tools and guidewire passage, have increased the success rate and reduced the main complications of hemorrhage and perforation to less than 2%. In malignant ampullary obstruction, endoscopic sphincterotomy allows access to deeper tissues for biopsy to increase the yield for diagnosis. In all forms of malignant obstruction, sphincterotomy may allow presurgical decompressive therapy alone or with prostheses or, in the nonoperative patient, it may allow definitive stent therapy.

MATERIALS AND PROCEDURES

Today a plethora of biliary stents are commercially available. They vary in shape (straight, monopigtail, or double-pigtail), length (5–20 cm), outside diameter (3–12F), and material (Teflon, polyethylene, or polyurethane).

Initially, stents of 6 to 7F size were utilized by either single or multiple placement. As larger channel endoscopes became available, the larger-sized endoprosthesis (10–12F) appeared to provide a longer duration of patency than the smaller size (7F) (Tytgat et al. 1986; Snady and Siegel 1985). The straight or Amsterdam stents have found wider acceptance than curved ones because they are easier to introduce and also produce better flow rates.

Over the past 16 years, endoscopes have improved in the areas of optics, durability, sterilization ability, and electrical grounding. Since 1981, several instruments with larger channels have been developed (Olympus JFIT, 3.7 mm; Olympus TJF, 4.2 mm [Olympus Corp. of America, 4 Nevada Dr., New Hyde Park, NY 11042]; Pentax FD34A, 4.2 mm [Pentax Corporation, 30 Ramland Rd., Orangeburg, NY 10962-2699]), allowing placement of larger stents.

Endoscopic endoprosthesis placement requires both endoscopic and radiological guidance. After the patient is lightly sedated, the duodenoscope is passed to the ampullary level, giving an adequate esophageal, gastric, and duodenal view; at this point, a biopsy is performed for obvious lesions. ERCP is performed for diagnosis and localization of biliary and pancreatic ducts. Occasionally, a prosthesis may be placed directly through a normal sphincter or obvious tumor by use of ampullary dilators, but usually a small sphincterotomy (6–8 mm) is accomplished to facilitate endoprosthesis placement. A thin wire guide (0.035 in. diameter) with a flexible tip is introduced into the common bile duct through the malignant obstruction, well into the above biliary system; care is taken to avoid penetration into small biliary ductules. Several special wire guides have been developed to aid in crossing the strictures.

The size and length of a prosthesis is determined in accordance with radiographs of the obstruction. The prosthesis is placed over the guide wire followed by a pusher tube that advances it into the proper position. The upper portion of the prosthesis is left well above the obstruction, while the lower portion remains in the duodenum, projecting 1.2 cm. The distal "flap" on the straight stents or the curved end of the pigtail stents allows them to remain without extrusion. Bile flow, sometimes of a dark or purulent nature, will be endoscopically obvious.

SUCCESS RATES

Results are similar once the procedure is mastered (Cotton 1984; Hagenmuller 1984; Classen and Hagenmuller 1984; Siegel 1985; Haber and Kortan 1985). The overall success rate of the procedure is around 90%. The highest success rate (95%–100%) has been achieved in treatment of ampullary tumors, whereas in mid common duct and bifurcation tumors it has been only 70% to 75%. Bifurcation tumors require attempts at placing prostheses into both lobes to reduce the risk of cholangitis. The procedure is only completed in approximately 30% of these cases; however, placement of even one stent may be helpful (Tytgat et al. 1976; Cotton 1986). The overall failure rate of approximately 10% is related to duodenal deformity or compression by tumor, difficulty with papillotomy, or failure to pass the stenotic biliary segment. Mortality rates directly related to the procedure approach 2%. The 30-day mortality rate for advanced cancer ranges from 10% to 20%, whereas a mean survival of six to eight months and disappearance of jaundice is noted in 70% to 90% of cases.

COMPLICATIONS

Complications may occur soon after endoscopic endoprosthesis placement or weeks to months later. Early complications, which are related to cholangitis, occur in about 10% of cases particularly when first attempts at placement are not successful (Cotton 1986). Tumor perforation, pancreatitis, and post-sphincterotomy bleeding are less frequent. Administration of antibiotics and close attention to equipment sterilization are recommended to prevent cholangitis; however, achievement of adequate biliary drainage remains the single most important therapeutic regimen. Cholangitis occurs in 25% to 40% of cases in which hilar tumors are not fully drained and in 8% to 15% of cases of mid duct obstruction (Cotton 1984; Tytgat et al. 1986). Placement of a stent with endoscopic evidence of bile flow and no subsequent alleviation of jaundice suggests primary liver disease or multiple metastases.

The major late complication, clogging of the stent by biliary sludge, occurs in 20% to 30% of cases. The clogging occurs within three to five months after the insertion and may be heralded by fever, chills, a decline in liver function, or malaise (Tytgat et al. 1986; Snady and Siegel 1985). With such complications, the stent must be replaced. Other rare but potential complications include dislodgement or breakage of the endoprosthesis or tumor overgrowth. Late duodenal obstruction (mean interval of 305 days) has been reported in 4% to 8% of pancreatic cancer patients with distal common bile duct obstruction and in 17% of patients with papillary carcinomas (Huibregtse and Tytgat 1983; Huibregtse et al. 1986). Endoscopic exchange of a blocked stent is usually unsuccessful in such cases of duodenal obstruction, and gastroenterostomy is recommended.

CONCLUSION

Adenocarcinoma of the pancreas is the underlying cause of most cases of malignancy-related obstructive jaundice. These lesions are not commonly resectable for cure; thus, endoscopic placement of a large-sized endoprosthesis is a realistic alternative to surgical bypass or to percutaneous stenting to relieve jaundice. The palliative effect for those with expected short longevity can be achieved with 90% success.

Surgical intervention should be recommended as the appropriate first step in some cases, including those involving young patients with potential longer survival, those with tumors other than adenocarcinomas of the pancreas or with ampullary carcinomas, and those with impending duodenal obstruction. For all others, endoscopic biliary drainage is preferred.

For early or late complications of sepsis caused by biliary obstruction, adequate drainage should be provided by available methods. Therefore, multiple endoscopic stent changes, transhepatic drainage, and/or surgical decompression may be used to palliate the obstruction and relieve jaundice. The goal of therapy in those patients with expected short survival is to alleviate their symptoms and reduce their hospitalization time as much as possible.

Further study in endoscopic therapy is needed. Use of laser technology, placement of radioactive wires (iridium), diathermy tumor therapy, and more investigation of the events of biliary clogging await clarification and potential clinical application. Indeed, this new wave of endoscopic applications has permanently altered the routine management of malignant obstructive jaundice.

REFERENCES

Arnesjo B, Bakkevold K. 1984. Assessment of resectability. In *Non-Surgical Biliary Drainage,* M Classen, J Geenen, K Kawai, eds., pp. 15–19. New York: Springer-Verlag.

Classen M, Hagenmuller F. 1984. Endoscopic biliary drainage. *Scand J Gastroenterol* 102 [Suppl 2]:76–83.

Cotton PB. 1984. Endoscopic methods for relief of malignant obstructive jaundice. *World J Surg* 8:854–861.

Cotton PB. 1986. Endoscopic biliary stents: Trick or treatment. *Gastrointest Endosc* 82: 364–365.

Edmondson HA, Peters RL. 1982. Neoplasms of the liver. In *Diseases of the Liver,* 5th ed., L Schiff, ER Schiff, eds., pp. 1101–1157. Philadelphia: J.B. Lippincott.

Fedusca WJ, Dent TL, Lindenauer SM. 1971. Results of palliative operations for carcinoma of the pancreas. *Arch Surg* 103:330–334.

Gudjonsson B. 1981. Pancreatic carcinoma: Diagnostic and therapeutic approach—A word of caution. *J Clin Gastroenterol* 3:301–305.

Haber GB, Kortan PP. 1985. Complications of endobiliary prostheses (abstract 176). *Gastrointest Endosc* 31:168.

Hagenmuller F. 1984. Results of endoscopic bilioduodenal drainage in malignant bile duct stenosis. In *Non-Surgical Biliary Drainage,* M Classen, J Geenen, K Kawai, eds., pp. 93–104. New York: Springer-Verlag.

Hermann RE, Vogt DP. 1983. Cancer of the pancreas. *Compr Ther* 9:66–74.

Huibregtse K, Tytgat GNJ. 1983. Endoscopic placement of biliary prosthesis. In *Advances in Gastrointestinal Endoscopy,* Vol. 1, pp. 219–231. London: Chapman and Hall.

Huibregtse R, Raton RM, Coerve PP, et al. 1986. Endoscopic palliative treatment in pancreatic cancer. *Gastrointest Endosc* 32:334–338.

Ihse I. 1982. Treatment of pancreatic cancer: Current status. *Scand J Gastroenterol* 17:449–453.

Kummerle F, Ruckert K. 1984. Surgical treatment of pancreatic cancer. *World J Surg* 8:889–894.

Kuperman AM. 1981. Cancer of the ampulla of Vater, bile duct and duodenum. Symposium on Liver, Spleen and Pancreas. *Surg Clin North Am* 61:99–106.

Longmire WP Jr. 1984. Cancer of the pancreas: Palliative operation, Whipple procedure, or total pancreatectomy. *World J Surg* 8:872–879.

Oi I. 1970. Fiberduodenoscopy and endoscopic pancreatocholangiography. *Gastrointest Endosc* 17:59–62.

Sarr MG, Cameron JL. 1984. Surgical palliation of unresectable carcinoma of the pancreas. *World J Surg* 8:906–918.

Siegel JH. 1985. Biliary stents to unblock the system. Postgraduate Course, The American Society for Gastrointestinal Endoscopy. B Charles, E Stark, eds., pp. 195–202.

Snady H, Siegel JH. 1985. The significance of endoscopically placed prostheses in the management of malignant obstructions: Effect response of single large caliber catheters (abstract). *Am J Gastroenterol* 80:853.

Tytgat GN, Huibregtse R, Bartelsman JF, et al. 1986. Endoscopic palliative therapy of gastrointestinal and biliary tumours with prostheses. *Clin Gastroenterol* 15:249–271.

van Heerden JA. 1984. Pancreatic resection for carcinoma of the pancreas: Whipple versus total pancreatectomy—an institutional perspective. *World J Surg* 8:880–888.

Annual Clinical Conference on Cancer, Vol. 30
Gastrointestinal Cancer: Current Approaches to Diagnosis and Treatment
© 1988 by The University of Texas System Cancer Center

28. Hepatocellular Carcinoma: Clinical Presentation, Etiology, and Prevention

Michael C. Kew

Although hepatocellular carcinoma (HCC) is uncommon in North America, one quarter of a million people worldwide develop and die from this tumor each year. Incidence alone qualifies HCC as one of the major malignant diseases in the world today. HCC occurs commonly (age-adjusted incidences of greater than 20/100,000/yr) throughout Africa south of the Sahara and in many parts of the Far East, the highest frequencies being recorded in Mozambique (103.8/100,000/yr in males), Taiwan, and southeast China (Waterhouse, Muir, and Powell 1977). Moderately high incidences (10–20/100,000/yr) are encountered in Japan, southern Europe, Switzerland, and Bulgaria. The tumor is uncommon or rare (less than 5 and usually less than 3/100,000/yr) in North America, Canada, Britain, Australia, New Zealand, Scandinavia, Israel, Latin America, India, Sri Lanka, and in South African Caucasians. In the remaining countries, there is either an intermediate frequency of HCC (5–9/100,000/yr in Poland, Germany, Romania, Austria, Belgium, Czechoslovakia, Hungary, France, and Yugoslavia) or the incidence has not been documented. In some low-risk regions, including North America, the incidence of HCC may be increasing (San Jose et al. 1965), and a definite increase has occurred in Japan.

In most parts of the world, HCC occurs predominantly in elderly or middle-aged people. Patients living in regions where the tumor incidence is low or moderate are usually in the sixth, seventh, or eighth decade of life (mean age from several studies ranges from 55 to 62 years) (Higginson 1963), and even Oriental patients are seldom young—only 5% of Hong Kong Chinese (Lai et al. 1981), 14% of Taiwanese (Sung, Wang, and Yu 1967), and 10% of Japanese patients (Okuda 1976) are less than 30 years of age (mean age of Oriental patients in various studies ranges from 50 to 57 years). The exception is African patients, in whom HCC often develops at a young age. For example, 50% of Mozambican Shangaans with this tumor are less than 30 years of age (mean age, 33 years) (Prates 1961).

Although HCC occurs more often in men than women throughout the world, male preponderance is more impressive in populations having a high incidence of the tumor (4–8:1) than in those with a low incidence (2–3:1) (Higginson 1963; Okuda 1976). In the latter, male predilection is observed mainly in the older age groups, whereas in patients aged less than 40 years, the sex distribution may be equal or the incidence in women may be even slightly higher. This phenomenon may be explained in part by the fact that the fibrolamellar variant of HCC (Craig et al. 1980) has a predilection to occur at a younger age and in females. Populations with an intermediate risk of HCC generally have a male:female ratio of HCC occurrence of about 4:1.

CLINICAL PRESENTATION

HCC presents clinically in many and diverse ways. The variety of the presentations stems partly from the different biologic characteristics of HCC in regions of high and low incidence of the tumor (Kew 1981) and partly from the wide range of paraneoplastic phenomena that occurs in HCC that may precede the local manifestations of the tumor (Kew and Dusheiko 1981).

HCC is insidious in onset and runs a silent course during its early stages, making early diagnosis difficult. The absence of pathognomonic symptoms and signs, the position of the liver deep to the lower ribs rendering it relatively inaccessible to the examining hand, and the dearth of specific changes in biochemical tests of hepatic function combine to further delay diagnosis. The resulting large tumor burden at the time that treatment can be instituted contributes in no small measure to the poor prognosis of HCC.

In spite of the advanced stage of the tumor when the patient is first seen, the history of symptoms is often short, sometimes remarkably so. This phenomenon is more evident in, although not confined to, patients in populations of high HCC incidence. In rural southern African blacks, for example, the mean duration of symptoms before diagnosis is only five weeks (Kew and Geddes 1982).

An important difference in the general mode of presentation of HCC between high- and low-risk regions concerns the relation of the tumor to cirrhosis. In countries in which HCC is uncommon (and also in Japan), the tumor frequently manifests against a background of clinically apparent cirrhosis or, less often, chronic hepatitis: a patient known for some years to have cirrhosis, usually alcoholic in origin, develops one or more new symptoms or signs that signal that a tumor has supervened in the cirrhotic liver. This sequence of events occurred in one quarter of British (Kew, Dos Santos, and Sherlock 1971) and one fifth of North American patients (Chlebowski et al. 1984). Alternatively, the patient may show all or some of the typical features of cirrhosis when he or she is first examined. It may be extremely difficult to recognize the presence of a small HCC in a patient with advanced cirrhosis, and these tumors may only be discovered at necropsy. By contrast, in countries in which HCC occurs commonly, the tumor usually develops in individuals who previously appeared to be healthy, even though cirrhosis is frequently found to coexist with the tumor (Alpert, Hutt, and Davidson 1969; Kew and Geddes 1982): the cirrhosis is either discovered coincidentally during the course of investigation of the symptoms attributable to the tumor or is detected at necropsy.

In countries where HCC is uncommon, important differences in the clinical presentation of the tumor between patients with and without coexisting cirrhosis have been described (Melia et al. 1984). These include a greater frequency of jaundice, ascites, and gastrointestinal hemorrhage in patients with cirrhosis.

Common Presentations

Abdominal pain is the most common symptom in HCC, occurring in 74% to 95% of patients in high-risk regions and 53% to 58% of those in low-risk regions. In one half of the former patients, pain is also the first symptom. The pain is generally felt in the right hypochondrium or epigastrium, although it occasionally occurs in the left hypochondrium, in the back, or lower in the abdomen. It is typically a constant, dull ache, which may, however, be aggravated in certain positions and by jolting. The pain tends to become more severe in the later stages of the disease, though in black and Chinese patients it is not infrequently severe from the outset.

Young African men with HCC not infrequently present with a short history of severe right hypochondrial pain, an enlarged and tender liver, and fever, a presentation which is difficult to distinguish clinically from that of patients with an amebic hepatic abscess. In an occasional Western patient, right hypochondrial pain accompanied by fever and mild jaundice might initially suggest a diagnosis of acute cholecystitis.

Patients may have their attention drawn to an upper abdominal mass by pain. Other patients may become aware of a mass in the absence of pain (this occurs in about one third of patients in North America) (Chlebowski et al. 1984). Increasing abdominal girth or generalized abdominal distention, resulting from ascites, is also noticed. In patients known to have cirrhosis, unexplained enlargement of the liver or the appearance of ascites (especially when this is blood stained) should alert the clinician to the possibility of HCC formation.

Anorexia, weakness, malaise, and weight loss vary in prominence in different reported series; however, they are almost invariably present in all populations during the late stages of the illness. Other nonspecific gastrointestinal symptoms—constipation, vomiting, indigestion—may also be present. Unexplained loss of weight in a cirrhotic patient may be the first evidence that a tumor has developed.

Unusual Presentations

Jaundice is an infrequent but important presenting complaint. In some patients, especially those already suffering from advanced cirrhosis, the jaundice is of the hepatocellular variety. This form of jaundice is usually mild, but it often deepens as the disease progresses. In the remainder, jaundice is related to obstruction caused by compression of the main intrahepatic bile ducts by the primary tumor, compression of the common hepatic duct by malignant glands in the porta hepatis, extensive infiltration of tumor into the biliary radicles with occlusion of the major ducts, or hemobilia (Kew and Paterson 1985).

A small number of patients present with a so-called acute surgical abdomen accompanied by shock and pallor. This complication, more common in regions of high incidence of HCC (Kew and Paterson 1985), is caused by an acute hemoperitoneum that results from rupture of the tumor. More commonly, the tumor ruptures later in the course of the disease and causes death.

Between 3% and 12% of patients with HCC experience bone pain, and in some, this may be the initial or sole symptom. Bone metastases most often affect the vertebrae (when they may be complicated by paraplegia or nerve root compression), ribs, femora, and skull bones (Kew and Paterson 1985). Pathological fractures may occur.

Acute respiratory symptoms are a rare initial complaint in patients with HCC. Less infrequently, these symptoms are present but are overshadowed by the other symptoms of the tumor. They are caused by multiple pulmonary metastases, a large pleural effusion, or a diaphragm markedly raised on the right. Very rarely, multiple tumor emboli to the pulmonary microvasculature may result in pulmonary arterial hypertension (Willett et al. 1984).

In spite of the wide variety of presentations possible with HCC, some patients are asymptomatic. This is more likely to occur in regions of low incidence (e.g., it occurred in 29% of patients in one study in North America) (Luna, Florence, and Johansen 1985).

Physical Findings

The physical findings in HCC obviously depend upon the stage of the disease at which the patient presents. Early in the disease course, the only abnormality may be a slightly or moderately enlarged liver. More frequently, however, the disease is far advanced when the patient is first seen and the physical signs are obvious.

Liver enlargement is the most frequent physical finding in patients with HCC, whether they are from regions of high or low incidence. However, hepatomegaly tends to be both more frequent and of greater degree in high-risk regions (91%–98% in black and Chinese patients) than in Western patients (56%–93%). The surface of the liver may be smooth, but more often it is irregular or even nodular. Although the liver may have focal or generalized tenderness, the tumor usually has a hard, stony consistency.

An hepatic arterial bruit, ascites, and splenomegaly are also frequent findings. A focal bruit may be heard over the tumorous liver in about 25% of patients. This bruit needs to be distinguished from that transmitted from the aorta compressed by the enlarged tumorous liver (which is heard in the midline and is soft and decrescendo). Ascites is present slightly more often in Western patients, probably reflecting the greater prevalence of well-established cirrhosis in these patients. The fluid may be blood stained. The spleen is enlarged in about one third of patients. In other patients, tense ascites or massive enlargement of the liver (especially the left lobe) may prevent an enlarged spleen from being felt.

Muscle wasting may already be apparent at the time of first admission to the hospital, particularly with large, rapidly growing tumors. As the disease runs its course, progressive wasting is the rule, and in the terminal stages the patients are often emaciated. Along with muscle wasting, persistent mild or moderate fever may be present in patients with HCC. Fever tends to be more common in high-risk populations (38% in blacks; 54% in Chinese), but is also seen in Western patients (10%–24%). Although low-grade fever may occur in patients with cirrhosis, finding a persistently raised temperature in a cirrhotic should suggest the possibility of HCC formation.

Patients with HCC also may be jaundiced when they are first seen. This is more likely in those in whom the tumor develops against the background of well-established cirrhosis. The jaundice is usually of slight or moderate degree when the patient is first seen, but it tends to become deeper with progression of the disease. In some patients the jaundice is caused by obstruction. Dilated veins may be present on the upper part of the anterior abdominal wall. Stigmata of chronic hepatic disease (e.g., gynecomastia, spider nevi) may also be seen.

HCC may invade and occlude the hepatic veins, producing the clinical picture of the Budd-Chiari syndrome with tense ascites and a uniformly enlarged and tender liver. In about two thirds of the patients with hepatic vein invasion, the tumor plug grows into the inferior vena cava, partially or completely occluding the lumen and causing the patient to develop gross pitting edema of the lower limbs (Kew and Paterson 1985). Occasionally, the tumor grows up the inferior vena cava into the right atrium.

Paraneoplastic Syndromes

HCC is capable of producing a large number and a great diversity of paraneoplastic phenomena (Kew and Dusheiko 1981). Most of these result in characteristic biochemical changes rather than clinically apparent syndromes. The latter are, however, important because they may precede the local manifestations of the tumor and draw the clinician's attention to the presence of HCC. The clinically important syndromes are hypoglycemia, erythrocytosis, and hypercalcemia. Rarer syndromes are feminization, porphyria cutanea tarda, carcinoid syndrome, hypertrophic osteoarthropathy, hypertension, and hyperthyroidism.

Hypoglycemia may take two forms in patients with HCC (McFadzean and Yeung 1969). The first and more common (type A) occurs during the last few weeks of life. Glycopenia is of moderate severity only and can easily be missed unless specifically sought; it is readily controlled. The second form of this complication (type B) is characterized by severe glycopenia that manifests early in the course of the disease. These patients frequently present with acute neuropsychiatric disturbances, confusion, convulsions, stupor, or coma, and the underlying tumor can easily be overlooked. The hypoglycemia is unresponsive to corticosteroids, thiazides, glugagon, and diazoxide, and carries a poor prognosis. Type B hypoglycemia occurs in 2% to 3% of patients with HCC (Kew and Paterson 1985). Another paraneoplastic syndrome, erythrocytosis (polycythemia), occurs in between 3% and 12% of patients with HCC. Its appearance in a patient known to have cirrhosis highly suggests that a tumor has developed. The third in this series of paraneoplastic syndromes has manifestations as dramatic as those of hypoglycemia. Hypercalcemia, whose prevalence has not been defined, has symptoms (confusion, weakness, malaise, depression, coma, anorexia, nausea, vomiting) that may readily mask those of the underlying tumor, causing it to be overlooked.

ETIOLOGY

The geographical distribution of HCC and the pattern of its occurrence in migrant populations suggest that this tumor is caused, in almost all instances, by one or more environmental agents. There is no evidence for a major inherited component in human HCC, although genetic, immunological, and nutritional factors may play a contributory role or act indirectly by increasing susceptibility to environmental carcinogens, and the individual's hormonal make-up may have a permissive role. Many chemicals, both naturally occurring and synthetic, can cause HCC in laboratory animals. But most of these are not encountered in day-to-day living, and very few can be incriminated in human HCC (Newberne 1984). Currently available evidence suggests that HCC is multifactorial and complex in origin. Three major etiologic associations—chronic hepatitis B virus (HBV) infection, cirrhosis, and aflatoxin ingestion—and several occasional ones have been identified. The biologic characteristics of HCC vary considerably in different parts of the world and in different populations (Kew 1981). One possible explanation for this phenomenon is that the etiology of the tumor varies geographically or culturally. Indeed, there is now persuasive evidence that the blend of causative factors differs substantially in different parts of the world but most obviously between populations having very high and low incidences of HCC.

Hepatitis B Virus Infection

There is compelling evidence that incriminates persistent HBV infection in the etiology of about 80% of cases of HCC worldwide (Beasley and Hwang 1984). This evidence can be summarized as follows: There is a close geographical parallel between the incidence of HCC and the prevalence of the HBV carrier state. In regions of high incidence, there are no exceptions to the correlation with a high HBV carrier rate, but in regions of low incidence, one or two possible exceptions (Greenland and Chile, each with a relatively high viral carrier rate and a low HCC incidence) have been reported. We have recently shown in southern African blacks that when the HBV carrier rate decreases as a result of urbanization, the incidence of HCC correspondingly decreases (Kew et al. 1986).

Most Chinese and blacks with HCC show serological markers of current HBV infection, and almost all of the remainder have markers of past infection. In low-incidence populations, a lesser but still significant proportion of patients show these markers. Persistent HBV infection precedes the development of the tumor by several to many years. Indeed, the carrier state in Chinese and blacks is established in the early years of childhood.

In a prospective study, Beasley and Hwang (1984) showed that Taiwanese male carriers of HBV have a lifetime relative risk of developing HCC of 217 and that 40% of these carriers will die from HCC, cirrhosis, or both. Institutionalized mentally retarded HBV carriers in California (North America) have recently been shown to have a similar (247) relative risk of developing HCC (Lohiya et al. 1985).

During the past few years, molecular hybridization and gene cloning techniques have been used to demonstrate that HBV DNA is integrated into the human genome in the malignant cells of most (but not all) patients with HBV-related HCC (Sherman and Shafritz 1984). Integration is known to precede the development of the tumor. Although the sequence of cellular events leading to human HCC is not yet understood, these findings are consistent with the idea, but do not prove, that HBV acts as a genotoxic initiator of hepatocarcinogenesis.

Indirect evidence for the hepatocarcinogenicity of HBV is provided by recent observations in the hepatotropic DNA (Hepadna) group of viruses (of which HBV is one). The American woodchuck, the Beechii ground squirrel, and the Peking duck have each been shown to be chronically infected with a virus that is morphologically and immunologically almost identical to HBV. Chronically infected woodchucks in particular, and the ground squirrel and Peking duck less frequently, develop an HCC that is very similar to that which develops in human HBV carriers.

Aflatoxin Ingestion

Evidence of chemical hepatocarcinogenicity in man often remains indirect because no biologic stigmata have been identified that can still be measured years after exposure. There is at present no unequivocal evidence that any single chemical causes human HCC (Newberne 1984). Nevertheless, data are available suggesting that aflatoxin B_1, a metabolite of the fungus *Aspergillus flavus,* may play, either in combination with HBV or independently, an etiologic role in this tumor.

Mycotoxins are produced by fungi that contaminate cereals and other foods stored under hot and humid conditions after harvesting. Aflatoxin B_1 is the most potent experimental hepatocarcinogen known to man (Linsell 1984). Field studies in several parts of Africa and the Far East have shown a direct correlation between high incidences of human HCC and contamination of foodstuffs by this mycotoxin (Newberne 1984; Linsell 1984). No correlation could, however, be found in studies in Hong Kong and Greece. Levels of aflatoxin M_1, a metabolite of aflatoxin B_1, excreted in the urine are much higher in inhabitants of HCC high-risk areas in China than they are in people living in low-risk areas (Harris and Sun 1984). Analyses in China (Wang et al. 1983) and Kenya (Bagshawe et al. 1975) have shown the geographical correlation between HCC incidence and mycotoxin intake to be closer than that between HCC incidence and the HBV carrier rate.

It has also been postulated that aflatoxin B_1, by virtue of its immunosuppressive properties, may cause HCC indirectly by making individuals exposed to it more susceptible to developing the HBV carrier state (Lutwick 1979). However, a study in Kenya showed similar prevalence rates of HBV markers in areas of high and low aflatoxin contamination (Bagshawe et al. 1975). Moreover, the HBV carrier state is established in blacks and Chinese in the early months of life before significant exposure to aflatoxin is likely.

Cirrhosis

The majority of patients who develop HCC in regions of low incidence do so against a background of long-standing cirrhosis (a few have chronic active hepatitis), and cirrhosis per se is without doubt the most important etiologic association of the tumor in these populations (Kew and Popper 1984). In low-risk populations, alcohol abuse has long been considered to be the commonest cause of the cirrhosis, which is complicated by HCC, and hence the major environmental factor involved in the pathogenesis of HCC. Micronodular cirrhosis, which is most often caused by excessive alcohol consumption, is complicated by malignant transformation in 3% to 10% of cases. However, macronodular cirrhosis may also occur with alcohol abuse, and when HCC develops in chronic alcoholics, this type of cirrhosis is likely to be present. Abstinence after the onset of alcoholic cirrhosis is associated with a higher frequency of macronodular cirrhosis and an increased risk of tumor formation (Lee 1966). The likelihood of malignant transformation is, in addition, related to the severity of the cirrhosis (Leevy, Gellene, and Ning 1964).

Alcohol has not been shown experimentally to be mutagenic and is unlikely to be an initiator of hepatocarcinogenesis; however, it could function as a promotor, acting in conjunction, for example, with HBV or with chemicals such as vinyl chloride. Alternatively, the apparent role of alcohol as a cocarcinogen could be explained by excessive alcohol's being a cause of cirrhosis.

The pathogenesis of malignant transformation in cirrhosis is not known, but two explanations have been suggested (Kew and Popper 1984). The first is that cirrhosis is itself a premalignant condition, that is, that hyperplasia leads to neoplasia in the absence of additional factors. The second possible explanation is that the accelerated hepatocyte turnover rate in cirrhosis renders these cells more susceptible to environmental carcinogens, that is, cirrhosis acts as a promotor.

Occasional etiologic associations of HCC include idiopathic hemochromatosis, Wilson's disease, cigarette smoking, oral contraceptive steroids, anabolic androgenic steroids, and α_1-antitrypsin deficiency.

PREVENTION

HCC generally has a grave prognosis. The tumor is seldom amenable to resection, is radioresistant, and is largely unresponsive to cancer chemotherapy. Prevention of HCC should therefore receive urgent attention. In practical terms, attempts at prevention of HCC will hinge on the elimination of two of the three major etiologic associations of the tumor—chronic HBV infection and aflatoxin contamination of staple foodstuffs. The latter, although theoretically feasible, has thus far been difficult to achieve in those Third World countries where aflatoxin contamination of staple foods is common and is thought to play a major etiologic role in HCC. Nevertheless, educational and intervention programs aimed at improving methods of storage of foods likely to be contaminated by molds should be continued or introduced in these countries.

Two HBV vaccines, one plasma derived and the other a recombinant yeast-derived vaccine, have recently become available and have proved to be effective in preventing HBV infection. Trials in neonates in areas of endemic HBV infection have shown that the vaccines will prevent the development of the HBV carrier state. If this virus proves to be the cause of 80% of HCC in the world, then successful vaccination programs targeted at newborn or very young babies should result ultimately in the elimination of the majority of cases of this tumor worldwide. However, until the HBV carrier state can be eradicated by vaccination, many millions of these carriers are at high risk of HCC formation, and attempts must continue to be made to treat the persistent viral infection. Presently available antiviral drugs, notably the interferons, are only effective in replicative infection and then only in a minority of affected patients. There is clearly a need for more effective anti-HBV drugs. For those carriers who have nonreplicative (and presumably integrative) HBV infection, programs of surveillance, aimed at the early detection of small resectable tumors, have been introduced in high-risk populations (so-called secondary prevention). Carriers have their serum α_1-fetoprotein concentrations measured and an ultrasonogram of the liver performed at three-month to six-month intervals as a screening procedure, and this has resulted in many resectable tumors being detected.

REFERENCES

Alpert ME, Hutt MSR, Davidson CS. 1969. Primary hepatoma in Uganda. *Am J Med* 46:794–802.

Bagshawe AF, Gacengi DM, Cameron CH, et al. 1975. Hepatitis B surface antigen and liver cancer: A population-based study in Kenya. *Br J Cancer* 31:581–584.

Beasley RP, Hwang LY. 1984. Hepatocellular carcinoma and hepatitis B virus. *Semin Liver Dis* 4:113–121.

Chlebowski RT, Tong M, Weissman J, et al. 1984. Hepatocellular carcinoma: Diagnostic and prognostic features in North American patients. *Cancer* 53:2701–2706.

Craig JR, Peters RL, Edmondson HA, et al. 1980. Fibrolamellar carcinoma of the liver: A tumor of adolescents and young adults with distinctive clinico-pathologic features. *Cancer* 46:372–379.

Harris CC, Sun TT. 1984. Multifactorial etiology of human liver cancer. *Carcinogenesis* 5:677–701.

Higginson J. 1963. The geographical pathology of primary liver cancer. *Cancer Res* 23:1624–1633.

Kew MC. 1981. Clinical and etiologic heterogeneity in hepatocellular carcinoma: Evidence from southern Africa. *Hepatology* 1:366–369.

Kew MC, Dos Santos HA, Sherlock S. 1971. Diagnosis of primary cancer of the liver. *Br Med J [Clin Res]* 4:408–411.

Kew MC, Dusheiko GM. 1981. Paraneoplastic manifestations of hepatocellular carcinoma. In *Frontiers in Liver Disease,* pp. 305–319. New York: Thieme-Stratton.

Kew MC, Geddes EW. 1982. Hepatocellular carcinoma in rural southern African blacks. *Medicine (Baltimore)* 61:98–108.

Kew MC, Kassianides C, Hodkinson J, et al. 1986. Hepatocellular carcinoma in urban-born blacks: Frequency and relation to hepatitis B virus infection. *Br Med J [Clin Res]* 293:1339–1341.

Kew MC, Paterson AC. 1985. Unusual clinical presentations of hepatocellular carcinoma. *Trop Gastroenterol* 6:10–22.

Kew MC, Popper H. 1984. Relationship between hepatocellular carcinoma and cirrhosis. *Semin Liver Dis* 4:136–146.

Lai CL, Lam KC, Wong KP, et al. 1981. Clinical features of hepatocellular carcinoma: Review of 211 patients in Hong Kong. *Cancer* 47:2746–2755.

Lee FI. 1966. Cirrhosis and hepatoma in alcoholics. *Gut* 17:77–85.

Leevy CM, Gellene R, Ning M. 1964. Primary liver cancer in cirrhosis of the alcoholic. *Ann NY Acad Sci* 114:1026–1040.

Linsell A. 1984. Liver cancer and mycotoxins. In *Virus-Associated Cancers in Africa,* AO Williams, GT O'Conor, GB De-The, CA Johnson, eds., pp. 161–165. Lyons, France: International Agency for Research on Cancer.

Lohiya G, Pirkle H, Hoefs J, et al. 1985. Hepatocellular carcinoma in young, mentally retarded HBsAg carriers without cirrhosis. *Hepatology* 5:824–826.

Luna G, Florence L, Johansen K. 1985. Hepatocellular carcinoma: A 5-year institutional experience. *Am J Surg* 149:591–594.

Lutwick LI. 1979. Relation between aflatoxin, hepatitis B virus and hepatocellular carcinoma. *Lancet* 1:755–757.

McFadzean AJS, Yeung RTT. 1969. Further observations on hypoglycemia in hepatocellular carcinoma. *Am J Med* 47:220–235.

Melia WM, Wilkinson ML, Portmann BC, et al. 1984. Hepatocellular carcinoma in the noncirrhotic liver: A comparison with that complicating cirrhosis. *Q J Med* 53:391–400.

Newberne PM. 1984. Chemical carcinogenesis: Mycotoxins and other chemicals to which humans are exposed. *Semin Liver Dis* 4:122–135.

Okuda K. 1976. Clinical aspects of hepatocellular carcinoma—Analysis of 134 cases. In *Hepatocellular Carcinoma*, K Okuda, RL Peters, eds., pp. 387–436. New York: John Wiley & Sons.

Prates MD. 1961. Cancer and cirrhosis of the liver in the Portuguese East African. *Acta Unio Internationale Contra Cancrum* 17:718–739.

San Jose D, Cady A, West M, et al. 1965. Primary carcinoma of the liver: Analysis of clinical and biochemical features of 80 cases. *Dig Dis Sci* 10:657–674.

Sherman M, Shafritz OA. 1984. Hepatitis B virus and hepatocellular carcinoma: Molecular biology and mechanistic considerations. *Semin Liver Dis* 4:98–112.

Sung JL, Wang TH, Yu JY. 1967. Clinical study of primary carcinoma of the liver in Taiwan. *Dig Dis Sci* 12:1036–1049.

Wang Y, Yeh P, Li W, et al. 1983. Correlation between geographical distribution of liver cancer and aflatoxin B_1 climate conditions. *Acta Sinica Series B* 431–437.

Waterhouse J, Muir C, Powell J. 1977. *Cancer Incidence in Five Continents*. Lyons, France: World Health Organization.

Willett IR, Sutherland RC, O'Rourke MF, et al. 1984. Pulmonary hypertension complicating hepatocellular carcinoma. *Gastroenterology* 87:1180–1184.

Annual Clinical Conference on Cancer, Vol. 30
Gastrointestinal Cancer: Current Approaches to Diagnosis and Treatment
© 1988 by The University of Texas System Cancer Center

29. Embolization of Neuroendocrine Hepatic Metastases

Sidney Wallace, C. Humberto Carrasco, Jaffer A. Ajani,
Chusilp Charnsangavej, and Naguib A. Samaan

Hepatic devascularization is a general term that includes arterial ligation, catheter-induced arterial injury, and drug-related arteritis as well as transcatheter hepatic artery embolization (HAE). The rationale for hepatic devascularization as a treatment modality for hepatic neoplasms is based on the existence of a dual blood supply to the normal liver via the hepatic artery (30%) and the portal vein (70%); 50% of the oxygen supply comes from each source (Segall 1923). Primary and secondary neoplasms, on the other hand, receive as much as 90% of their blood supply from the hepatic artery with complementary but less contribution from the portal vein (Breedis and Young 1954; Healey and Sheena 1963; Bierman et al. 1951; Lin, Hagerstrand, and Lunderquist 1984; Ekelund, Lin, and Jeppsson 1984). Therefore, occlusive therapy delivered to the hepatic artery almost selectively affects the neoplasm.

The concept of treating liver tumors by interrupting their hepatic arterial supply was first suggested by Markowitz (1952). Gelin et al. (1968) demonstrated a 90% decrease in tumor blood flow and a 35% to 40% decrease in flow in the normal liver parenchyma following hepatic artery ligation. In a patient with gastric carcinoma metastatic to the liver, Mori et al. (1966) noted selective destruction of the tumor without damage to the liver following inadvertent interruption of flow in the hepatic artery. Varying results of hepatic artery ligation in the management of hepatic neoplasms have been reported, but the effects of surgical ligation are usually short-lived because of intrahepatic and extrahepatic collaterals that develop to reconstitute flow.

HEPATIC ARTERY EMBOLIZATION

Occlusion of the more peripheral branches of the hepatic arteries through emboliza-tion with small particles lasts longer than surgical occlusion; it causes varying de-grees of necrosis of hepatic neoplasms by depriving them of their arterial blood supply. The normal liver parenchyma is protected from infarction by the portal vein and the collateral arterial supply. The collateral circulation that develops after occlu-sion of any portion of the hepatic arterial system also determines, at least in part, the degree of necrosis of the hepatic neoplasms. The more peripheral the occlusion, the less effective is the collateral circulation and, therefore, the greater is the tumor necrosis. It is also possible that some neoplasms are more sensitive to ischemia than others. Complete necrosis of hepatic neoplasms does not usually occur following the initial HAE.

Sequential peripheral unilobar embolization is our preferred approach. The first step is peripheral embolization of one lobe, using 100 to 200 mg of polyvinyl alcohol foam particles (Ivalon) 150 μm to 250 μm in diameter; one month later, the patient returns for embolization of the remaining lobe. If prominent collaterals have developed in the previously embolized lobe, these are also occluded. Two to three months after the initial embolization, a third angiographic procedure is performed to occlude the residual or recanalized arteries and any remaining intrahepatic or extrahepatic collaterals. Subsequent HAE can be performed at three- to six-month intervals, depending on the patient's clinical status and the vessels available.

At The University of Texas M. D. Anderson Hospital and Tumor Institute at Houston, more than 500 patients with inoperable primary and secondary hepatic neoplasms have been treated by HAE. Some of the patients were sequentially embolized on as many as 12 occasions. The post-HAE syndrome consists of nausea, vomiting, adynamic ileus, fever, and pain. Liver function studies, usually abnormal before embolization, become more abnormal immediately following the procedure. All of the above usually resolve within five to seven days but may last as long as two to three weeks. The pain is due in part to cystic artery embolization, which is usually self-limited and decreases as collateral circulation develops. However, cholecystectomy was necessary in 2 of the more-than-500 patients. Nonspecific gas formation, produced by air injected with the embolic material and the necrosis of the ischemic neoplasm, lasts from days to months and is visible especially by computerized tomography. HAE was complicated by two hepatic abscesses. The spleen in six patients and the pancreas in two were embolized unintentionally. Patients with the splenic infarcts, which were discovered on follow-up scanning procedures, were asymptomatic. One of the two pancreatic complications resulted in acute pancreatitis. These unfortunate incidents were due to technical errors.

In a review of the first 310 patients treated by HAE, we observed that 18 patients died of hepatorenal failure in the immediate postembolization period (within 30 days after the procedure). All 18 patients had (1) replacement of more than 50% of the liver by tumor, (2) a serum lactic dehydrogenase level above 425 mU/ml, (3) a serum glutamic oxaloacetic transaminase level of more than 100 mU/ml, and (4) a serum bilirubin level above 2 mg/dl. These conditions were seen in only 2 of the 292 patients who survived the immediate postembolization period. Therefore, we believe that HAE is contraindicated in patients in whom *all* four of the above criteria are present. HAE is also contraindicated in the face of intrinsic occlusion of the portal vein, usually by a tumor thrombus, which directs portal flow away from the liver (Charnsangavej, unpublished data).

NEUROENDOCRINE TUMORS

In an attempt to create a unified concept, Pearse suggested that neuroendocrine, or APUD, cells are diffusely distributed in many organs and systems and include cells of the anterior pituitary gland, the parafollicular thyroid cells, the chromaffin cells of the adrenal medulla and the extraadrenal paraganglia, the enterochromaffin and peptide-secreting cells of the gastrointestinal tract and pancreatic islet cells, and the Feyrter cells of the tracheobronchial tree (Pearse 1974; Temple, Sugarbaker, and Ketcham 1981). The acronym APUD was derived from their most prominent features, i.e., the fluorogenic amine content, *a*mine *p*recursor *u*ptake, and the presence of amino acid *d*ecarboxylase.

Numerous polypeptides with neurotransmitter and regulatory functions have been found in the endocrine cells of the gut and in the pancreatic islet cells of Langerhans, the gastroenteropancreatic endocrine axis. Digestive peptides of the gut include, in the stomach, gastrin, adrenocorticotropic hormone-like polypeptides, somatostatin, serotonin, and vasoactive intestinal polypeptides; in the duodenum and jejunum, cholecystokinin, gastric-inhibitory polypeptide, gastrin, glucagon, motilin, somatostatin, secretin, substance P, serotonin, vasoactive intestinal polypeptide, and bombesin; in the small and large bowels, glucagon, neurotensin, serotonin, and bombesin. Peptides of the pancreas include insulin, glucagon, somatostatin, and pancreatic polypeptide (Weiland 1986).

The APUD cells and their corresponding neoplasms, *apudomas*, are closely related in terms of their biosynthetic mechanisms, their histochemical and ultrastructural features, and possibly their embryological origin (Pearse 1974; Temple, Sugarbaker, and Ketcham 1981; Weiland 1986; Welbourn 1977; Gould et al. 1979; Pearse and Polak 1971). Apudomas may produce abnormal quantities of amines or peptide hormones that may be identical to the secretory products of their nonneoplastic counterparts. Apudomas may be benign or malignant; hyperplasia is included among them because of the functional resemblance. These neoplasms also form part of the multiple endocrine neoplasia (MEN) syndromes. Generally, apudomas grow slowly, and even after metastasizing, they are associated with prolonged survival.

Treatment for localized apudomas is surgical resection. In case of incurable disease, tumor "debulking" procedures may offer significant palliation because of the tumor's slow growth and the direct relationship existing between the tumor mass and the amount of pharmacologically active substances secreted by the functioning apudomas (Moertel et al. 1961; Jager and Polk 1977; Friesen 1982). Surgical excision of the end organ of the endocrine complex (such as gastrectomy and adrenalectomy for gastrin-secreting and ACTH-secreting apudomas, respectively) is sometimes performed for its palliative effect.

The medical management of unresectable apudomas involves cytotoxic chemotherapy directed against the primary tumor and its metastases. Antihormonal therapy plays an important role in the management of certain pharmacologically active apudomas.

Hepatic metastases constitute an important factor in the survival of patients with apudomas, and several methods have been used in their treatment. A reduction in the bulk of the hormone-secreting hepatic metastases may offer significant clinical improvement to patients with syndromes whose clinical symptoms are determined by the secondary tumors in the liver. Partial hepatectomy or enucleation of hepatic metastases has resulted in relief of symptoms associated with metastatic neuroendocrine tumors. Hepatic devascularization has decreased the size of hepatic metastases and resulted in clinical improvement. Chemotherapy and immunotherapy have added to the clinical management of neuroendocrine hepatic metastases, and the combination of hepatic devascularization and chemotherapy has interesting potential. These various treatments will be discussed as they apply to specific neuroendocrine neoplasms, carcinoids, and pancreatic islet cell tumors.

CARCINOIDS

Carcinoids are relatively rare neuroendocrine neoplasms that usually originate in the appendix, small bowel, rectum, and bronchi and less frequently in the stomach, duodenum, biliary tract, pancreas, and ovary (Godwin 1975). These tumors were originally considered to be benign, but we now know that extraappendiceal carcinoids, particularly those arising in the small bowel, are frequently malignant (Davis, Moertel, and McIlrath 1973). Malignant carcinoids may secrete pharmacologically active substances such as serotonin, kallikrein, substance P, and prostaglandins, which have been implicated in producing the carcinoid syndrome. Its symptoms are cutaneous flushing, diarrhea, and wheezing, and may less frequently include fibrosis of the pulmonic and tricuspid valves, arthropathy, psychiatric symptoms, and pellagra-like dermatitis (Davis, Moertel, and McIlrath 1973; Moertel 1983, Feldman 1986). At least some of the secreting products are metabolized by the liver during the first pass; as a result, gastrointestinal carcinoids almost never produce the carcinoid syndrome unless hepatic metastases are present (Wilson 1959).

Palliative Therapy

Pharmacological Blocking Agents

The carcinoid syndrome may be extremely incapacitating; therefore, various forms of palliative therapy have been attempted to relieve it. Although many pharmacological agents, including adrenergic blockers, kinin and serotonin antagonists (cyproheptadine), and corticosteroids, have been used to neutralize the effects of the active substances secreted, success with them has been limited (Moertel 1983). Control of the carcinoid syndrome by a somatostatin analogue is most encouraging, but thus far it has produced little change in the size and extent of the hepatic metastases (Kvols et al. 1986).

Hepatic Resection

Because hepatic metastases usually determine the occurrence of the carcinoid syndrome and may also determine the length of survival, it is logical that antineoplastic therapy be directed primarily against the liver metastases. Surgical resection of the hepatic metastases appears to be the best palliative treatment for localized disease. Of course, these metastases must be amenable, by extent and distribution, to anatomic segmental or lobar resection or even to more limited wedge resections. Therefore, this approach entails highly selective application (Wilson 1959; Stephen and Grahame-Smith 1972; Martin et al. 1983).

Chemotherapy and Immunotherapy

In patients with unresectable hepatic metastases, interferon and chemotherapeutic agents have yielded relatively low response rates (Schein et al. 1973; Mengel and Shaffer 1973; Solomon, Sonoda, and Patterson 1976; Chernicoff et al. 1979; Moertel and Hanley 1979; Moertel, Hanley, and Johnson 1980; Kelsen et al. 1982; Ajani et al. 1983; Moertel et al. 1984; Engstrom et al. 1984; Bukowski et al. 1983; Oberg, Funa, and Alm 1983; Funa et al. 1983). The best reported results have been achieved with a combination of methotrexate and cyclophosphamide, which induced a response in 6 of 11 patients (Mengel and Shaffer 1973). However, this same drug combination did not result in many responses in a larger series (Moertel et al. 1984). The combination of 5-fluorouracil (5-FU) and streptozotocin administered at 6- and 10-week intervals yielded response rates of 33% in 42 patients (Moertel and Hanley 1979) and 22% in 86 patients (Engstrom et al. 1984). The combination of streptozotocin and doxorubicin resulted in 4 responses in a group of 10 patients (Kelsen et al. 1982). A four-agent program of 5-FU, streptozotocin, doxorubicin, and cyclophosphamide has achieved responses in 7 of 20 patients (Bukowski, et al. 1983). All six patients treated with interferon by Oberg et al. showed symptomatic improvement and reduction in 5-hydroxyindoleacetic acid (5-HIAA) excretion, but long-term results are not yet available (Oberg, Funa, and Alm 1983; Funa et al. 1983; Strayer et al. 1984).

Hepatic Devascularization

Hepatic Artery Ligation

The present technique of hepatic artery ligation consists of interruption of the hepatic artery distal to the origin of the gastroduodenal artery and, when present, the aberrant hepatic arteries, as well as division of the round, triangular, and falciform ligaments of the liver and the gastrohepatic omentum. Any other palpable arteries supplying the liver are transected, and the gallbladder is removed.

In a review of the literature through 1982, Moertel found 32 cases of surgical ligation of the hepatic artery for treatment of the carcinoid syndrome caused by unresectable hepatic metastases. Eighteen patients (56%) experienced striking improvement or complete clinical remission, whereas seven (22%) died in the postoperative period (Madding, Kennedy, and Sogemeier 1970; Aune and Schistad 1972; McDermott and Hensle 1974; Jugdutt, Watanabe, and Turner 1975; Edelman, Boutelier, and deMontalier 1978; Bricot, Boutboul, and LeTreut 1981).

In another series reported by Martin et al. (1983) of 10 patients with metastatic carcinoid tumors who underwent ligation of the hepatic artery, 8 showed symptomatic improvement; in addition, the urinary excretion of 5-HIAA dropped to less than 50% of the pretreatment levels. The median duration of response was five months. There was one postoperative death.

Hepatic Artery Embolization

In order to prolong the remission of the carcinoid syndrome by embolization of the hepatic artery (Doyon et al. 1975; Allison, Modlin, and Jenkins 1977; Pueyo et al.

1978; Henry et al. 1980; Lunderquist et al. 1982; Maton et al. 1983; Carrasco, Chuang, and Wallace 1983; Martensson et al. 1984; Stockman et al. 1984; Mitty et al. 1985; Carrasco et al. 1986), we have performed periodic or sequential embolization in 25 patients with this disease (Carrasco, Chuang, and Wallace 1983; Carrasco et al. 1986). In all 25 patients, there was histological documentation of primary or metastatic carcinoids and elevated urinary excretion of 5-HIAA. We excluded any patients who did not have an elevated urinary excretion of 5-HIAA. Fifteen patients were men and 10 were women; the median age was 58 years (range, 23–69). The sites of the primary neoplasms were the small bowel (16 patients), the bronchus (4 patients), colon (1 patient), and pancreas (1 patient). The primary site was unknown in three patients. In 24 patients, the median duration of symptoms before HAE was one year (range, 1 month–20 years); in 1 patient it was not documented. Extraabdominal metastases were present in three patients with bronchial carcinoids and in four patients with gastrointestinal carcinoids. Ten patients had right-sided cardiac valvulopathy. Eight patients had received chemotherapy in combination with or after the start of embolotherapy.

The first HAE was limited to one lobe in 21 patients and encompassed both lobes in the remaining 4 patients. Subsequent embolizations were performed to both hepatic lobes in all 19 patients in whom the procedure was repeated. Embolization was performed through collateral vessels—inferior phrenic, gastroduodenal, inferior pancreaticoduodenal, intercostals, lumbar, and internal mammary arteries—in four patients because previous embolization had partially or completely occluded the main branches of the hepatic artery. Seventy-nine embolizations were performed in the 25 patients, ranging from one to eight (median, three) embolizations per patient. Six patients underwent a single embolization, and the remainder were embolized at intervals of one to three months for the first two to three times; subsequently, the intervals varied, depending on the clinical response.

Results. A response was defined as symptomatic improvement of the carcinoid syndrome. In addition, follow-up hepatic angiography in 19 patients, computerized tomography in nine patients, and urinary 5-HIAA measurements in 19 patients were available for comparison with the preembolization studies and were correlated with a symptomatic response.

Twenty-three of the 25 patients could be evaluated. Twenty of the 23 (87%) experienced symptomatic improvement and were considered responders, one patient (4%) did not respond, and two patients (9%) died of complications from embolization (fig. 29.1). The two patients who could not be evaluated had undergone a single episode of HAE and were subsequently lost to follow-up. The median follow-up time for the 21 evaluable patients who survived the procedure was 16 months (range, 1–50 months). Responses were subjectively categorized as excellent in 14 of the 20 responding patients (70%) and moderate in 6 (30%). The symptomatic response could be objectively correlated with hepatic imaging or urine 5-HIAA in 18 patients. The extent of the hepatic metastases decreased in 17 of those 18, and the urine 5-HIAA values decreased after embolization in all 18 responders; the mean of the lowest value was 41% (range, 8%–67%) of the preembolization level. Objective documentation of the response by either hepatic imaging or urinary

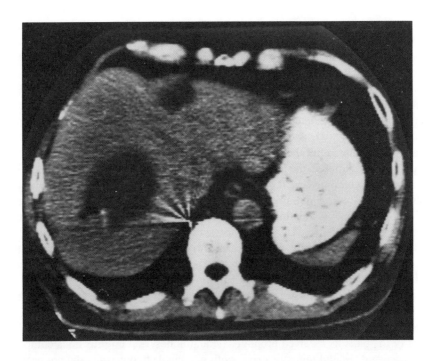

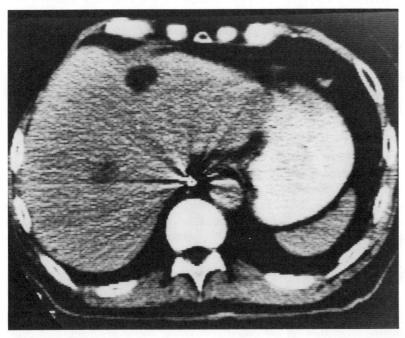

Fig. 29.1. Carcinoid metastatic to the liver (A) and after three embolizations, nine months later (B).

5-HIAA excretion testing was not available for two responders, both of whom were lost to follow-up one month after their first embolization.

Four of the 20 responders experienced a recurrence of symptoms an average of 14 months (range, 9–23 months) after the first embolization. These patients had not been embolized for a mean of 9 months (range, 8–11 months) before relapse. One patient who also received intraarterial chemotherapy in conjunction with embolization could not be evaluated. Fifteen patients are alive at a median of 16 months (range, 1–50 months), and eight patients died at a median of 8 months (range, 5 days–22 months) after their first embolization.

All patients suffered the postembolization syndrome consisting of abdominal pain, nausea, vomiting and fever, usually lasting from 3 to 10 days after the first embolization. These symptoms, however, decreased in severity with subsequent embolization so that by the third episode most of the patients had an uneventful postembolization course. The first embolization also precipitated episodes of intense flushing in most of the patients; five also experienced hypertensive crises that usually did not last beyond the procedure. These five patients required administration of antihypertensive agents to control the hypertension.

Comment. Our patients were not routinely premedicated to counteract the effects of the active substances released during the embolization. However, some of the patients were being treated with cyproheptadine at the time of the embolization. None of the patients received prophylactic antibiotics, and no infectious complications occurred. Bradykininergic crises with intractable hypotension did not occur in any of our patients. Infarction of the gallbladder was probably responsible for most of the pain experienced by our patients in the postembolization period, but this pain appeared to be self-limiting and otherwise well-tolerated. Two patients whose hepatic function was already severely impaired by metastatic disease died of hepatic failure worsened by embolization within seven days of the procedure. In retrospect, these two patients should not have been candidates for embolization because of their extensive metastatic disease.

Hepatic Devascularization and Chemotherapy

The results of hepatic artery embolization compare favorably with those achieved by surgical hepatic devascularization. More recently, occlusion of the hepatic artery by surgical ligation or embolization combined with systemic chemotherapy (doxorubicin, dacarbazine, 5-FU, and streptozotocin) was reported to result in striking or complete symptomatic relief of the carcinoid syndrome in 9 of 10 patients (Moertel et al. 1985; Murray-Lyons et al. 1970; Gulesseran, Lawton, and Condon 1972; Kune and Goldstein 1974; Sparks et al. 1975; Melia et al. 1982). The median duration of response was 6+ months.

PANCREATIC ISLET CELL TUMORS

Endocrine syndromes are associated with tumors of the pancreatic islet cells, including gastrinomas, the insulin-producing tumors, as well as vasoactive intestinal polypeptide-, glucagon-, and somatostatin-secreting tumors. A single tumor may produce more than one hormone of pancreatic islet cell origin plus those hormones not usually attributed to the pancreas, i.e., adrenocorticotropic hormone (ACTH), antidiuretic hormone (ADH), parathyroid hormone, 5-OH tryptophan or 5-OH trypamine, and thyrocalcitonin. Other endocrinopathies that involve the parathyroid, pituitary, and adrenal glands occur in conjunction with islet cell tumors as part of multiple glandular disorders (MEN) in families.

The management of hepatic metastases from pancreatic islet cell tumors requires decreasing both hormone production and tumor cell population by debulking the neoplasm and administering antihormonal therapy in a fashion similar to that discussed with the carcinoids. Surgical hepatic resection of functioning metastases should be performed in the presence of local disease. Multiple hepatic metastases necessitate intraarterial or systemic chemotherapy, hepatic devascularization (ligation or embolization), or a combination of the two (Moertel et al. 1985; Bonfils, Mignon, and Gratton 1979; McCarthy and Jensen 1985; Maton et al. 1985; Ellison et al. 1985; Ellison 1986).

Chemotherapy

Streptozotocin, which destroys pancreatic beta cells, is employed alone or in combination as the mainstay of treatment for islet cell carcinoma of the pancreas. In a randomized study, the Eastern Cooperative Oncology Group (ECOG) found that the combination of 5-FU and streptozotocin yielded a 63% objective response rate (complete response rate, 37%) with a 17-month median duration of response and a 26-month median survival time. These results were superior to those of streptozotocin alone, which produced a 36% objective response rate (12% complete response rate) and a 16.5-month median survival time. Significant toxicity included nausea, vomiting, hepatotoxicity, and nephrotoxicity. The ECOG is now comparing streptozotocin and 5-FU versus streptozotocin and doxorubicin versus chlorozotocin (2-chloroethyl analogue of streptozotocin) alone. The combination of doxorubicin and dacarbazine is also undergoing trials (Moertel et al. 1985; Bonfils, Mignon, and Gratton 1979; McCarthy and Jensen 1985; Maton et al. 1985; Ellison et al. 1985; Ellison 1986; Schutt 1986).

Hepatic Artery Embolization

At UT M. D. Anderson Hospital, 22 patients with pancreatic islet cell carcinoma with hepatic metastases were treated by HAE. The tumors of 11 were documented to be secreting—9 gastrinomas and 2 glucagonomas. Twelve of the patients were men and 10 were women; the median age was 53 years (range, 23–78). Twelve patients had previously received chemotherapy and two had had radiation therapy. Two patients were not available for follow-up. Of the 20 evaluable patients with hepatic metastases from pancreatic islet cell carcinoma, 16 (80%) responded; there were also endocrine syndrome responses. In one patient with a glucagonoma and diffuse hepatic metastases, the migratory necrolytic erythema cleared almost completely within one week after HAE of one lobe of the liver with Ivalon (150 mg).

In preparation for embolization, blocking agents, i.e., antihormonal agents, must be given to prevent the ill-effects of a sudden outpouring of endocrine. This became graphically apparent in a patient with metastatic gastrinoma. Four days following hepatic artery embolization, her gastrin levels were markedly elevated and a previously known duodenal ulcer perforated. At present, we initiate nasogastric suction and administer cimetidine or ranitidine prior to embolization.

CONCLUSION

Hepatic artery embolization provides the most effective treatment for the diffuse hepatic metastases from neuroendocrine neoplasms and their associated syndromes. This procedure not only yields the highest response rates but also, when repeated periodically, maintains clinical remission for prolonged periods. In view of the symptomatic improvement of the endocrine syndrome associated with the use of somatostatin analogue, as reported by Kvols et al. (1986), combining this treatment with HAE should prove interesting. Surgery, if feasible, or chemotherapy still must be considered to treat the primary carcinoid or pancreatic neoplasm once the hepatic metastases have been controlled. However, the eventual occlusion of the main trunks of the hepatic artery and its collaterals will not allow the embolization to be continued indefinitely. Search for a more effective combination of chemotherapeutic agents is still necessary.

REFERENCES

Ajani JA, Legha SS, Karlin DA, et al. 1983. Combination chemotherapy of metastatic carcinoid tumors with 5-FU, adriamycin and Cytoxan (FAC) and 5-FU, adriamycin, mitomycin, and methyl-CCNU (FAMMe) (abstract). *Proceedings of the American Association for Cancer Research* 2:124.

Allison DJ, Modlin IM, Jenkins WJ. 1977. Treatment of carcinoid liver metastases by hepatic artery embolisation. *Lancet* 2:1323–1325.

Aune S, Schistad G. 1972. Carcinoid liver metastases treated with hepatic dearterialization. *Am J Surg* 123:715–717.

Bierman HR, Byron RL, Kelley KH, et al. 1951. Studies on the blood supply of tumors in man: Arteriography in vivo. *JNCI* 12:107–131.

Bonfils S, Mignon M, Gratton J. 1979. Cimetidine treatment of acute and chronic Zollinger-Ellison syndrome. *World J Surg* 3:597–604.

Breedis C, Young G. 1954. The blood supply of neoplasms in the liver. *Am J Pathol* 30:969–985.

Bricot R, Boutboul R, LeTreut YP. 1981. La devascularisation hepatique dans les metastases de tumeurs carcinoides: À propos de deux cas. *J Chir (Paris)* 118:25–28.

Bukowski RM, Stephens R, Oishi N, et al. 1983. Phase II trial of 5FU, adriamycin, cyclophosphamide, and streptozotocin (FAC-S) in metastatic carcinoid (abstract). *Proceedings of the American Association of Clinical Oncology* 2:130.

Carrasco CH, Charnsangavej C, Ajani J, et al. 1986. The carcinoid syndrome: Palliation by hepatic artery embolization. *AJR* 147:149–154.

Carrasco CH, Chuang VP, Wallace S. 1983. Apudomas metastatic to the liver: Treatment by hepatic artery embolization. *Radiology* 149:79–83.

Chernicoff D, Bukowski RM, Groppe CW, et al. 1979. Combination chemotherapy for islet cell carcinoma and metastatic carcinoid tumors with 5-fluorouracil and streptozotocin. *Cancer Treat Rep* 63:795–796.

Davis Z, Moertel CG, McIlrath DC. 1973. The malignant carcinoid syndrome. *Surg Gynecol Obstet* 137:637–644.

Doyon D, Mouzon A, Holler A, et al. 1975. L'embolisation arterielle hepatique: Interet de cette technique dans les tumeurs malignes hepatiques te notamment les metastases de tumores carcinoides (abstract). *Nouv Presse Med* 4:1971.

Edelman G, Boutelier PH, de Montalier H. 1978. Traitement des metastases carcinoidiennes par ligature de l'artere hepatique: À propos de deux cas personnels. *Chirurgie* 104: 300–310.

Ekelund L, Lin G, Jeppsson B. 1984. Blood supply of experimental liver tumors after intra-arterial embolization with Gelfoam powder and absolute ethanol. *Cardiovasc Intervent Radiol* 7:234–239.

Ellison EC. 1986. The current role of surgery in the Zollinger-Ellison syndrome (abstract). In *Gastrointestinal Endocrine Tumors: A Symposium for Medical and Surgical Oncologists.* Houston: The University of Texas System Cancer Center.

Ellison EC, O'Dorisio TM, Woltering EA, et al. 1985. Suppression of gastrin and gastric acid secretion in the Zollinger-Ellison syndrome by long acting somatostatin (SMs 201-995). *Scand J Gastroenterol* 21 (Suppl 119):206–211.

Engstrom PF, Lavin PT, Moertel CG, et al. 1984. Streptozotocin plus fluorouracil versus doxorubicin therapy for metastatic carcinoid tumor. *J Clin Oncol* 2:1255–1259.

Feldman JM. 1986. Pathophysiology and diagnosis of carcinoid tumors (abstract). In *Gastrointestinal Endocrine Tumors: A Symposium for Medical and Surgical Oncologists.* Houston: The University of Texas System Cancer Center.

Friesen SR. 1982. Tumors of the endocrine pancreas. *N Engl J Med* 306:580–590.

Funa K, Alm GV, Ronnblom L, et al. Evaluation of the natural killer cell-interferon system with mid-gut carcinoid tumors treated with leukocyte interferon. *Clin Exp Immunol* 53:716–724.

Gelin LE, Lewis DH, Nilsson L. 1968. Liver blood flow in man during abdominal surgery. *Acta Hepatosplenol* 15:21.

Godwin JD. 1975. Carcinoid tumors: An analysis of 2837 cases. *Cancer* 36:560–569.

Gould VE, Memoli V, Chejfec G, et al. 1979. The APUD cell system and its neoplasms: Observations on the significance and limitations of the concept. *Surg Clin North Am* 59: 93–108.

Gulesserian HP, Lawton RL, Condon RE. 1972. Hepatic artery ligation and cytotoxic infusion in treatment of liver metastases. *Arch Surg* 105:280–285.

Healey JE, Sheena KS. 1963. Vascular patterns in metastatic liver tumors. *Surg Forum* 14:121–122.

Henry JF, Di Marino V, Grisoli J, et al. 1980. Embolisation de l'artere hepatique propre pour metastases carcinoidiennes: Recul de 4 ans (abstract). *Nouv Presse Med* 9:1388.

Jager RM, Polk HC Jr. 1977. Carcinoid apudomas. *Curr Probl Cancer* 1:1–53.

Judgutt BI, Watanabe M, Turner FW. 1975. Hepatic artery ligation in treatment of carcinoid syndrome. *Can Med Assoc J* 112:325–327.

Kelsen DP, Chegn E, Kemeny N, et al. Streptozotocin and adriamycin in the treatment of APUD tumors (carcinoid, islet cell and medullary carcinomas of the thyroid) (abstract). *Proceedings of the American Association of Cancer Research* 23:433.

Kune GA, Goldstein J. 1974. Malignant liver carcinoid: The place of surgery and chemotherapy. Review and case presentation. *Med J Aust* 2:777–780.

Kvols LK, Moertel CG, Schutt AT, et al. 1986. Treatment of the malignant carcinoid syndrome: Evaluation of a long acting somatostatin analogue. *N Engl J Med* 315:663–666.

Lin G, Hagerstrand I, Lunderquist A. 1984. Portal blood supply of liver metastases. *AJR* 143:53–55.

Lunderquist A, Ericsson M, Nobin A, et al. 1982. Gelfoam powder embolization of the hepatic artery in liver metastases of carcinoid tumors. *Radiologe* 22:65–70.

McCarthy DM, Jensen RT. 1985. Zollinger-Ellison syndrome: Current issues. In *Hormone-*

Producing Tumors of the Gastrointestinal Tract, S Cohen, RD Soloway, eds., pp. 25–55. Contemporary Issues in Gastroenterology, Vol. 5. New York: Churchill Livingstone.

McDermott WV, Hensle TW. 1974. Metastatic carcinoid to the liver treated by hepatic de-arterialization. Ann Surg 180:305–308.

Madding GF, Kennedy PA, Sogemeier E. 1970. Hepatic artery ligation for metastatic tumor in the liver. Am J Surg 120:95–96.

Markowitz J. 1952. The hepatic artery. Surg Gynecol Obstet 95:644–646.

Martensson H, Noben A, Bengmark S, et al. 1984. Embolization of the liver in the management of metastatic carcinoid tumors. J Surg Oncol 27:152–158.

Martin JK, Moertel CG, Adson MA, et al. 1983. Surgical treatment of functioning metastatic carcinoid tumors. Arch Surg 118:537–542.

Maton P, O'Dorisio TM, Howe BA, et al. 1985. Effect of a long acting somatostatin analogue (SMS 201-995) in a patient with pancreatic cholera. N Engl J Med 312:17–21.

Maton PN, Camilleri M, Griffin G, et al. 1983. Role of hepatic arterial embolization in the carcinoid syndrome. Br Med J 287:932–935.

Melia WM, Nunnerley HB, Johnson PJ, et al. 1982. Use of arterial devascularization and cytotoxic drugs in 30 patients with carcinoid syndrome. Br J Cancer 46:331–339.

Mengel CE, Shaffer RD. 1973. The carcinoid syndrome. In Cancer Medicine, JF Holland, E Frei, eds., pp. 1584–1593. Philadelphia: Lea & Febiger.

Mitty HA, Warner RRP, Newman LA, et al. 1985. Control of carcinoid syndrome with hepatic artery embolization. Radiology 155:623–626.

Moertel CG. 1983. Treatment of the carcinoid tumor and the malignant carcinoid syndrome. J Clin Oncol 1:727–740.

Moertel CG, Hanley JA. 1979. Combination chemotherapy trials in metastatic carcinoid tumor and the malignant carcinoid syndrome. Cancer Clin Trials 2:327–334.

Moertel CG, Hanley JA, Johnson LA. 1980. Streptozotocin alone compared with streptozotocin plus fluorouracil in the treatment of advanced islet cell carcinoma. N Engl J Med 303:1189–1194.

Moertel CG, May GR, Martin JK, et al. 1985. Sequential hepatic artery occlusion (HAO) and chemotherapy for metastatic carcinoid and islet cell carcinoma (ICC) (abstract). Proceedings of the American Society of Clinical Oncology 4:80.

Moertel CG, O'Connell MJ, Reitemeier RJ, et al. 1984. Evaluation of combined cyclophosphamide and methotrexate therapy in the treatment of metastatic carcinoid tumor and the malignant carcinoid syndrome. Cancer Treat Rep 68:665–667.

Moertel CG, Sauer WG, Dockerty MD, et al. 1961. Life history of the carcinoid tumor of the small intestine. Cancer 14:901–912.

Mori W, Masada M, Miyanaga T. 1966. Hepatic artery ligation and tumor necrosis in the liver. Surgery 59:359.

Murray-Lyons IM, Parsons VA, Blendis LM, et al. 1970. Treatment of secondary hepatic tumors by ligation of hepatic artery and infusion of cytotoxic drugs. Lancet 2:172–175.

Oberg K, Funa K, Alm G. 1983. Effects of leukocyte interferon on clinical symptoms and hormone levels in patients with mid-gut carcinoid tumors and carcinoid syndrome. N Engl J Med 309:129–133.

Pearse AGE. 1974. The APUD cell concept and its implication in pathology. Pathol Annu 9:27–41.

Pearse AGE, Polak JM. 1971. Neural crest origin of the endocrine polypeptide (APUD) cells of the gastrointestinal tract and pancreas. Gut 12:783–788.

Pueyo I, Jimenez JR, Hernandez J, et al. 1978. Carcinoid syndrome treated by hepatic embolization. AJR 131:511–513.

Schein P, Kahn P, Gordon P, et al. 1973. Streptozotocin for malignant insulinomas and carcinoid tumor. Arch Intern Med 132:555–561.

Schutt AJ. 1986. Chemotherapy of gut hormone tumors (abstract). In Gastrointestinal Endocrine Tumors. A Symposium for Medical and Surgical Oncologists. Houston: The University of Texas System Cancer Center.

Segall HN. 1923. An experimental anatomical investigation of the blood and bile channels of the liver. *Surg Gynecol Obstet* 37:152–178.

Solomon A, Sonoda T, Patterson FK. 1976. Response of metastatic malignant carcinoid tumor to adriamycin (NSC-123127). *Cancer Treat Rep* 60:273–276.

Sparks FC, Mosher MB, Hallaner WC, et al. 1975. Hepatic artery ligation and postoperative chemotherapy for hepatic metastases: Clinical and pathophysiological results. *Cancer* 35:1074–1082.

Stephen JL, Grahame-Smith DG. 1972. Treatment of the carcinoid syndrome by local removal of hepatic metastases. *Proc R Soc Med* 65:444–445.

Stockman F, Von Romatowski HJ, Reimold WV, et al. 1984. Hepatic artery embolization for treatment of endocrine gastrointestinal tumors with liver metastases. *Z Gastroenterol* 22:652–660.

Strayer DR, Carter WA, Brodsky I, et al. 1984. Carcinoid tumor response to fibroblast interferon (letter). *JAMA* 251:1682–1683.

Temple WJ, Sugarbaker EV, Ketchan AS. 1981. The APUD system and its apudomas. *International Advances in Surgical Oncology* 4:255–276.

Weiland LH. 1986. Endocrine tumors of the gastrointestinal tract (abstract). In *Gastrointestinal Endocrine Tumors. A Symposium for Medical and Surgical Oncologists.* Houston: The University of Texas System Cancer Center.

Welbourn RB. 1977. Current status of the apudomas. *Ann Surg* 185:1–12.

Wilson H. 1959. The malignant carcinoid syndrome: Massive liver resection for symptomatic relief. *Ann Surg* 25:567–570.

GASTRIC CANCER

Annual Clinical Conference on Cancer, Vol. 30
Gastrointestinal Cancer: Current Approaches to Diagnosis and Treatment
© 1988 by The University of Texas System Cancer Center

30. Gastric Cancer and Its Precursors: Clinical Implications to Be Drawn from Morphological Changes

Grant N. Stemmermann

In this chapter I describe the anatomic changes that are associated with an increased risk of gastric cancer and summarize the diagnostic opportunities that they imply. I then describe those pathological characteristics of gastric cancer that may influence treatment for the patients who are its victims.

PRECURSOR STATES

Epidemiological studies have identified three forms of gastritis that favor the development of cancer in the antrum and corpus of the stomach (table 30.1).

The first of these, type A gastritis, is an atrophic gastritis of the oxyntic, or acid-producing, mucosa of the corpus of the stomach (Kaplan and Rigler 1947; Mossbech and Videbaek 1950; Segal and Samloff 1973; Strickland and Mackay 1973; Correa 1984). This autoimmune disease affects adults who have pernicious anemia and is frequently present asymptomatically among their siblings (Samloff et al. 1986). It is characterized by severe atrophy of the oxyntic glands, increased cell turnover (Deschner, Winawer, and Lipkin 1972), focal intestinal metaplasia (Stemmermann, Hayashi, and Teruya 1984), antral-cell metaplasia of the corpus (Samloff et al. 1982), and the accumulation of dense collections of lymphocytes and plasma cells in the lamina propria. The decreased mass of the corpus chief cells results in lower serum levels of pepsinogen group I (PG I) since production of this substance is confined to these cells (Samloff 1971). The serum levels of pepsinogen group II (PG II) are less likely to be lowered because this substance is also produced in the antrum (Samloff and Liebman 1973) and, in addition, may be produced by metaplastic antral cells in the atrophic corpus. The distorted relationship between these two aspartic proteinases is the basis of a test that offers maximal specificity and sensitivity in the diagnosis of this disease—a PG I:PG II ratio <2.0 (Samloff et al. 1982). Other features of this disease are hypergastrinemia and the appearance of parietal-cell antibodies (Correa 1984; Walsh 1981; Samloff et al. 1982). The ultimate confirmation of this state rests with a mucosal biopsy of the proximal greater curvature of the gastric corpus. The typical histological changes of autoimmune atrophic gastritis must be present to justify this diagnosis. The greater curvature is the preferred biopsy site because proximal extension of antral gastritis (see below) along the lesser curvature may obscure the differences between these two forms of gastritis.

Table 30.1. *Precursors of Cancer of the Gastric Antrum and Corpus*

Patient Characteristics	Precursor		
	Type A Gastritis: Atrophic	Type B Gastritis: Environmental	Subtotal Gastrectomy
Geographic association	Northern Europe	Japan, Korea, Polynesia, Eastern Europe, Chile, Colombia	Not applicable
Family association	Genetic	Environmental	None
Superficial gastritis	Severe	Severe	Severe
Atrophic gastritis	Corpus	Antrum	Inconstant
Intestinal metaplasia	Corpus	Antrum and corpus	Inconstant
PG I:PG II	<2.0 (98%)	<2.0 (35%)	Not applicable
Serum gastrin	>100 pg/ml (90%)	Not elevated	Not elevated
Associated ulcers	None	Increased risk GU in early stages	History of DU
Hyperplastic polyps	Uncommon	Uncommon	Common

Abbreviations: PG, pepsinogen group; GU, gastric ulcer; DU, duodenal ulcer.

The gastric cancers that accompany type A gastritis may develop in the intestinalized corpus or the nonintestinalized antrum. It has been proposed that the increased cancer risk in these patients stems from the in vivo formation of carcinogenic nitroso compounds in the hypochlorhydric stomach (Mirvish 1975). If autoimmune gastritis of the corpus is known to exist, screening for gastric cancer at five-year intervals appears to be justified. This time interval is based on the observation that untreated early carcinomas discovered in screening programs average 38 months between diagnosis and dissemination and 77 months between diagnosis and death of the patient (Oshima et al. 1980). Thus, cancers that develop between examinations probably have not disseminated in the interval.

Atrophic antral gastritis, type B gastritis, is the most common precursor of gastric cancer in countries at high risk for this malignancy and has been termed environmental gastritis (Correa 1984). It begins on the lesser curvature of the antrum and at the antrocorpus junction and is characterized by the replacement of antral glands with those lined by cells resembling small intestinal epithelium (Stemmermann and Hayashi 1968). As the process expands, the intestinalized mucosa may come to line the entire antrum and extend into the corpus, replacing oxyntic mucosa as well.

There are distinct differences between the intestinalized cells of the stomach and the cells of the normal small bowel (table 30.2), and electronmicroscopy shows that some intestinalized cells are clearly dysplastic (Stemmermann, Hayashi, and Teruya 1984). Differences in mucus content, enzyme production and the presence of Paneth cells have been used to distinguish between two types of intestinalized gastric mucosa—complete and incomplete (Matsukura et al. 1980). Briefly, the complete form is characterized by the presence of Paneth cells, alkaline phosphatase, and alcian blue-positive mucin, while the incomplete form lacks Paneth cells and contains iron-diamine-positive mucin and lencine amino peptidase. Some observers attribute an increased cancer risk to the presence of "colonic type" mucins in the intestinalized mucosa (Teglbjaerg and Nielson 1978; Segura and Montero 1983). However, the same cells that produce colonic type mucins also produce small-intestinal disaccharidases; hence one should not conclude that these cells have differentiated in a colonic direction. Both Matsukura et al. (1980) and Jass (1984) assign an increased cancer risk to the presence of incomplete intestinal metaplasia. It should be noted, however, that Jass differs from Matsukura in his use of the term "incomplete," since he puts greater stress upon mucous histochemistry as a distinguishing characteristic. Whatever criterion is used, however, the importance of this distinction is reduced by the following: (1) The majority of small gastric cancers (i.e., <5 mm in diameter) arise at the antrocorpus junction (Oohara et al. 1982; Nagayo 1975), where the metaplastic process is most likely to be complete (Matsukura et al. 1980); and (2) although Paneth cells are good markers for complete metaplasia, they are also commonly found in areas of adenomatous dysplasia.

Because intestinal metaplasia can be produced experimentally by known carcinogens (Matsukura et al. 1979; Watanabe 1978) and because metaplastic cells demonstrate ultrastructural evidence of dysplastic changes, extensive intestinal metaplasia should not be taken lightly. If antral gastritis is sufficiently extensive, it may also be associated with a PG I:II ratio <2.0 (Maki et al. 1983; Stemmermann, Samloff,

Table 30.2. *Differences Between Epithelium of Small Bowel and that of Intestinal Metaplasia*

Histological Features	Normal Small Intestine	Stomach Intestinal Metaplasia
Microscopic structure	Crypts and villi	Glands, no villi
Glycocalyceal enzymes	Uniformly found in all cells	Random cell-to-cell deletion
	Throughout duodenum and jejunum	Site-dependent deletion within stomach
"Bushy" microvilli	Absent	May be present
Cytoplasmic mucus	Uniformly alcian blue-positive	Site-dependent variation between alcian blue- and high-iron diamine-positive
Mucous-Paneth cell hybrids	Absent	Present
Intracytoplasmic cysts with microvilli	Absent	Present
Cilia	Absent	May be present and dysplastic
Paneth cell distribution	All glands	Site-dependent deletion
Paneth cell location	Crypts	Basal or superior aspects if atypia present
Paneth cell DNA synthesis	Absent or infrequent	Common

and Hayashi in press). Once a diagnosis of severe antral gastritis has been established, either by endoscopy or serum pepsinogen analysis, screening at five-year intervals appears to offer the best means of detecting early cancers.

National populations at high risk for gastric cancer are also at high risk for gastric ulcer, probably because both conditions develop in areas of intestinal metaplasia at the antrocorpus junction. Nagayo (1975) has noted that 49 of 58 small gastric cancers (i.e., <5 mm in diameter) (84.5%) are accompanied by gastric ulcer and that 23 of the 58 tumors (39.7%) border an actual or healed ulcer. In vitro and in vivo studies of the morphology and cell kinetics of the mucosa at ulcer margins and of regenerating epithelia indicate that the marginal mucosa contains an increased number of cells in the S phase of the mitotic cycle, while regenerating epithelial cells contain few S-phase cells (Stemmermann, Hayashi, and Taki 1977). If the risk of cancer induction is proportional to the number of cells in the S phase, biopsies of the intact mucosa at the ulcer margin are more likely to be positive than those taken from the ulcer base. In countries without mass screening, most stage I, or early, tumors are found incidently after resection for a chronic recurring gastric ulcer.

Gastroenterostomies, whether gastroduodenal or gastrojejunal, are associated with severe reflux gastritis in the gastric remnant (Dixon et al. 1986). Hyperplastic polyps are commonly found on the gastric side of the stoma (Stemmermann and Hayashi 1979; Koga, Watanabe, and Enjoji 1979), as early as seven years postgastrectomy. Although these may undergo malignant change, the presence of carcinoma may be obscured by severe hemorrhagic gastritis. The risk of acquiring gastric cancer after subtotal gastrectomy for benign disease is actually reduced up to 20 years following establishment of the gastroenterostomy, but is greatly increased at 25 years postgastrectomy (Stalsberg and Taksdal 1971; Caygill et al. 1986). This suggests that endoscopic screening at five-year intervals can be delayed until 20 to 25 years postgastrectomy but, when performed, it should include both quadrant biopsies of the stoma and random biopsies of the gastric remnant.

Carcinoma of the cardia is emerging as one of the more common gastric cancers among otherwise low-risk U.S. whites (Wang, Antonioli, and Goldman 1986; Kalish et al. 1984), in parallel with adenocarcinomas of the distal esophagus arising in metaplastic Barrett's epithelium. The two tumor sites share an association with hiatus hernia and heavy smoking, and neither is associated with significant atrophic gastritis of the antrum or corpus. Cancers of the cardia may be associated with hyperplasia of surface and foveolar cells similar to that seen in hyperplastic polyps of the stomach. Also present may be severe superficial gastritis similar to that found with the hypersecretory state associated with duodenal ulcer (Correa 1984), and many patients with cardia cancers have a history of prior peptic ulcer. Such patients may well have a serum PG I in excess of 100 μg/L (Samloff, Secrist, and Passaro 1976; Samloff et al. 1986). Patients who fit this pattern, especially if they combine the habit of heavy cigarette smoking with a high-grade hiatus hernia, may constitute a select group that might be subject to screening at five-year intervals.

GASTRIC CANCER PATHOLOGY

Lauren (1965) divided gastric cancer into two basic types, intestinal and diffuse. This simple classification has superseded more complicated, and possibly more accurate, histological groupings. This system gives good inter- and intraobserver reproducibility and is consistent in predicting patterns of metastatic spread, as noted in table 30.3 (Stemmermann 1977). The intestinal form is characterized by distinct gland formation and a scanty supporting stroma. All exophytic growths and most ulcerating tumors arising in areas of intestinal metaplasia fall into this category. Diffuse tumors consist of scattered, nonpolarized cells. Often such tumor cells, especially in the more superficial aspects, assume a signet-ring configuration. Diffuse cancers usually have a dense collagenous stroma in the submucosa and muscularis propria.

The diffuse cancers are most common in women, in patients under 50 years of age, and in populations at low risk for acquiring gastric cancer. It is this tumor that appears to be related to blood type A (Correa et al. 1973). Most gastric metastases to the female genital tract occur in the premenopausal period (Stemmermann 1961); hence, they are likely to be diffuse in type. Gastric intestinal tumors are more likely to spread to the liver, forming discrete space-occupying lesions. Hepatic metastases from diffuse cancers seldom form discrete masses, but extend from the porta hepatis

Table 30.3. Patterns of Metastatic Spread at Autopsy According to Histological Type of Gastric Carcinoma

Histological Type	Total	Liver		Adrenal		Lung		Skeleton		Female Genitalia[a]	
		No.	(%)	No.	(%)	No.	(%)	No.	(%)	No.	(%)
Intestinal	85	43	(50.6)	14	(16.5)	29	(34.1)	7	(8.2)	3	(13.0)
Diffuse	82	16	(19.5)	23	(28.0)	34	(41.5)	16	(19.5)	27	(57.5)
Mixed/other	23	6	(26.1)	6	(26.1)	11	(47.8)	2	(8.7)	3	(42.9)
Total	190	65	(34.2)	43	(22.6)	74	(38.9)	25	(13.2)	33	(42.9)

Source: Stemmermann 1977.

[a]Based on cases in 77 women (intestinal−23, diffuse−47, mixed/other−7).

into the liver substance via the portal connective tissue; hence, they may be associated with obstructive jaundice.

Ultrastructural studies indicate that the majority of gastric cancers are composed of cells that have the characteristics of intestinal epithelium but that one-third appear to be of gastric origin (Sasano et al. 1969). Histochemical studies of the mucins in cancer cells show marked variations in the types of mucins produced among the various tumors and even within the same tumor (Stemmermann 1967). Approximately two thirds of tumors produce enzymes that are normally encountered in the intestine rather than the stomach, suggesting that these tumors arose from areas of intestinal metaplasia. Conversely, one third of gastric cancers contain PG II and one tenth of these contain PG I (Stemmermann, Samloff, and Hayashi 1985). It seems reasonable to assume that these pepsinogen-producing cells are of gastric rather than intestinal origin.

The most important factors used to stage gastric cancer are the depth of invasion (T), the presence, number, and location of regional lymph node metastases (N), and the presence of distant spread (M). The current TNM system, together with the survival expectations at each stage, is shown in table 30.4. These data are derived from the latest Japanese data (Miwa et al. 1984).

The Japanese Research Society for Gastric Cancer (Miwa 1978) provides the largest body of survival data of patients treated for gastric cancer. These data indicate that, although tumor size is inversely related to survival, large tumors (e.g., >8 cm) have a favorable prognosis if confined to submucosa and mucosa, while few patients with small tumors that have penetrated the serosa survive five years. The location of the tumor in the stomach also influences survival. Tumors of the cardia and proximal stomach area were associated with a 23.8% five-year survival rate in this series as compared with a 52.6% rate for tumors of the corpus-antral junction and the proximal antrum. These differences in survival rate are widened if the postoperative mortality is compared for proximal cancer (8%) with that of tumors in distal segments of the stomach (3% to 4%).

Tumors classified as intestinal according to the Lauren criteria are associated with better survival than are tumors classified as diffuse (Stemmermann and Brown 1974; Wronkowski, Stemmermann, and Rellahan 1977). Women with diffuse tumors survive longer than men with diffuse tumors, but this difference is confined to patients with stages II and III cancer, since the prognosis for both sexes is good at stage I and uniformly poor at stage IV.

A recent Surveillance, Epidemiology, and End Results (SEER) study (Young, Ries, and Pollack 1984) indicates that in the United States, Japanese are more likely to be five-year survivors than are whites. Although this difference holds true for gastric tumors at every stage, it is greatest for stages I and II. Since it is reasonable to assume that the two races share comparable levels of medical care, the speed of progression from early to advanced cancer may be influenced by as yet unidentified genetic factors.

Table 30.4. TNM Staging System for Gastric Cancer

Stage	T	N	M	Estimated 5-Year Survival Rate
IA	T1—Tumor penetrates mucosa or submucosa	N0—No lymph node metastases	M0—No distant metastases	99%
IB	T2—Tumor invades muscularis propria or subserosa	N0	M0	88%
	T1—	N1—Node ≤3 cm from primary	M0	
II	T1—	N2—Regional nodes >3 cm from primary	M0	70%
	T2—	N1	M0	
	T3—Penetrates serosa but no contiguous organ	N0	M0	
IIIA	T2—	N2	M0	48%
	T3—	N1	M0	
	T4—Invades contiguous structure	N0	M0	36%
IIIB	T3—	N2	M0	24%
	T4—	N1	M0	
IV	Any T	Any N	M1—Distant metastases	10%
	T4—	N2	M0	

Source: Adapted from Miwa et al. 1984.

SUMMARY

The population of North America is generally at low risk for gastric cancer; hence, mass screening to discover early gastric cancer is not likely to be cost effective. Selective screening at five-year intervals of persons at exceptionally high risk may, however, be cost-effective. Such high-risk groups include: (1) patients with pernicious anemia and any of their siblings who have biopsy-proven autoimmune gastritis; (2) patients who have had a gastroenterostomy longer than 20 years; (3) immigrants older than 50 from high-risk countries (e.g., Japan, Korea, eastern Europe, Colombia, Chile); (4) persons with biopsy-proven antral gastritis and extensive intestinal metaplasia or a serum PG I : PG II ratio <2.0; (5) heavy smokers with high-grade hiatus hernia; and (6) persons with chronic, recurring gastric ulcers.

The depth of tumor invasion, the number and location of positive lymph nodes, and the presence of distant metastases are the best guides for predicting five-year survival rates. Other factors that affect survival are the histological type of the tumor (intestinal forms are more favorable than diffuse types), the location of the tumor (tumors of the cardia are less favorable than cancers of the antrum), and race: at every stage, more U.S. Japanese than U.S. whites survive five years.

REFERENCES

Caygill CPJ, Hill MJ, Kirkham JS, et al. 1986. Mortality from gastric cancer following gastric surgery for peptic ulcer. *Lancet* 1 : 929–931.

Correa P. 1984. Chronic gastritis and gastric cancer. In *Precursors of Gastric Cancer*, SC Ming, ed., pp. 105–116. New York: Praeger.

Correa P, Sasano N, Stemmermann GN, et al. 1973. Pathology of gastric carcinoma in Japanese populations: Comparison between Miyagi Prefecture, Japan, and Hawaii. *JNCI* 51 : 1449–1459.

Deschner EE, Winawer SJ, Lipkin M. 1972. Patterns of nucleic acid and protein synthesis in normal human gastric mucosa and atrophic gastritis. *JNCI* 48 : 1567–1574.

Dixon MF, O'Connor HJ, Axon ATR, et al. 1986. Reflux gastritis: Distinct histopathologic entity. *J Clin Pathol* 79 : 524–530.

Jass JR. 1984. Role of intestinal metaplasia in the histogenesis of gastric cancer. In *Precursors of Gastric Cancer*, SC Ming, ed., pp. 167–193. New York: Praeger.

Kalish RJ, Clancy PE, Orringer MB, et al. 1984. Clinical epidemiologic comparison between adenocarcinomas arising in Barrett's esophageal mucosa and in the gastric cardia. *Gastroenterology* 86 : 461–467.

Kaplan HS, Rigler LG. 1947. Pernicious anemia and susceptibility to gastric neoplasms. *J Lab Clin Med* 32 : 644–653.

Koga S, Watanabe H, Enjoji M. 1979. Stomal polypoid hypertrophic gastritis. A polypoid gastric lesion at gastroenterostomy site. *Cancer* 43 : 647–657.

Lauren P. 1965. The two main types of intestinal and diffuse gastric cancer. *Acta Pathol Microbiol Scand* 64 : 31–49.

Maki K, Chang LM, Ichinose M, et al. 1983. Relationship between the endoscopic type of glandular border by Congo red test and the serum pepsinogen level and gastric acid-pepsin analysis (Japanese with English summary). *Gastroenterological Endoscopy* 25 : 1920–1927.

Matsukura N, Kawachi T, Sugimura T, et al. 1979. Induction of intestinal metaplasia and carcinoma of the glandular stomach of rats by N-alkyl-N'-nitro-N-nitroso guanadines. *Gann* 70 : 181–185.

Matsukura N, Suzuki K, Kawachi T, et al. 1980. Distribution of marker enzymes and mucin in intestinal metaplasia of the stomach and relation of complete to incomplete types of metaplasia to minute gastric cancer. *JNCI* 65:231–236.

Mirvish SS. 1975. Formation of *N*-nitroso compounds: Chemistry, kinetics and in vivo occurrence. *Toxicol Appl Pharmacol* 31:325–351.

Miwa K. 1978. *The Report of Treatment Results of Stomach Cancer in Japan (1963–1966)*. Tokyo: Japanese Research Society for Gastric Cancer, National Cancer Center.

Miwa K. 1984. Evaluation of the TNM classification of stomach cancer and proposal for its regional stage grouping. *Jpn J Clin Oncol* 14:385–410.

Mossbech J, Videbaek A. 1950. Mortality from and risk of gastric carcinoma among patients with pernicious anemia. *Br Med J* 2:390–401.

Nagayo T. 1975. Microscopical cancer of the stomach. A study on histogenesis of gastric carcinoma. *Int J Cancer* 16:52–60.

Oohara T, Tohma H, Takazoe K, et al. 1982. Minute gastric cancer less than 5 mm in diameter. *Cancer* 50:801–810.

Oshima A, Fujimoto I, Hiraoka T, et al. 1980. Evaluation of interval trials in stomach cancer. *U.S.-Japan Cooperative Research Program: Seminar on Epidemiology and Chemical-Radiation Carcinogenesis*. Hawaii, March 3–6.

Samloff IM. 1971. Cellular localization of group I pepsinogens in human gastric mucosa by immunofluorescence. *Gastroenterology* 61:185–188.

Samloff IM, Liebman WM. 1973. Cellular localization of the group II pepsinogen in human stomach by immunofluorescence. *Gastroenterology* 65:36–42.

Samloff IM, Secrist DM, Passaro E. 1976. Serum group I pepsinogen levels and their relation to gastric acid secretion in patients with and without recurrent ulcer. *Gastroenterology* 70:309–313.

Samloff IM, Stemmermann GN, Heilbrun LK, et al. 1986. Elevated serum pepsinogen I and II as risk factors for duodenal and gastric ulcer. *Gastroenterology* 90:570–576.

Samloff IM, Varis K, Ihamaki T, et al. 1982. Relationships among serum pepsinogen I, serum pepsinogen II and gastric mucosal histology. A study of relatives with pernicious anemia. *Gastroenterology* 83:204–209.

Sasano N, Nakamura K, Arai M, et al. 1969. Ultrastructural cell patterns in human gastric carcinoma compared with non-neoplastic gastric mucosa. *JNCI* 43:783–802.

Segal HL, Samloff IM. 1973. Gastric cancer: Increased frequency in patients with achlorhydria. *Am J Dig Dis* 18:295–299.

Segura DI, Montero C. 1983. Histochemical characterization of different types of intestinal metaplasia in gastric mucosa. *Cancer* 52:498–503.

Stalsberg H, Taksdal S. 1971. Stomach cancer following gastric surgery for benign conditions. *Lancet* 2:1175–1177.

Stemmermann GN. 1961. Extrapelvic carcinoma metastatic to the uterus. *Am J Obstet Gynecol* 82:1261–1266.

Stemmermann G. 1967. Comparative study of histochemical patterns in non-neoplastic and neoplastic epithelium. *JNCI* 39:375–383.

Stemmermann GN. 1977. Gastric cancer in Hawaiian Japanese. *Gann* 68:525–535.

Stemmermann GN, Brown CA. 1974. A survival study of intestinal and diffuse types of gastric cancer. *Cancer* 33:1190–1195.

Stemmermann G, Hayashi T. 1968. Intestinal metaplasia of the gastric mucosa: A gross and microscopic study of its distribution in various disease states. *JNCI* 41:627–634.

Stemmermann GN, Hayashi T. 1979. Hyperplastic polyps of gastric mucosa at gastroenterostomy stomas. *Am J Clin Pathol* 71:341–345.

Stemmermann GN, Hayashi T, Taki M. 1977. A study of the morphology and kinetics of epithelial migration in response to gastric ulceration: A new approach to the ulcer-cancer question. In *Pathophysiology of Carcinogenesis in Digestive Organs*, E Farber et al., eds., pp. 37–47. Baltimore: University Park Press.

Stemmermann G, Hayashi T, Teruya S. 1984. The dysplastic nature of intestinal metaplasia in the stomach. In *Precursors of Gastric Cancer,* SC Ming, ed., pp. 155–166. New York: Praeger.

Stemmermann GN, Samloff IM, Hayashi T. 1985. Pepsinogens I and II in carcinoma of the stomach: An immunohistochemical study. *Appl Pathol* 3:159–163.

Strickland RG, MacKay IR. 1973. A reappraisal of the nature and significance of chronic atrophic gastritis. *Am J Dig Dis* 18:426–440.

Teglbjaerg PS, Nielson HO. 1978. "Small intestine type" and "colonic type" intestinal metaplasia of the human stomach. *Acta Pathol Microbiol Scand* 86:351–355.

Walsh JH. 1981. Functional and provocative tests for gastroduodenal disorders. *J Clin Gastroenterol* 2 (Suppl 2):73–78.

Wang HH, Antonioli DA, Goldman H. 1986. Comparative features of esophageal and gastric adenocarcinomas: Recent changes in type and frequency. *Hum Pathol* 17:482–487.

Watanabe H. 1978. Experimentally induced intestinal metaplasia in Wistar rats by x-ray irradiation. *Gastroenterology* 75:796–799.

Wronkowski Z, Stemmermann G, Rellahan W. 1977. Stomach carcinoma among Caucasians and Hawaiians in Hawaii. *Cancer* 39:2310–2316.

Young JL, Ries LG, Pollack ES. 1984. Cancer patient survival among ethnic groups in the United States. *JNCI* 73:341–352.

Annual Clinical Conference on Cancer, Vol. 30
Gastrointestinal Cancer: Current Approaches to Diagnosis and Treatment
© 1988 by The University of Texas System Cancer Center

31. Current Issues in the Treatment of Patients with Gastric Cancer

Robert J. Mayer

The incidence and mortality rates for gastric adenocarcinoma have decreased remarkably during the past 50 years for reasons that elude definitive explanation. Nonetheless, stomach cancer represents the eighth most common cause of cancer-related mortality in the United States with more than 14,000 Americans being expected to die of this condition each year (Silverberg and Lubera 1986).

RECENT CHANGES IN PATHOLOGICAL PATTERNS

The decreasing frequency of gastric cancer has necessitated a reexamination of two features previously associated with this malignancy: the relative frequency of certain pathological subtypes and the anatomic location of the tumor. Whereas approximately 95% of stomach tumors have been thought to be adenocarcinomas (Macdonald, Cohn, and Gunderson 1985) and 4% to 5% lymphomas (Shiu et al. 1986), the proportion of gastric lymphomas compared with gastric adenocarcinomas appears to be rising (Macon 1979). It seems likely that 7% to 8% of gastric cancers are now lymphomas and that adenocarcinomas represent closer to 90%. Since the prognosis and treatment for gastric adenocarcinomas and lymphomas are considerably different, this change in the relative appearance of the two neoplasms underscores the importance of establishing a correct histological diagnosis. The two diseases are difficult to distinguish clinically because they both are most often detected during the sixth decade of life, present with epigastric pain, early satiety, and generalized fatigue, are usually characterized by ulceration, and reveal a ragged, thickened mucosal pattern when radiographic studies are performed. A biopsy at the time of gastroscopy or laparotomy is required to make the distinction; the failure of a gastroscopic biopsy to detect lymphoma should not be interpreted as conclusive, however, since superficial biopsies may not reveal the more deeply situated lymphoid infiltration.

Gastric adenocarcinoma is generally believed to arise more often in the antrum of the stomach than in the body or cardia and in the lesser curvature more often than the greater curvature (Macdonald, Cohn, and Gunderson 1985). Recent pathological surveys (Antonioli and Goldman 1982; Cady and Choe 1980) comparing the anatomic location of stomach cancer at single institutions in the United States during successive time periods have indicated that the number of distal gastric cancers has decreased more rapidly than the number of proximal lesions (table 31.1). Ac-

Table 31.1. *Changing Anatomic Distribution of Gastric Adenocarcinoma at the Lahey Clinic*

Location of Gastric Cancer	1940–1949		1950–1959		1960–1969	
	No.	%	No.	%	No.	%
Distal	286	64	217	56	106	46
Body	70	16	61	16	48	21
Proximal	90	20	111	29	79	34
Total	446		389		233	

Source: Adapted from Cady and Choe 1980.

cordingly, a greater proportion of stomach cancers are now being detected in the gastric body and cardia than were previously reported.

The prognosis for patients who have gastric adenocarcinomas is influenced by the histological appearance of the neoplasm. Tumors that have an intestinal (i.e., glandular) architecture are less aggressive biologically than those that have a less differentiated structure (Ribeiro et al. 1981). Proximal gastric cancers are more frequently composed of poorly differentiated tumor cells than are distal lesions (Antonioli and Goldman 1982). Thus, the change in the anatomic location of gastric cancers has led to a relative increase in the appearance of the more virulent pathological subtype of the disease leading to a more ominous clinical outcome.

SURGERY

The surgical resection of all detectable tumor is the only curative treatment presently available to patients who have gastric cancer. Such a complete resection, in which all surgical margins are microscopically tumor-free, is possible in only 25% to 30% of patients (Adashek, Sanger, and Longmire 1979; Dupont et al. 1978; Weed, Nuessle, and Ochsner 1981). The effectiveness of surgical intervention is dependent on the degree of invasion and the extent of tumor spread. Carcinomas located in the distal portion of the stomach are optimally treated by subtotal gastrectomy and resection of adjacent lymph nodes. Adenocarcinomas of the esophagogastric junction require transection of the distal esophagus several centimeters above the tumor and anastomosis of the distal esophagus to the gastric remnant. Tumors of the body of the stomach are resected by total or near-total gastrectomy. Those patients who do not have peritoneal implants, ascites, or extensive liver metastases but who have tumors that are considered to be surgically incurable should still be considered for an attempt at resecting the primary lesion because reducing the residual tumor burden offers the best form of palliation and may improve the potential for subsequent chemotherapy, radiation therapy, or both.

The prognosis following complete resection is negatively correlated with the depth of tumor penetration through the stomach wall, regional lymph node involvement, poorly differentiated histology, and vascular invasion (Bedikian et al. 1984). For the majority of patients in the United States, the prognosis is poor: the five-year

Table 31.2. *Five-Year Survival Rate of Patients after Curative Resection for Gastric Cancer*

Tumor Location	Survival Rate (%)	
	Lymph Nodes Negative	Lymph Nodes Positive
Distal, midstomach	46	20
Proximal, total stomach	13	6

Source: Douglass and Nava 1985.

survival rate following complete resection is approximately 25% for those with distal lesions and less than 10% for those with proximal tumors (Buchholz, Welch, and Malt 1978; Douglass and Nava 1985). These estimates can be further refined by including in the analysis the presence or absence of regional lymph node involvement (Douglass and Nava 1985). The probability for five-year survival for patients who have undergone the total resection of a distal cancer falls from 46% to 20% if nodal spread is present; after a proximal lesion has been completely removed, nodal involvement results in a decrease in the five-year survival rate from 13% to 6% (table 31.2). Tumor can recur as long as eight years following surgery (Serlin et al. 1977).

RADIATION THERAPY

Gastric adenocarcinoma is a relatively radioresistant tumor. For this reason, doses of external-beam radiation in excess of the tolerance of such surrounding structures as bowel mucosa and spinal cord are required to achieve adequate control of the primary tumor. This toxicity has limited the role of radiation to palliation of pain and to adjunctive therapy in combination with surgery and chemotherapy.

Controlled studies have not been performed to determine whether radiotherapy can prolong survival after an operative resection performed for a potentially curable lesion. The incorporation of radiation therapy into such a postsurgical program is worthy of study, since the majority of recurrences in patients who have undergone the total removal of a gastric cancer have been reported to occur in the epigastrium within an area that could be encompassed by a radiation treatment portal (Gunderson and Sosin 1982).

For patients with unresectable disease that is limited to the epigastrium, a comparative trial has shown that treatment with 3,500–4,000 cGy did not improve survival, although survival was prolonged slightly when both 5-fluorouracil (5-FU) and irradiation were administered (Moertel et al. 1969). In more recent prospectively randomized studies of patients with unresectable gastric cancer, no significant benefit has been observed when radiation therapy (maximum doses of 4,000 cGy [Klaassen et al. 1985] or 5,000 cGy [Gastrointestinal Tumor Study Group 1982b]) has been added to 5-FU alone (Klaassen et al. 1985) or to 5-FU combined with semustine (methyl-CCNU) (Gastrointestinal Tumor Study Group 1982b). The efficacy of external-beam radiotherapy is marginal at best.

CHEMOTHERAPY

Treatment of Advanced Disease

Experience during the past decade with chemotherapy as treatment for patients with disseminated gastric adenocarcinoma has led to cautious optimism. Each of several drugs, acting by different cytotoxic mechanisms, has, when used as a single agent, been associated with greater than 50% reductions in measurable tumor mass (i.e., partial response) in more than 15% of patients (table 31.3). These responses, however, are generally short-lived and are rarely associated with the complete disappearance of previously measurable lesions.

5-FU has been studied more extensively than any other agent in the treatment of gastric cancer, producing response rates ranging from 3% to greater than 40% (Comis and Carter 1974). This variation presumably reflects the variety of drug doses and schedules employed, the lack of uniformity in establishing response criteria, and differences in patient selection. Mitomycin C, doxorubicin, cisplatin, and carmustine (BCNU) appear each to have independent activity against gastric adenocarcinoma similar to that of 5-FU (table 31.3). The efficacy of both doxorubicin and cisplatin is particularly noteworthy, since neither drug is useful in managing such other gastrointestinal malignancies as colorectal and pancreatic carcinomas.

Combinations of the drugs that are active as single agents against gastric cancer have increased the rate (table 31.4) and usually prolonged the duration of response observed when any of the compounds have been used alone. Response rates in the 30% to 45% range have been reported after administering such combinations, with these responses lasting for six to nine months. Combining 5-FU with a nitrosourea

Table 31.3. *Chemotherapy for Gastric Carcinoma: Single-Agent Activity*

Drug	No. Responses/ No. Patients	No. Responses	Study
5-Fluorouracil	92/420	22	Comis and Carter 1974 Moertel et al. 1976b
Mitomycin C	63/211	30	Comis and Carter 1974
Doxorubicin	52/258	20	Levi et al. 1986 Wadler, Green, and Muggia 1985
Cisplatin	14/64	22	Aabo, Pedersen, and Rorth 1985 Lacave et al. 1985 Leichman et al. 1984
Carmustine (BCNU)	10/56	18	Moertel 1973 Moertel et al. 1976b
Semustine (methyl-CCNU)	5/48	10	Engstrom et al. 1976 Moertel et al. 1976a

Table 31.4. Chemotherapy in Gastric Carcinoma: Activity of Drug Combinations

Drugs	No. Responses/ No. Patients	Percent Response	Study
5-Fluorouracil + semustine (Methyl-CCNU)	20/62	30	Moertel and Lavin 1979 Moertel et al. 1976a
5-Fluorouracil + carmustine (BCNU)	16/52	31	Kovach et al. 1974 Schnitzler et al. 1986
5-Fluorouracil + mitomycin C	24/79	39	Krauss, Sonada, and Solomon 1979 Moertel and Lavin 1979
5-Fluorouracil + doxorubicin + mitomycin C (FAM)	115/348	33	Wadler, Green, and Muggia 1985
5-Fluorouracil + doxorubicin + semustine (Methyl-CCNU) (FAMe)	14/41	34	Gastrointestinal Tumor Study Group, 1979 Gastrointestinal Tumor Study Group, 1982a Gastrointestinal Tumor Study Group, 1984
5-Fluorouracil + doxorubicin + cisplatin (FAP)	32/79	40	Moertel et al. 1986 Wagener et al. 1985 Woolley et al. 1981
5-Fluorouracil + doxorubicin + carmustine (BCNU) (FAB)	76/177	43	Levi, Dalley, and Aroney 1979 Levi et al. 1986 Lopez et al. 1986 Schnitzler et al. 1986

such as carmustine (BCNU) or semustine (methyl-CCNU) or with mitomycin C has proven to be moderately effective, but the best results to date have emerged from clinical trials in which 5-FU has been combined with doxorubicin and mitomycin C (FAM), with doxorubicin and semustine (FAMe), with doxorubicin and cisplatin (FAP), or with doxorubicin and carmustine (FAB). These drug regimens are surprisingly well tolerated—an important consideration in the treatment of patients who are often malnourished and debilitated—and may usually be administered on an outpatient basis.

It remains uncertain whether any of these three-drug combinations is superior to the others in terms of the probability of disease regression. The heterogeneity of patients in regard to prior treatment, performance status, and site of measurable disease as well as the variations in response criteria and dose schedules among the different studies makes such a comparison difficult. For example, following the initial observation from Georgetown University (Macdonald et al. 1979) of a 50% response rate in 36 patients treated with FAM, other groups observed "objective" disease regressions in as few as 8% (Biran and Sulkes 1984) to as many as 55% (Bitran et al. 1979) of apparently similar patients. When the Georgetown investigators expanded their experience with FAM to 62 previously untreated patients with gastric cancer, the response rate fell slightly to 42% (Macdonald et al. 1980). A recent compilation of data from 348 patients treated with FAM revealed a response rate of 33% (Wadler, Green, and Muggia 1985).

Additionally, few prospectively randomized trials have been conducted that have adequately compared the effects of these various drug combinations on similar patients. The results of those studies that have been completed are conflicting; using median survival time and response rate as measures of efficacy, the Eastern Cooperative Oncology Group (ECOG) found FAM to be superior to FAMe (Douglass et al. 1984) while the Gastrointestinal Tumor Study Group (GITSG) (whose FAM regimen differed somewhat in the dose schedule of 5-FU) reached the opposite conclusion (Gastrointestinal Tumor Study Group 1984). Subsequently, GITSG has reported FAP to be more effective than FAMe and comparable in activity to a new combination under investigation that includes 5-FU, doxorubicin, and triazinate (Bruckner and Stablein 1986).

Recently, the notion that combination chemotherapy is superior to single-agent treatment for patients with advanced gastric cancer has been challenged. Investigators from the North Central Cancer Treatment Group (NCCTG) randomly assigned 151 patients with gastric cancer to receive 5-FU alone, 5-FU in combination with doxorubicin, or FAM (Cullinan et al. 1985). No difference was observed in terms of time to disease progression, and the investigators concluded that both doxorubicin combinations only enhanced toxicity and cost but did not provide sufficient benefit over 5-FU alone to justify their continued use. Although this report engendered widespread publicity and controversy throughout the oncology community, a critical analysis of the findings reveals response rates for patients with measurable lesions of 39% for FAM, 27% for the 5-FU–doxorubicin combination, and 18% for single-agent 5-FU—similar to those previously observed by others (tables

31.3 and 31.4). Additionally, when workers in Australia subsequently compared single-agent doxorubicin to the FAB regimen in 187 patients with advanced gastric cancer, they also found that the response rate was greater in patients who had received the drug combination (40% vs. 13%) but that the tumor regressions were not of sufficient magnitude to affect overall survival (Levi et al. 1986).

Both of these important clinical trials (table 31.5) appear to show that the 50% to 90% reduction in measurable tumor mass that has characterized almost all the responses following treatment with available drug combinations, while achievable in almost half of patients, is inadequate, suggesting that survival benefit will not be improved upon unless complete responses can be attained. Such improvement may require more intensive treatment programs, causing potentially more severe toxic events. One such program under investigation, developed by Klein and colleagues in West Germany, has added high doses of methotrexate with leucovorin factor rescue to 5-FU and doxorubicin in a treatment program called "FAMTX" (Klein et al. 1983). Initial uncontrolled experiences with this regimen in 167 patients treated at a single West German institution (Klein, Dias Wickramanayake, and Farrokh 1986) and by members of the European Organization for Research and Treatment of Cancer (Wils et al. 1986) have suggested a 49% response rate; more important, 21 of 167 (13%) of the treated patients were believed to have achieved not merely a partial response but the complete disappearance of all measurable tumor (table 31.6). These provocative data are encouraging, but the overall importance of FAMTX as treatment for patients with gastric cancer cannot be determined until a prospective comparison is made with an established drug combination such as FAM or with single-agent 5-FU. The impact of complete disease regression on both response duration and overall survival will presumably emerge from such a trial.

Adjuvant Chemotherapy

Metastases eventually develop in more than two thirds of patients who undergo the complete surgical removal of a gastric carcinoma, suggesting that most gastric cancers have spread microscopically before the primary lesion is resected. The identification of drugs active against this malignancy has led to trials in which combination chemotherapy has been administered as an adjuvant to surgical intervention. Although the use of 5-FU and mitomycin, either singly (Fujimoto et al. 1977; Nakajima et al. 1980) or in combination (Nakajima et al. 1980), has been reported to favorably influence survival rates in patients with gastric cancer in Japan, clinical trials in the United States have produced conflicting outcomes. Prospectively randomized studies conducted by the Veterans Administration Surgical Oncology Group failed to demonstrate benefit when patients treated with either thio-TEPA (VA Cooperative Surgical Adjuvant Group 1965) or 5-fluorodeoxyuridine (Serlin et al. 1969) were compared with nontreated control groups. The apparent finding that the combination of 5-FU and semustine (methyl-CCNU) was significantly more effective than semustine alone against advanced gastric cancer (Moertel et al. 1976a) led to separate controlled evaluations of this two-drug program by GITSG (Gastrointestinal Tumor Study Group 1982c), ECOG (Engstrom et al. 1985), and the Vet-

Table 31.5. *Phase III Trials Comparing Single-Agent Chemotherapy with Drug Combinations in Patients with Advanced Gastric Cancer*

| Study | Study Design | No. Evaluable Patients | Responses in Patients with Measurable Disease | | Median Survival (wk) | Percent Surviving after 60 Weeks |
			No.	(%)		
NCCTG (Cullinan et al. 1985)	5-FU + doxorubicin + mitomycin C	51	5/13	(39)	35	22
	vs.					
	5-FU + doxorubicin	49	3/11	(27)	28	22
	vs.					
	5-FU	51	2/11	(18)	35	19
Sydney Cooperative Oncology Group (Levi et al. 1986)	5-FU + doxorubicin + carmustine	94	30/75	(40)	33	16
	vs.					
	5-FU	93	9/70	(13)	19	12

Abbreviations: NCCTG, North Central Cancer Treatment Group; 5-FU, 5-fluorouracil.

Table 31.6. *Phase II Experience with FAMTX in Patients with Advanced Gastric Cancer*

Study	No. of Treated Patients	Responding Patients		Complete-Responding Patients	
		No.	(%)	No.	(%)
Klein, Dias Wickramanayake, and Farrokh 1986	100	59	(59)	12	(12)
EORTC (Wils et al. 1986)	67	22	(33)	9	(13)

Abbreviations: FAMTX, 5-fluorouracil, doxorubicin, methotrexate plus Leucovorin factor rescue; EORTC, European Organization for Research and Treatment of Cancer.

erans Administration Surgical Oncology Group (Higgins et al. 1983) in the adjuvant setting. After these three trials were begun, however, additional experience with the 5-FU and semustine combination in patients with advanced disease showed it to be no better than 5-FU alone (Moertel et al. 1979).

The published results of the three adjuvant trials employing the 5-FU and semustine combination are shown in table 31.7. One of these studies, that conducted by GITSG, demonstrated a statistically significant survival advantage for the patients who received treatment. After an additional 52 months of follow-up, 19% more of the treatment group remain alive than the control cohort (unpublished data). The results of the other two trials failed to suggest any benefit for postoperative 5-FU and semustine.

Satisfactory explanations have not been offered to account for the discrepancy created by these differing therapeutic outcomes. All three studies were initiated at about the same time (1974–1975) and had similar experimental designs (i.e., treatment vs. control). The chemotherapy dose schedules in the GITSG and ECOG trials were identical. It is possible that the GITSG investigators required closer prospective scrutiny of the operative and pathology reports in their protocol than did their colleagues in ECOG and the VA Surgical Oncology Group. Additionally, it is conceivable that GITSG avoided the inappropriate inclusion of patients whose resection margins contained tumor cells because of the concomitant availability of a parallel study for patients with locally unresectable gastric cancer (Gastrointestinal Tumor Study Group 1982b). It is clear, however, that the prognosis for patients randomized to the nontreatment (i.e., control) cohort in the GITSG study was similar to that for patients in the other two trials (table 31.7), indicating that the difference between the two experimental groups in the GITSG trial was related to the improved outcome for the patients who received adjuvant therapy. Furthermore, the prognostic advantage for the patients in the treatment cohort of the GITSG trial continued to be evident when the data were analyzed in terms of such prospectively stratified factors as nodal status and anatomic location of tumor (i.e., distal vs. proximal). Nonetheless, the apparent efficacy of adjuvant chemotherapy shown in the GITSG trial remains unconfirmed by any other American experience, and the concept of adjuvant

Table 31.7. Adjuvant Gastric Cancer Trials: 5-Fluorouracil Plus Semustine (Methyl-CCNU) Versus Control

Study	Median Follow-up Time (mo)	Total Pts. Alive/ Total Pts. Evaluable		Control Pts. Alive/ Control Pts. Evaluable		Treated Pts. Alive/ Treated Pts. Evaluable		? Adjuvant Effect
		No.	(%)	No.	(%)	No.	(%)	
GITSG (Gastrointestinal Tumor Study Group, 1982c)	48	73/142	(51)	31/71	(44)	42/71	(59)	+
ECOG (Engstrom et al. 1985)	64	72/180	(40)	38/89	(43)	34/91	(37)	—
VA Surgical Oncology Group (Higgins et al. 1983)	48	62/134	(46)	32/68	(47)	30/66	(46)	—

Abbreviation: ECOG, Eastern Cooperative Oncology Group.

treatment for patients following the resection of a gastric cancer should continue to be regarded as investigational.

Several areas of study seem worth examining in future trials, including perioperative chemotherapy, radiation therapy, intraperitoneal chemotherapy, or the inclusion of cisplatin or a combination of mitomycin C, doxorubicin, and cisplatin into adjuvant chemotherapy regimens. Many successful adjuvant programs in Japan have initiated treatment with chemotherapy either intraoperatively or shortly after the time of surgery. This contrasts markedly with the practice in the United States where chemotherapy does not usually commence until four to six weeks after surgery, owing to concern for adequate healing of the anastomosis. Such a delay may possibly lead to a doubling in the number of residual tumor cells (Douglass 1985). Since the potential for controlling such minimal residual disease may be compromised by delaying the start of chemotherapy, it would seem appropriate to design a trial that would prospectively explore the feasibility and possible benefit of perioperative treatment. Another possible approach to adjuvant gastric therapy would address the problem of the high frequency of peritoneal and regional recurrences after a complete resection (Gunderson and Sosin 1982). Previous attempts at examining the benefit of adjuvant external-beam irradiation combined with chemotherapy have been compromised by an insufficient radiation dose (Dent et al. 1979) or patient evaluability problems brought about by a "prerandomization" process (Moertel et al. 1984). The issue of adjuvant radiation in the setting of "minimal residual disease" merits further study. The high likelihood of patients with gastric cancer developing peritoneal metastases would suggest that the postoperative period is an ideal time to explore the value of intraperitoneal chemotherapy. Last, the 5-FU and semustine adjuvant chemotherapy programs were designed before the activity of mitomycin C, doxorubicin, and cisplatin against advanced gastric cancer had been recognized. Single-agent mitomycin C has been reported to be an effective adjuvant, not just in studies from Japan but also in a recent report from Spanish investigators (Alcobendas et al. 1983). An international cooperative group is presently conducting a controlled trial to determine the value of FAM as adjuvant treatment (Schein, Coombes, and Chilvers 1986). Drug combinations such as FAP, FAB (table 31.4), and possibly "FAMTX" (table 31.6), perhaps more active than FAM in terms of effecting transient responses in patients with metastatic disease, would appear appropriate for inclusion in future controlled adjuvant programs.

SUMMARY

The falling incidence of gastric cancer in the United States has resulted in a relative increase of gastric lymphoma among stomach malignancies and has also been associated with a greater decrease in distal than in proximal carcinomas. Surgery remains the only curative treatment for patients with gastric carcinoma. However, the greater proportion of patients with proximal lesions and a diffuse pathological pattern in recent years has lessened the efficacy of this therapeutic approach. In patients with locally unresectable disease, the benefit of adding radiation therapy to chemotherapy has not been clearly established. Although combination chemotherapy enhances response rates over those achieved by single-agent treatment, complete responses are rare and any survival advantage with presently examined drug combinations is marginal. In the United States, adjuvant therapy following a "curative" resection remains an investigational concept.

REFERENCES

Aabo K, Pedersen H, Rorth M. 1985. Cisplatin in the treatment of advanced gastric carcinoma: A phase II study. *Cancer Treat Rep* 69:449–450.

Adashek K, Sanger J, Longmire WP Jr. 1979. Cancer of the stomach. Review of consecutive ten year intervals. *Ann Surg* 189:6–10.

Alcobendas F, Milla A, Estape J, et al. 1983. Mitomycin-C as an adjuvant in resected gastric cancer. *Ann Surg* 198:13–17.

Antonioli DA, Goldman H. 1982. Changes in the location and type of gastric adenocarcinoma. *Cancer* 50:775–781.

Bedikian AY, Chen TT, Khankhanian N, et al. 1984. The natural history of gastric cancer and prognostic factors influencing survival. *J Clin Oncol* 2:305–310.

Biran H, Sulkes A. 1984. A possible dose response relationship in "FAM" chemotherapy for advanced gastric cancer (abstract). *Proceedings of the American Society of Clinical Oncology* 3:132.

Bitran JD, Desser RK, Kozloff MF, et al. 1979. Treatment of metastatic pancreatic and gastric adenocarcinomas with 5-fluorouracil, adriamycin, and mitomycin C (FAM). *Cancer Treat Rep* 63:2049–2051.

Bruckner HW, Stablein DM. 1986. A randomized study of 5-fluorouracil (F) and doxorubicin (A) with semustine (Me), *cis*-platinum (P), or triazinate (T) for treatment of advanced gastric cancer (abstract). *Proceedings of the American Society of Clinical Oncology* 5:90.

Buchholtz TW, Welch CE, Malt RA. 1978. Clinical correlates of resectability and survival in gastric carcinoma. *Ann Surg* 188:711–715.

Cady B, Choe DS. 1980. Changing patterns of gastric cancer. In *Third International Symposium on Detection and Prevention of Cancer*, HE Nieburgs, ed., pp. 2041–2049. New York: Dekker.

Comis RL, Carter SK. 1974. A review of chemotherapy in gastric cancer. *Cancer* 34:1576–1586.

Cullinan SA, Moertel CG, Fleming TR, et al. 1985. A comparison of three chemotherapeutic regimens in the treatment of advanced pancreatic and gastric carcinoma: Fluorouracil vs. fluorouracil and doxorubicin vs. fluorouracil, doxorubicin, and mitomycin. *JAMA* 253:2061–2067.

Dent DM, Werner ID, Novis B, et al. 1979. Prospective randomized trial of combined onocological therapy for gastric carcinoma. *Cancer* 44:385–391.

Douglass HO Jr. 1985. Gastric cancer: Overview of current therapies. *Semin Oncol* 12 (Suppl 4):57–62.

Douglass HO Jr, Lavin PT, Goudsmit A, et al. 1984. An Eastern Cooperative Oncology Group evaluation of combinations of methyl-CCNU, mitomycin C, adriamycin, and 5-fluorouracil in advanced measurable gastric cancer (EST 2277). *J Clin Oncol* 2:1372–1381.

Douglass HO Jr, Nava HR. 1985. Gastric adenocarcinoma: Management of the primary disease. *Semin Oncol* 12:32–45.

Dupont JB Jr, Lee JR, Burton GR, Cohn I Jr. 1978. Adenocarcinoma of the stomach: Review of 1,497 cases. *Cancer* 41:941–947.

Engstrom PF, Catalano RB, Creech RH. 1976. Phase II study of methyl-CCNU (NSC-95441) in advanced gastrointestinal cancer. *Cancer Treat Rep* 60:285–287.

Engstrom PF, Lavin PT, Douglass HO Jr, et al. 1985. Postoperative adjuvant 5-fluorouracil plus methyl-CCNU therapy for gastric cancer patients. Eastern Cooperative Oncology Group Study (EST 3275). *Cancer* 55:1868–1873.

Fujimoto S, Akao T, Itoh B, et al. 1977. Protracted oral chemotherapy with fluorinated pyrimidines as an adjuvant to surgical treatment for stomach cancer. *Ann Surg* 185: 462–466.

Gastrointestinal Tumor Study Group. 1979. Randomized study of combination chemotherapy studies in advanced gastric cancer. *Cancer Treat Rep* 63:1871–1876.

Gastrointestinal Tumor Study Group. 1982a. A comparative clinical assessment of combination chemotherapy in the management of advanced gastric cancer. *Cancer* 49:1362–1366.

Gastrointestinal Tumor Study Group. 1982b. A comparison of combination chemotherapy and combined modality therapy for locally advanced gastric cancer. *Cancer* 49: 1771–1777.

Gastrointestinal Tumor Study Group. 1982c. Controlled trial of adjuvant chemotherapy following curative resection for gastric cancer. *Cancer* 49:1116–1122.

Gastrointestinal Tumor Study Group. 1984. Randomized study of combination chemotherapy in unresectable gastric cancer. *Cancer* 53:13–17.

Gunderson LL, Sosin H. 1982. Adenocarcinoma of the stomach: Areas of failure in a re-operation series (second or symptomatic look). Clinicopathologic correlation and implications for adjuvant therapy. *Int J Radiat Oncol Biol Phys* 8:1–11.

Higgins GA, Amadeo JH, Smith DE, et al. 1983. Efficacy of prolonged intermittent therapy with combined 5-FU and methyl-CCNU following resection for gastric carcinoma. A Veterans Administration Surgical Oncology Group report. *Cancer* 52:1105–1112.

Klaassen DJ, MacIntyre JM, Catton GE, et al. 1985. Treatment of locally unresectable cancer of the stomach and pancreas: A randomized comparison of 5-fluorouracil alone with radiation plus concurrent and maintenance 5-fluorouracil—An Eastern Cooperative Oncology Group study. *J Clin Oncol* 3:373–378.

Klein HO, Dias Wickramanayake P, Dieterle F, et al. 1983. High-dose MTX/5-FU and adriamycin for gastric cancer. *Semin Oncol* 10 (Suppl 2):29–31.

Klein HO, Dias Wickramanayake P, Farrokh GR. 1986. 5-Fluorouracil (5-FU), adriamycin (ADM), and methotrexate (MTX): A combination protocol (FAMTX) for treatment of metastasized stomach cancer (abstract). *Proceedings of the American Society of Clinical Oncology* 5:84.

Kovach JS, Moertel CG, Schutt AJ, et al. 1974. A controlled study of 1-3-*bis*-(2-chlorethyl)-1-nitrosourea and 5-fluorouracil therapy for advanced gastric and pancreatic cancer. *Cancer* 33:563–567.

Krauss S, Sonada T, Solomon A. 1979. Treatment of advanced gastrointestinal cancer with 5-fluorouracil and mitomycin-C. *Cancer* 43:1598–1603.

Lacave AJ, Wils J, Diaz-Rubio E, et al. 1985. *Cis*-platinum as second-line chemotherapy in advanced gastric adenocarcinoma. A phase II study of the EORTC Gastrointestinal Tract Cancer Cooperative Group. *Eur J Cancer Clin Oncol* 21:1321–1324.

Leichman L, McDonald B, Dindogru A, et al. 1984. Cisplatin: An active drug in the treatment of disseminated gastric cancer. *Cancer* 53:18–22.

Levi JA, Dalley DN, Aroney RS. 1979. Improved combination chemotherapy in advanced gastric cancer. *Br Med J* 2:1471–1473.

Levi JA, Fox RM, Tattersall MH, et al. 1986. Analysis of a prospectively randomized comparison of doxorubicin versus 5-fluorouracil, doxorubicin, and BCNU in advanced gastric cancer: Implications for future studies. *J Clin Oncol* 4:1348–1355.

Lopez M, DiLauro L, Papaldo P, et al. 1986. Treatment of advanced measurable gastric carcinoma with 5-fluorouracil, adriamycin, and BCNU. *Oncology* 43:288–291.

Macdonald JS, Cohn I Jr, Gunderson LL. 1985. Cancer of the stomach. In *Cancer: Principles and Practice of Oncology,* 2 ed., VT Devita Jr, S Hellman, SA Rosenberg, eds., pp. 659–690. Philadelphia: J. B. Lippincott.

Macdonald JS, Schein PS, Woolley PV, et al. 1980. 5-Fluorouracil, doxorubicin, and mitomycin (FAM) combination chemotherapy for advanced gastric cancer. *Ann Intern Med* 93:533–536.

Macdonald JS, Woolley PV, Smythe T, et al. 1979. 5-Fluorouracil, adriamycin, and mitomycin C (FAM) combination chemotherapy in the treatment of advanced gastric cancer. *Cancer* 44:42–47.

Macon WL IV. 1979. Gastric lymphoma vs. adenocarcinoma: A diagnostic problem. *Arch Surg* 114:305–306.

Moertel CG. 1973. Therapy of advanced gastrointestinal cancer with the nitrosoureas. *Cancer Chemother Rep* Pt III 4:27–34.

Moertel CG, Childs DS, O'Fallon JR, et al. 1984. Combined 5-fluorouracil and radiation therapy as a surgical adjuvant for poor prognosis gastric carcinoma. *J Clin Oncol* 2:1249–1254.

Moertel CG, Childs DS Jr, Reitemeier RJ, et al. 1969. Combined 5-fluorouracil and supervoltage radiation therapy of locally unresectable gastrointestinal cancer. *Lancet* 2:865–867.

Moertel CG, Engstrom P, Lavin PT, et al. 1979. Chemotherapy of gastric and pancreatic carcinoma: A controlled evaluation of combination of 5-fluorouracil with nitrosoureas and lactones. *Surgery* 85:509–513.

Moertel CG, Lavin PT. 1979. Phase II-III chemotherapy studies in advanced gastric cancer. *Cancer Treat Rep* 63:1863–1869.

Moertel CG, Mittelman JA, Bakemeier RJ, et al. 1976a. Sequential and combination chemotherapy of advanced gastric cancer. *Cancer* 38:678–682.

Moertel CG, Rubin J, O'Connell MJ, et al. 1986. A phase II study of combined 5-fluorouracil, doxorubicin, and cisplatin in the treatment of advanced upper gastrointestinal adenocarcinomas. *J Clin Oncol* 4:1053–1057.

Moertel CG, Schutt AJ, Reitemeier RJ, et al. 1976b. Therapy for gastrointestinal cancer with the nitrosoureas alone and in drug combinations. *Cancer Treat Rep* 60:729–732.

Nakajima T, Fukami A, Takagi K, et al. 1980. Adjuvant chemotherapy with mitomycin C, and with a multi-drug combination of mitomycin C, 5-fluorouracil, and cytosine arabinoside after curative resection of gastric cancer. *Jpn J Clin Oncol* 10:187–194.

Ribiero MM, Sarmento JA, Simoes MA, Bastos J. 1981. Prognostic significance of Lauren and Ming classifications and other pathologic parameters in gastric carcinoma. *Cancer* 47:780–784.

Schein PS, Coombes RC, Chilvers C. 1986. A controlled trial of FAM (5-FU, doxorubicin, and mitomycin-C) chemotherapy as adjunctive treatment for resected gastric carcinoma (abstract). *Proceedings of the American Society of Clinical Oncology* 5:79.

Schnitzler G, Queisser W, Heim ME, et al. 1986. Phase III study of 5-FU and carmustine versus 5-FU, carmustine, and doxorubicin in advanced gastric cancer. *Cancer Treat Rep* 70:477–479.

Serlin O, Keehn RJ, Higgins GA Jr, et al. 1977. Factors related to survival following resection for gastric carcinoma: Analysis of 903 cases. *Cancer* 40:1318–1329.

Serlin O, Wolkoff JS, Amadeo JM, et al. 1969. Use of 5-fluorodeoxyuridine (FUDR) as an adjuvant to the surgical management of carcinoma of the stomach. *Cancer* 24:223–228.

Shiu MH, Nisce LZ, Pinna A, et al. 1986. Recent results of multimodal therapy of gastric lymphoma. *Cancer* 58:1389–1399.

Silverberg E, Lubera J. 1986. Cancer statistics, 1986. *CA* 36:9–25.

VA Cooperative Surgical Adjuvant Group. 1965. Use of thio-TEPA as an adjuvant to the surgical management of carcinoma of the stomach. *Cancer* 18:291–297.

Wadler S, Green M, Muggia F. 1985. The role of anthracyclines in the treatment of gastric cancer. *Cancer Treat Rev* 12:105–132.

Wagener DJTh, Yap SH, Wobbes T, et al. 1985. Phase II trial of 5-fluorouracil, adriamycin and cisplatin (FAP) in advanced gastric cancer. *Cancer Chemother Pharmacol* 15:86–87.

Weed TE, Nuessle W, Ochsner A. 1981. Carcinoma of the stomach. Why are we failing to improve survival? *Ann Surg* 193:407–413.

Wils J, Bleiberg H, Dalesio O, et al. 1986. An EORTC gastrointestinal group evaluation of the combination of sequential methotrexate and 5-fluorouracil, combined with adriamycin in advanced measurable gastric cancer. *J Clin Oncol* 4:1799–1803.

Woolley P, Smith F, Estevez R, et al. 1981. A phase II trial of 5-FU, adriamycin, and cisplatin (FAP) in advanced gastric cancer (abstract). *Proceedings of the American Society of Clinical Oncology* 22:455.

JOANNE VANDENBERGE HILL AWARD AND WILLIAM O. RUSSELL LECTURESHIP IN ANATOMIC PATHOLOGY

Annual Clinical Conference on Cancer, Vol. 30
Gastrointestinal Cancer: Current Approaches to Diagnosis and Treatment
© 1988 by The University of Texas System Cancer Center

32. Premalignancy and Dysplasia in the Gastrointestinal Tract: Detection, Diagnosis, and Implications

Robert H. Riddell

"Premalignancy" is a very broad term that needs further definition. Conceptually, it most simply means a condition, disease, or lesion—some factor—that increases an individual's likelihood of developing a malignancy, compared with a control population without that factor. Examples of such factors are age, as in colorectal carcinoma; or sex, as in the vast male predominance of adenocarcinoma complicating Barrett's esophagus; and the presence of a ureterosigmoidostomy, for cancer of the large bowel. Some diseases have a well-documented familial/hereditary component. Environmental factors may also be invoked, as in the association of combined alcohol and tobacco use with the genesis of squamous carcinoma of the esophagus.

Another aspect of premalignancy is that a variety of benign *diseases* and *conditions* are known to predispose to gastrointestinal malignancy. In the stomach, for instance, these include pernicious anemia and possibly the postgastrectomy stomach. Familial adenomatous polyposis coli can be associated with periampullary carcinomas, and celiac sprue predisposes to lymphomas and carcinomas of the small intestine and possibly squamous carcinoma of the esophagus. Inflammatory bowel disease, particularly ulcerative colitis, predisposes to adenocarcinoma of the colorectum.

The final level at which we may look at premalignancy is in premalignant *lesions*. These primarily are the adenomas wherever they occur in the gastrointestinal tract. But dysplasia, which is particularly prevalent in those diseases characterized by long-standing chronic inflammation, is also encompassed here.

The subtitle of this chapter involves a separate concept, namely, the practical side—how dysplasia and possibly early invasive carcinoma can be detected and the implications of that detection for patient management. Currently, the pathological stage at which gastrointestinal carcinoma is first seen is purely a matter of chance: one patient will be seen relatively early in the course of disease and fortunately be cured, whereas another will present with disseminated disease and soon die. It is hoped that early detection will result in an increased cure rate and not just longer survival times, as the latter might only reflect such intrinsic biases as lead-time bias. It is important to realize that to date no trial has proven the benefit of a surveillance program; however, convincing studies may never be carried out because of the potential difficulties in randomizing patients with any form of "premalignancy" to an appropriate control arm.

Clinical strategies for early detection are surprisingly limited and will be discussed below. Nevertheless, it is important to separate whether one is searching primarily for premalignant as opposed to early invasive lesions. If the end point of clinical surveillance studies is the latter, the likelihood of advanced lesions and thus of mortality from disseminated disease will of course be much greater.

In this chapter, I shall use the model of colorectal carcinoma, as it embraces the spectrum of changes found in the gastrointestinal tract.

PREMALIGNANT LESIONS

If most carcinomas really did arise "de novo," there would be little point in searching for preinvasive lesions. In the case of adenocarcinoma of the large intestine, there is considerable evidence that most tumors likely originate in adenomas. What, then, is an adenoma?

Adenomas

An adenoma is a benign proliferation of neoplastic epithelium. It can be readily identified by the presence of enlarged cells containing enlarged, usually hyperchromatic nuclei that produce a pseudostratified ("picket fence") appearance. This is also a typical morphological description of dysplasia and it is therefore necessary to compare and contrast these in a little more detail below. Thus, any well-defined polypoid lesion located in the gastrointestinal tract and composed of epithelium of this type is by definition an adenoma, with rare exceptions as discussed below.

Adenomas have a virtually identical morphology whether they occur in the large intestine, small intestine, or stomach. Further, in the large bowel it is well documented that adenomas are more likely to have an associated invasive adenocarcinoma (i.e., infiltration into the submucosa), the likelihood related to increasing lesion size, increasing dysplasia, and the presence of a villous component (Muto, Bussey, and Morson 1975). Although these correlations are useful, they do not help in deciding whether an individual adenoma encountered clinically does or does not have an associated invasive carcinoma. Only resection of the polyp and histological examination of the specimen will determine this point. Nevertheless, one of the most interesting features of adenomas is that there needs to be about 5 mm of adenoma for invasion to occur. Beneath this figure, invasion is extremely rare and can still be "written up."

Gilbertson and Nelms's 1978 report of a 25-year series of over 21,000 patients examined by sigmoidoscopy strongly suggests that adenomas predispose to carcinoma. In this series, any polyps that were found were removed. Initially, 27 patients were found to have cancer. During the follow-up period, between 85 and 100 cases of cancer were expected, but only 5 were found. One of these cancers infiltrated into the muscularis propria but the other four only reached the submucosa. It would therefore appear that removal of incidental polyps, presumably including most adenomas, is effective in preventing subsequent rectosigmoid carcinoma. Nevertheless, even this study was not controlled and subject to a variety of biases.

Adenomas of any gastrointestinal location are predisposed to invade. But we remain relatively ignorant about which adenomas are most likely to grow and which of those that do grow ultimately become invasive. Further, our knowledge of the time frames involved is sadly inadequate. For example, Vatn and Stalsberg in 1982 demonstrated a peak of adenomas in Oslo women in their 50s, which seemed not to be translated into a later carcinoma peak at all in their series.

The practical implication is that once a patient has developed an adenoma in any organ, malignant potential should be assumed and regular follow-up instituted. The means and intervals of follow-up will vary, but air-contrast barium studies or endoscopy should probably be performed every two to three years.

Follow-up of Patients with Proven Adenomas or Carcinomas

The follow-up of patients who have or had proven adenomas or in whom carcinoma was treated depends on a variety of features and will vary markedly depending upon such factors as the organ involved, the feasibility of carrying out further intervention in a particular patient if a lesion is found, and the prevalence of carcinoma in the population under consideration. A North American in whom a gastric adenoma has been removed is almost certainly at a much lower risk of developing a gastric carcinoma than a counterpart in areas of the world with a high prevalence of gastric carcinoma such as Japan, Scandinavia, or Italy; the intensity of follow-up may therefore differ markedly on a geographic basis.

Assuming a patient who had carcinoma has been cured, surveillance is aimed solely at preventing the development of another potentially lethal tumor. But how often should that surveillance be carried out? This question is much discussed for the gamut of adenomas and carcinomas, but it is virtually impossible to answer. One reply is: the more frequent the surveillance, the less likely the development of a lethal tumor but the greater the usage of manpower. The problem might be better posed as the likelihood of adenoma, invasive carcinoma, or lethal invasive carcinoma vis-à-vis surveillance, say, every six months, year, or two, three, or five years. Once such figures are generated, further attention can be given to the economic factors involved.

"Familial" Carcinoma of the Large Bowel

The familial diseases of the large bowel are best exemplified by the hereditary polyposis syndromes, namely, familial adenomatous polyposis coli and the much less common juvenile polyps and Peutz-Jeghers syndrome. The possibly familial nature of nonfamilial (sporadic) carcinoma of the large bowel is surprisingly neglected, particularly since strategies engendered by such findings might lessen the number of patients who present with advanced disease.

Lovett, for example, examined the death certificates of relatives of colorectal carcinoma patients and found that 7% to 10% of probands' parents, 16% of probands' brothers, and 18% of probands' sisters had died of the disease (Lovett 1976). Assuming an overall mortality in this disease of about 50% would imply that these figures could be doubled. Thus, perhaps one in three siblings of patients with carcinoma of the large bowel might themselves develop the disease. Regular surveillance of such relatives should be seriously considered; it could even be argued that routine management and follow-up in patients with carcinoma of the large bowel should include routine investigation of siblings and any living parents. It remains to be seen whether the offspring of these patients are at similarly high risk.

It should also be remembered that there are a variety of hereditary syndromes, admittedly all relatively uncommon, that tend to be characterized by the development of colon cancer. The cancer in these cases usually occurs on the right side and at an earlier age than in the general population: patients are frequently still in their 40s. These syndromes include cancer family syndrome, or hereditary adenocarcinomatosis, in which carcinoma of the right colon occurs in association with gastric, uterine, ovarian, or breast carcinoma, often in combination; hereditary gastrocolonic cancer, in which double primary tumors occur in either or both organs; hereditary colorectal cancer, in which family members develop carcinoma (frequently at the same site in the colon); and Muir's, or Torre's, syndrome, in which there is also an association with skin appendage tumors.

It could therefore also be argued that the routine family history that is taken (from any patient in any setting, not simply in gastroenterological contexts) should include not only what relatives have died of, but careful inquiry as to whether any relatives, living or dead, ever developed colorectal carcinoma. The clinical implication is that, because these patients and their families may be at increased risk for colorectal cancer, they should all have the option of undergoing regular surveillance. In families in which the colorectal carcinoma tends to manifest itself at an early age, surveillance should probably begin at least 5 and perhaps 10 years before the age at which clinically apparent disease is expected. On occasion, an adenoma is found at the precise site (e.g., cecal pole) at which a carcinoma developed in a first-degree relative.

Dysplasia

Dysplasia in the gastrointestinal tract can be defined as an unequivocally neoplastic proliferation essentially equivalent to an adenoma. All equivocal or regenerative lesions are excluded. Dysplasia usually occurs as background to a long-standing inflammatory disease and may be the superficial part of an invasive carcinoma (Riddell et al. 1983).

Dysplasia Versus Adenomas

Microscopic Differences.   As mentioned above, the cytological factors by which adenomas and areas of dysplasia are identified are identical. Virtually all of the variations that have been described in dysplasia occur in adenomas and carcinomas from time to time. However, it is in the converse situation where difficulties arise, for some carcinomas—the so-called minimal-deviation carcinomas—are characterized by surprisingly little nuclear change. These carcinomas tend to arise from mucosae that also tend to show lesions of a similar minimal deviation, so minimal in fact that it would be considered indefinite for dysplasia by current classification systems. Thus, even though this mucosa is exhibiting its potential to invade, it is difficult or impossible to categorize it histologically as dysplastic. Resection would not be considered unless an endoscopic (macroscopically visible) lesion led to such consideration. Minimal-deviation carcinomas are fortunately uncommon, but the diagnostic situation they present does bespeak a weakness of the classification systems.

In inflammatory conditions such as ulcerative colitis, however, a second difference becomes apparent. Adenomatous glands are readily distinguishable from adjacent "control" nonneoplastic crypts. In familial adenomatous polyposis coli, in fact, even single crypts are clearly different from their nonneoplastic counterparts.

In other inflammatory disorders with malignant potential such as Barrett's esophagus or inflammatory bowel disease, on the other hand, the change from nonneoplastic to neoplastic may be part of a spectrum, and normal crypts may not be available for comparison. Because a spectrum of changes exists between normal and dysplastic, any divisions within the spectrum are necessarily arbitrary and subjective. Biopsies taken to assess for dysplasia can thus be categorized as negative, indefinite, or positive (Riddell et al. 1983). Those that are positive will look essentially like adenomas, and those that are negative will resemble the normal mucosa. The indefinite group is that part of the spectrum wherein one is uncertain whether progression from negative to positive is occurring, or whether changes are stable. Rebiopsy over several months and on several occasions may be necessary to establish the stability of these lesions or whether adjacent areas of unequivocal dysplasia are also present.

As noted above, regenerative changes are not dysplastic changes. This statement covers the gamut of regenerative changes seen in inflammatory conditions. But because the actively regenerating stage is characterized by enlarged vesicular nuclei with prominent eosinophilic nucleoli, confusion with neoplastic change can readily occur. Once these changes are recognized, though, such confusion is largely eliminated (Riddell et al. 1983).

Macroscopic/Endoscopic Differences. Dysplasia sometimes occurs as raised areas evident as plaques or irregular areas of nodularity. The latter are often poorly circumscribed. This is in marked contrast to adenomas, which are invariably well circumscribed and pedunculated, broad based, or sessile. There are three distinct clinical implications in this difference in appearance.

First, when surveillance is being carried out to detect dysplasia, the gross appearances of the lesion being sought must be borne in mind and deliberately sought. The subtle nature of the lesions may otherwise lead to their being overlooked.

Second, it must be remembered that any adenoma over about 3 mm in diameter and any form of dysplasia might directly give rise to invasive carcinoma or actually be the superficial part of such a tumor. Unless the lesion is removed, it remains uncertain whether such transformation has actually occurred. It should be recognized that transformation to invasive carcinoma can occur in the absence of in situ carcinoma. The original concept of invasive carcinoma arising through different stages of dysplasia—as from mild to moderate to severe dysplasia, with in situ carcinoma preceding invasive carcinoma—has now given way to the concept that any dysplastic epithelium can directly give rise to infiltrating carcinoma, without an in situ phase. Fortunately, the chance of invasive carcinoma being present in adenomas is reasonably well known; however, there is a lack of data regarding the likelihood of invasive carcinoma in areas of dysplasia in different anatomic locations, and regarding the likelihood within a given location according to association with different diseases.

Third, the question of whether adenomas can exist, alone or with dysplasia, in situations in which dysplasia is expected needs to be examined. In ulcerative colitis, for instance, lesions indistinguishable from adenomas by all criteria appear to be relatively common. Also, the endoscopic excision of these lesions as if they were simple adenomas appears to be safe and is not apparently associated with an excess of carcinoma either in the lesion itself or in the remainder of that organ. Whether adenomas occur in excess in inflammatory bowel disease and whether their growth is potentiated by the underlying disease are unclear.

Clinical Implications.   Whether dysplasia or adenoma is the diagnosis affects the clinician's treatment strategy. Some clinicians and pathologists view the problem with relative indifference. Given an endoscopic biopsy showing features of dysplasia, the pathologist has the option of calling the lesion an adenoma or dysplasia. If there is little or no clinical information, or if the pathologist is unfamiliar with the concept, described by Blackstone et al. (1981), of dysplasia-associated lesions or masses, the lesion will be *reported* as an adenoma. If the clinician is unfamiliar with the concept of dysplasia-associated lesions or masses, it is possible that the lesion will be *treated* as an adenoma. However, if the pathologist reports dysplasia, the clinician immediately begins to consider whether colectomy is the appropriate strategy.

WHY ARE LESS THAN 100% OF CANCERS ASSOCIATED WITH ADENOMAS OR DYSPLASIA?

That all cases of carcinoma are not accompanied by dysplasia is well known. A variety of factors are involved in whether or to what degree premalignancy is found with colorectal malignancy; together these may be summarized as follows and apply to both "usual" carcinomas and those associated with inflammatory conditions.

1. In the usual variants of colorectal carcinoma, it is well documented that the chance of finding an adenomatous margin is a size-dependent phenomenon and decreases markedly with increasing size of the tumor. This is related to the fact that as carcinomas enlarge, they destroy any associated adenomatous or dysplastic component.
2. The highest incidence of an adenomatous component associated with colorectal carcinoma occurs when carcinoma has been found during endoscopic excision of adenomas.
3. As carcinomas increase in size, the pathologist is unlikely to increase commensurately the number of blocks taken, so that an adenomatous component may be missed.
4. The histological appearance of mucosal and submucosal tumor may be identical. This will cause problems for pathologists demanding a difference or morpho-

logical change when invasion occurs from a dysplastic/adenomatous lesion. At the opposite end of the spectrum, an extremely high-grade adenomatous/ dysplastic component might be interpreted as in situ carcinoma as if in situ carcinoma were a subcategory of carcinoma rather than of high-grade dysplasia. Interpretation as the former would clearly give rise to a lower figure of dysplasia/ adenoma.

5. Some poorly differentiated carcinomas, if examined by electron microscopy, silver staining, or immunocytochemistry, prove to be poorly differentiated carcinoid tumors. Carcinoid tumors do not appear to arise from classic dysplasia. Some are accompanied by endocrine cell hyperplasia of glands, sometimes with minimal atypia; others arise from endocrine cells in the lamina propria (these cells exist normally in the stomach, appendix, and large intestine). Under the latter circumstances, there may be hyperplasia of the endocrine cells, and in some cases it may be impossible to distinguish endocrine cell hyperplasia of the lamina propria from invasion of the lamina propria by tumor.

Implications for Patient Management

It should be recognized that surveillance in low-grade dysplasia is a definite management *decision* in a lesion that can directly give rise to invasive carcinoma and may therefore have already exerted that potential. Further, these carcinomas are sometimes not recognized clinically in patients with inflammatory disorders.

That there is a distinction between a first, "diagnostic," endoscopic examination and subsequent "surveillance" endoscopy is worth observing. This difference is particularly important if dysplasia is found. Dysplasia discovered on first endoscopy is likely to be much more serious because the length of time it has been present is unknown and the likelihood of an underlying invasive component is greater (Fuson et al. 1980).

GASTROINTESTINAL DYSPLASIA OUTSIDE THE LARGE INTESTINE

Although the classic descriptions of dysplasia are found in inflammatory bowel disease, dysplasia does occur in other sites in the gastrointestinal tract. Perhaps the most interesting of these other occurrences is Barrett's esophagus in which, however, the significance of dysplasia is even more poorly documented than in inflammatory bowel disease (Riddell 1985; Haggitt and Dean 1985; Lee 1985). In both diseases, we do not know how likely an accompanying invasive carcinoma is when either low-grade or high-grade dysplasia has been found, but the incidence almost certainly rises if an endoscopic lesion was detected and probably rises even more if that discovery was on first endoscopy. However, Barrett's esophagus is unique in that, of all the precancerous lesions occurring in the gastrointestinal tract, it is the only one in which the precipitating disease (gastroesophageal reflux in this case) can be arrested (by an antireflux operation). It is therefore interesting to speculate whether the removal of the underlying driving force could be accompanied by reversal of dysplasia or equivocal findings. Examples of regrowth squamous epithelium over typical Barrett's mucosa do occur in this disease (Skinner et al. 1983).

AIDS IN THE DIAGNOSIS OF DYSPLASIA

The classification system for dysplasia in inflammatory bowel disease (Riddell et al. 1983) has been adopted and used with success at many hospitals (Allen, Biggart, and Pyper 1985; Rosenstock et al. 1985). Some newer techniques for the assessment of dysplasia, including the use of mucins (Ehsanullah et al. 1985), lectins (in binding assays, particularly using peanut lectin agglutinin [Boland et al. 1984]), or other epithelial markers, now seem less specific than originally thought (Allen et al. 1985). However, it seems that measurement of DNA content using flow cytometry may be of value for determining which patients who have ulcerative colitis with dysplasia are likely to develop carcinoma (Hammarberg, Slezak, and Tribuhait 1984). Assay of tissue enzymes such as lactic dehydrogenase or glucose 6-phosphate dehydrogenase may also be of value (Vatn et al. 1984). Preliminary findings with these markers have been promising, but confirmatory studies are required.

More recently, work has been carried out on oncogenes and which of their products might be expressed preferentially in adenomas and carcinomas. To date, there has been virtually no work done on the potential of those products as markers in dysplasia.

CLINICAL STRATEGIES FOR EARLY DETECTION

Strategies for the early detection of invasive carcinoma are surprisingly straight-forward and fall into one of five categories. These are (1) to do nothing, which can be advocated in patients in whom surgery or further surgery would not be contemplated even if anything were found; (2) to institute regular surveillance and biopsy, carried out in patients in whom there has been no evidence of dysplasia; (3) to pursue biopsy at short intervals (e.g., every one to three months), indicated in patients with suspicious or possibly dysplastic lesions, for confirmation; (4) to remove the driving force of the disease, which could be contemplated in patients with Barrett's esophagus, possibly even in those Barrett's esophagus patients with low-grade dysplasia; and (5) to excise the diseased organ, for example, colectomy in ulcerative colitis and esophagectomy in Barrett's esophagus with dysplasia.

One of the most challenging aspects of managing gastrointestinal diseases today is when to change the mode of follow-up from one of these categories to another, particularly when the choice will entail local surgery. Similarly, it is imperative at this juncture to know whether one is dealing with cancer prevention (i.e., the detection of premalignant diseases) or whether detection of early invasive cancer may be acceptable. The latter may only be acceptable if the early discovery is by pathology; unfortunately, we are still not at the stage at which this determination can be guaranteed.

PRACTICAL INTERPRETATION OF DYSPLASIA ON BIOPSY

How to interpret gastrointestinal dysplasia can perhaps best be demonstrated by an imaginary slide that reveals features of typical low-grade dysplasia/tubular adenoma. The patient is an otherwise healthy, 55-year-old man and you (the pathologist) are asked to both make a histological diagnosis and make a recommendation to the clinician regarding further management or definitive treatment. The biopsy, in turn, represents one of the following:

1. Mucosa taken 29 cm from the incisors
2. One of three small polyps in the gastric antrum
3. Material from immediately proximal to a gastroenterostomy anastomosis line
4. A 3-mm polyp in the duodenal bulb
5. A 2-cm periampullary mass
6. An annular lesion in the ascending colon
7. A mucosal irregularity in the ascending colon, in the additional context of a 20-year history of ulcerative colitis
8. A 3-mm polyp in the sigmoid colon
9. An 8-cm villous lesion in the rectum

The corresponding diagnoses and recommendations would be:

1. This clearly is Barrett's esophagus with low-grade dysplasia, and one might well consider esophagectomy.

   This is perhaps the most difficult answer to formulate logically. Because the lesion is unequivocally neoplastic, there is a small but significant chance that an occult underlying carcinoma may already be present. Anecdotal evidence suggests that there is carcinoma in no more than 5% to 10% of cases. Options therefore are (a) resection of columnar esophageal mucosa, with primary anastomoses, (b) antireflux operation and follow-up (removal of the driving force), (c) maximal medical therapy to keep the pH of refluxed contents as high as possible (removal of the driving force), (d) continuation of surveillance until high-grade dysplasia or intramucosal carcinoma is found on biopsy, accepting the slightly increased chance of death due to invasive carcinoma, and (e) removal of all the dysplastic area endoscopically, by multiple large-particle ("jumbo") biopsies or by laser or other destructive treatment.

   There have been no data to suggest that any one of these modes of management is significantly (or even anecdotally) better than any of the others in preventing or reducing long-term mortality from esophageal adenocarcinoma. All of these options have to be weighed against the known 3% to 15% mortality from esophagectomy. The ultimate decision will therefore depend on a combination of a variety of factors and will have to be individualized for each patient.

2. This is a simple adenoma. That a carcinoma might be present elsewhere in the stomach cannot be excluded. Antrectomy should not be recommended, and follow-up should consist of periodic gastroscopy.

3. In the postgastrectomy stomach, this would be dysplasia, assuming the biopsy was a random one. Which management strategy would be best is not properly documented, but in this clinical circumstance it seems reasonable in North America to wait for demonstration of carcinoma invading the lamina propria or submucosa before resection is contemplated. The interval between dysplasia and cancer is probably very long, and there is no evidence that further gastrectomy in a patient who has already lost part of his stomach is of any value. However, in countries with a high incidence of this disease, a more aggressive approach may be warranted.

4. This also is an adenoma. In a young patient, the possibility of associated familial adenomatous polyposis coli would also need to be considered.

5. This is likely an invasive carcinoma, but that diagnosis cannot be made from this slide. However, the mass is clearly neoplastic. In all likelihood, the best surgical approach is to open the duodenum and try to remove the mass locally; should the mass prove to be simply an adenoma, local excision would be curative. If an underlying invasive carcinoma were suspected, intraoperative needle biopsy and frozen-section analysis could be undertaken; if invasion was thus demonstrated, a Whipple-type procedure could be used.

6. The lesion clinically would appear to be a carcinoma. We have demonstrated in this biopsy that the tissue is neoplastic; although invasive carcinoma is not demonstrated, it is quite reasonable to proceed directly to colectomy, as such an endoscopic lesion could not be excised by any other method.

7. Given the 20-year history of ulcerative colitis, this is likely a dysplasia-associated lesion or mass with an underlying risk (in the vicinity of 50%–67%) of invasive carcinoma. There would therefore be a very strong indication for total colectomy.

8. This is a simple tubular adenoma.

9. As in the above case of a periampullary mass, the presence of an underlying carcinoma cannot be determined until the lesion is completely excised. Complete local excision, when it is possible, followed by histological assessment for invasive carcinoma is probably the best management strategy, as unnecessary proctectomy is not carried out.

SUMMARY

In summary, dysplastic mucosa is essentially identical to adenomatous mucosa but differs from the latter in that macroscopically/endoscopically it occurs in flat mucosa or, if raised above the adjacent mucosa, forms an irregular and often nodular lesion that is unlike typical tubular or villous adenomas. Pathogenetically, the transition from normal to dysplastic perhaps takes place at an appreciably slower rate than the transition from normal to adenomatous. In many instances, this is reflected morphologically by the presence of a spectrum of changes between normal and dysplastic mucosa, whereas the all-or-none presence of dysplastic mucosa is the single most important criterion on which the diagnosis of adenoma is based. Because of this spectrum, biopsies can be subjectively categorized as negative, indefinite, or positive for dysplasia. Typical regenerative changes are considered negative for dysplasia. Low-grade dysplasia contains nuclei limited to the basal halves of involved cells; when nuclei are largely present in the upper halves of the cells, or dysplastic changes are accompanied by structural abnormalities such as back-to-back (gland-within-gland) appearance, the dysplasia is arbitrarily termed high grade.

Because dysplastic lesions may overlie invasive carcinoma, such lesions are followed knowing this risk; more usually, resection of the involved organ should be considered, or, in the columnar-lined (Barrett's) esophagus, removal of the driving force by reduction of acid reflux. Biopsies that show changes indefinite for dysplasia should lead to early rebiopsy to ensure that unequivocal dysplasia or carcinoma is not present in the adjacent mucosa; future biopsies may establish the morphological stability of the lesion. Whatever the clinical decision, it is based on balancing a variety of risks and benefits, both of continued surveillance and other forms of intervention.

REFERENCES

Allen DC, Biggart JD, Orchin JC, et al. 1985. An immunoperoxidase study of epithelial marker antigens in ulcerative colitis with dysplasia and carcinoma. *J Clin Pathol* 38:18–29.

Allen DC, Biggart JD, Pyper PC. 1985. Large bowel mucosal dysplasia and carcinoma in ulcerative colitis. *J Clin Pathol* 38:30–43.

Blackstone MO, Riddell RH, Rogers BHG, et al. 1981. Dysplasia-associated lesion or mass (DALM) detected by colonoscopy in long-standing ulcerative colitis: An indication for colectomy. *Gastroenterology* 80:366–374.

Boland CR, Lance P, Levin B, et al. 1984. Abnormal goblet cell glycoconjugates in rectal biopsies associated with an increased risk of neoplasia in patients with ulcerative colitis: Early results of a prospective study. *Gut* 25:1364–1371.

Ehsanullah M, Naunton Morgan M, Filipe MI, et al. 1985. Sialomucins in the assessment of dysplasia and cancer-risk patients with ulcerative colitis treated with colectomy and ileo-rectal anastomosis. *Histopathology* 9:223–235.

Fuson JA, Farmer RG, Hawk A, et al. 1980. Endoscopic surveillance for cancer in chronic ulcerative colitis. *Am J Gastroenterol* 73:120–126.

Gilbertson VA, Nelms JM. 1978. The prevention of invasive cancer of the rectum. *Cancer* 41:1137–1139.

Haggitt RC, Dean PJ. 1985. Dysplasia and regression in Barrett's esophagus. In *Barrett's Esophagus: Pathophysiology, Diagnosis and Management*, SJ Spechler, RK Goyal, eds., pp. 143–152. New York: Elsevier.

Hammarberg C, Slezak P, Tribukait B. 1984. Early detection of malignancy in ulcerative colitis. A flow-cytometric DNA study. *Cancer* 53:291–295.

Lee RG. 1985. Dysplasia in Barrett's esophagus. A clinicopathological study of 6 patients. *Am J Surg Pathol* 9:845–852.

Lovett E. 1976. Family studies in cancer of the colon and rectum. *Br J Surg* 63:13–18.

Muto T, Bussey HJR, Morson BC. 1975. The evolution of cancer of the colon and rectum. *Cancer* 36:2251–2270.

Riddell RH. 1985. Dysplasia and regression in Barrett's esophagus. In *Barrett's Esophagus: Pathophysiology, Diagnosis and Management*, SJ Spechler, RK Goyal, eds., pp. 143–152. New York: Elsevier.

Riddell RH, Goldman H, Ransohoff DR, et al. 1983. Dysplasia in inflammatory bowel disease: Standardized classification with provisional clinical applications. *Hum Pathol* 14:931–968.

Rosenstock E, Farmer RG, Petras R, et al. 1985. Surveillance for colonic carcinoma in ulcerative colitis. *Gastroenterology* 89:1342–1346.

Skinner DB, Walther BC, Riddell RH, et al. 1983. Barrett's esophagus. Comparison of benign and malignant cases. *Ann Surg* 198:554–565.

Vatn MH, Elgjo K, Norheim A, et al. 1984. Measurement of enzyme activity in colonic biopsies: A test for premalignancy in ulcerative colitis? *Scand J Gastroenterol* 19:889–892.

Vatn MH, Stalsberg H. 1982. The prevalence of polyps of the large intestine in Oslo: An autopsy study. *Cancer* 49:819–825.

JEFFREY A. GOTTLIEB MEMORIAL LECTURE

Annual Clinical Conference on Cancer, Vol. 30
Gastrointestinal Cancer: Current Approaches to Diagnosis and Treatment
© 1988 by The University of Texas System Cancer Center

33. Cisplatin in the Management of Solid Tumors

Lawrence H. Einhorn

Cis-diamminedichloroplatinum (cisplatin), one of the most valuable chemotherapy agents in the treatment of disseminated solid tumors, was the first heavy metal and the first inorganic compound ever to be evaluated as an antineoplastic agent. Its history is fascinating, not just in itself but also for phase I and phase II studies in general. In 1965, during experiments on the effects of electric dipoles on cellular growth, it was noticed that the cell division of *Escherichia coli* was inhibited near a platinum electrode (Rosenberg, VanCamp, and Krigas 1965). After attempts to explain this phenomenon, these investigators subsequently isolated a metal complex—cisplatin. Afterward, this drug was found to be active in preclinical systems and was evaluated in the early 1970s in phase I trials. Although the purpose of a phase I study is to determine if toxicity is manageable, rather than to elucidate therapeutic efficacy, cisplatin's phase I studies discouraged most investigators because of the severe gastrointestinal and renal toxicity it demonstrated and the lack of evidence of any meaningful therapeutic benefit. However, this scenario was dramatically changed once cisplatin was found to be extremely active in testicular cancer (Higby et al. 1974). At the same time, it began to be appreciated that cisplatin renal damage, like other heavy metal nephrotoxicity, could be significantly ameliorated. Two steps were necessary: first, to make certain that the patient was well hydrated before beginning cisplatin therapy and, second, to ensure that urinary excretion of the drug was adequate to prevent accumulation in the proximal tubules, ordinarily accomplished by saline hydration with or without mannitol diuresis. In more recent years, effective antiemetic regimens have likewise greatly mitigated the nausea and vomiting. Once a disease was found in which it was effective and once toxicity was more manageable, cisplatin underwent widespread evaluation. Physicians used it to treat a variety of different tumor types and, some thought, better patient populations. It would have been difficult to predict in 1973 the high level of activity and the widespread use cisplatin would have 10 to 15 years later, and indeed this is a lesson for those evaluating phase I and phase II studies in general. This drug was dangerously close to being ignored, but through the diligent research and persistence of individual investigators, cisplatin has assumed a major role in the management of solid tumors.

The mechanism of action of cisplatin still remains somewhat uncertain. Clearly, the major intracellular site of action is DNA. Inhibition of DNA synthesis by cisplatin is probably accomplished by alteration in the DNA template. An integral part of this activity is thought to be the ability of the *cis* isomer to form intrastrand (and perhaps, less important, interstrand) crosslinks, usually between guanine-

guanine groups (Lippard 1982). Cisplatin has interesting synergism with a variety of other compounds. For example, in L1210 leukemia, cisplatin and 5-fluorouracil (5-FU) produced a 60% cure rate, whereas either agent alone was virtually inactive (Schabel et al. 1979). In P338 leukemia, neither cisplatin nor etoposide reduced tumor burden greater than 1 log as a single agent; however, a 7-log reduction and a 30% cure rate were seen when the two drugs were used in combination (Schabel et al. 1979). These two examples of cisplatin synergism are among the most dramatic examples of drug interactions in preclinical systems. The prediction of synergism with cisplatin and etoposide has been realized in the clinic as well as with studies of cisplatin and etoposide in testicular cancer and small cell lung cancer. Likewise, cisplatin and 5-FU have produced seemingly synergistic clinical results in head and neck cancer and possibly several forms of gastrointestinal cancer as well.

TOXICITY OF CISPLATIN

When cisplatin was initially undergoing clinical trials, it was believed that the ultimate dose-limiting toxicity was going to be nephrotoxicity. Clearly, this is not the situation. Nephrotoxicity can be prevented relatively easily by appropriate hydration. However, what becomes the dose-limiting toxicity is the cumulative neuromuscular toxicity associated with cisplatin. This is similar to the neuromuscular toxicity and especially the peripheral neuropathy that is seen with other heavy metals such as lead. The other dose-limiting toxicity is the chronic anorexia, nausea, and vomiting associated with repetitive courses of cisplatin.

Cisplatin induces nausea and vomiting in almost all patients. However, numerous trials have shown this bothersome side effect reduced by such various drugs as cannabinoids (Vincent et al. 1983), dexamethasone (Seigel and Longo 1981), and metoclopramide (Gralla et al. 1981). At Indiana University, my colleagues and I have not employed metoclopramide in young patients (predominantly testicular cancer patients) because of the high incidence of extrapyramidal side effects associated with this agent in this setting. Our primary antiemetic strategy has been to combine antiemetics, usually dexamethasone, chlorpromazine, and lorazepam. Lorazepam is of value because of its amnestic capabilities. Many patients have anticipatory nausea and vomiting, which this particular drug combats.

In addition to the previously mentioned nephrotoxicity, hypomagnesemia occurs in a substantial number of patients who receive cisplatin, though only rarely is this of any clinical significance (Schilsky and Anderson 1979). Renal wasting of magnesium appears to be the primary mechanism. Magnesium replacement does not prevent the occurrence of hypomagnesemia, though it helps. In patients with concurrent symptomatic hypocalcemia, serum magnesium levels must be corrected before calcium levels will normalize. Peripheral neuropathy, which has developed as a major dose-limiting toxicity, is more common in patients who have had repetitive courses of cisplatin. Other forms of neurotoxicity reported have included tinnitus and weakness in the lower extremities.

Cisplatin also has an effect on fertility because it causes testicular atrophy and impaired spermatogenesis. Cisplatin combination chemotherapy's effect on gonadal function of patients with disseminated testicular cancer was reported by Drasga et al. in 1983. All patients treated with cisplatin combination chemotherapy develop significant oligospermia; however, recovery of sperm counts begins one and one-half to two years after starting therapy. Approximately 50% to 60% of the patients after two years will have a normal sperm count. In our studies, we have now had 32 patients who have fathered normal, healthy children after being cured of their disseminated testicular cancer with cisplatin combination chemotherapy. Other forms of cisplatin toxicity include alopecia, myelosuppression, and Raynaud's phenomenon. Although these can be bothersome to the patient and to the physician taking care of the patient, they are rarely of and by themselves reason for cessation of therapy.

Despite the fact that nephrotoxicity is not the major problem that it was predicted to be in 1973 with cisplatin, it still does cause some clinical difficulty. Recently, diethyldithiocarbamate (DDTC) was found to inhibit cisplatin nephrotoxicity in animal models without interfering with tumor response (Qazi et al. 1986). DDTC is now undergoing clinical trials.

CLINICAL USE

As mentioned above, cisplatin has shown significant activity in many different neoplasms. It is clearly the most active single agent in the treatment of testicular cancer. It is also as active, if not more active, than any other single agent in the treatment of bladder cancer, ovarian carcinoma, and head and neck cancer. In many other neoplasms, it also has activity as a single agent or as part of a combination chemotherapy regimen.

Testicular Cancer

Cisplatin has truly revolutionized the therapeutic strategy and cure rate in testicular cancer. In the entire field of medical oncology, no comparable drug has so dramatically altered the cure rate of a neoplasm. Ten years ago, prior to the widespread use of cisplatin in testicular cancer, the cure rate for stage I disease (confined to the testis alone) was 90%; for stage II disease (testis and retroperitoneal lymph nodes), 50%; and for stage III (disseminated disease), an abysmal 5% to 10%. Because of cisplatin combination chemotherapy and successful strategies that have been developed based upon the success of this drug, the present cure rates are 98% to 100% for stage I and stage II disease and 80% for stage III disease (Einhorn 1981).

The original study evaluating cisplatin combination chemotherapy at Indiana University was done between 1974 and 1976. In this study, the already established two-drug regimen of vinblastine and bleomycin was combined with the then new and experimental cisplatin (PVB) (Einhorn and Donohue 1977). In this original study, 47 patients with disseminated disease were treated with cisplatin (20 mg/m^2) for five consecutive days, vinblastine (0.2 mg/kg) on day 1 and day 2, and bleomycin (30 units) by i.v. push weekly. Courses were given every three weeks for a total of four courses followed by maintenance vinblastine at a dosage of 0.3 mg/kg for a total of two years of therapy. Thirty-three of 47 patients (70%) achieved complete remission, and the remaining 14 patients achieved partial remission. Of those 14 patients who achieved only partial remission, five were rendered disease free by surgical resection of residual disease, a strategy that has been widely employed in many institutions in the management of testicular cancer (Einhorn et al. 1981). These patients now have a minimum follow-up of 10 years. Thirty of 47 (64%) were alive five years after their diagnosis, and 27 of 47 (57%) are currently disease free.

The second-generation PVB study done at Indiana University was carried out from 1976 to 1978. In this study, we became convinced of the major therapeutic activity of cisplatin but were concerned about the hematologic and neuromuscular toxicity caused by the high doses of vinblastine. We therefore randomized 78 consecutive patients into two groups. All received identical dosages of cisplatin and bleomycin, but one group received the original 0.4 mg/kg of vinblastine and the other a 25% reduction (0.3 mg/kg). As expected, reducing the vinblastine significantly reduced the neuromuscular and hematologic toxicity. Overall, 52 of 78 (67%) have been continuously disease free (minimum follow-up, eight years) and are clearly cured of their disease, and 57 of 78 (73%) are currently disease free. Of these, five patients were cured with salvage chemotherapy consisting of cisplatin and etoposide (Hainsworth et al. 1985). Based upon the results of this study, in 1978 we permanently abandoned the 0.4 mg/kg dosage of vinblastine in favor of the 25% reduction because of identical cure rates and significant reduction in treatment-related morbidity (Einhorn and Williams 1980).

Next, we began a study of maintenance therapy in conjunction with the Southeastern Cancer Study Group. In testis cancer, cisplatin combination chemotherapy is so effective and serum markers such as human chorionic gonadotropin and alpha fetoprotein so accurate in identifying when complete remission is achieved, we wanted to verify that maintenance vinblastine as it had been used in two previous studies was warranted. Therefore, all patients who achieved a complete remission with cisplatin, vinblastine (0.3 mg/kg), and bleomycin and those patients who were rendered disease free following surgical resection of teratoma were randomized. They received traditional maintenance therapy with 0.3 mg/kg of vinblastine or no further therapy whatsoever (12 weeks of PVB induction therapy and then no further treatment). One hundred thirteen patients entered this random prospective study. After a minimum follow-up of five years, we found that 12% of patients with maintenance therapy had relapsed and only 7% without had (Einhorn et al. 1981). We believe that this patient population is large enough and has been followed long enough to say that optimal cure rates can be achieved in disseminated testicular cancer with merely 12 weeks of remission induction therapy and that maintenance therapy is unnecessary.

It was interesting for us to note the results of sequential PVB studies with the same investigators at a single institution (table 33.1). The cure rate rose from 57% with the first study to 80% in a study carried out from 1978 to 1981. This progress was made with the identical chemotherapy, as opposed to a new, innovative, more aggressive treatment. Study 1 was our original study, study 2 determined that we could lower the vinblastine dosage, and study 3 ascertained that maintenance vinblastine was not necessary. If our third testicular cancer study had utilized a new, innovative, more aggressive treatment and we had compared our results with histori-

Table 33.1. *Sequential Cisplatin, Vinblastine, and Bleomycin Studies at Indiana University*

Study	N	Complete Remission No.	(%)	NED with Surgery No.	(%)	NED at Present No.	(%)
1 (1974–1976)	47	33	(70)	5	(11)	27	(57)
2 (1976–1978)	78	51	(65)	13	(17)	57	(73)
3 (1978–1981)	147	92	(63)	31	(21)	117	(80)

Abbreviation: NED, no evidence of disease.

Table 33.2. *Vinblastine and Etoposide Compared in Induction Therapy*

	Cisplatin and Bleomycin with			
	Vinblastine		Etoposide	
Variable	No.	(%)	No.	(%)
No. of patients	116		121	
Complete remission	73	(63)	69	(57)
NED with surgery	13	(11)	25	(21)
Total NED	86	(74)	94	(78)

Abbreviation: NED, no evidence of disease.

cal controls, we would have erroneously concluded that our results represented a therapeutic advance. Instead, our use of identical chemotherapy emphasizes the obvious flaws in utilizing historical controls, even when the new data and the controls are from a single institution.

Despite the significant cure rate with PVB-based chemotherapy, there remained patients who were not cured with this chemotherapy. Starting in 1978, we began salvage chemotherapy studies in these patients with cisplatin and etoposide (Williams et al. 1980). Overall, 25% to 30% of these patients were cured with second-line chemotherapy, which fulfilled the prophecy of cisplatin's synergism with etoposide (Schabel et al. 1979).

Based on the high success rate with second-line chemotherapy, from 1981 to 1984 we performed our fourth study, also in conjunction with the Southeastern Cancer Study Group. In this study, we randomized patients with disseminated testicular cancer to receive standard PVB therapy over 12 weeks or to receive cisplatin, etoposide, and bleomycin as initial induction therapy. Both remission induction regimens were 12 weeks, and the therapeutic results were basically identical (table 33.2). However, there was a major statistically significant reduction in neuromuscular toxicity with the substitution of etoposide for vinblastine. Therefore, since 1984, standard chemotherapy at Indiana University has consisted of cisplatin, etoposide, and bleomycin. Of special interest in this study is that patients who had advanced disseminated disease treated with etoposide had a survival rate significantly better statistically than that of those receiving vinblastine.

Bladder Cancer

In the treatment of metastatic bladder cancer, cisplatin has been the most widely used single agent in the United States. Overall, in the literature, 90 of 314 patients have responded (29% response rate) with a median remission duration of six months. This translates to definite palliation of symptoms and perhaps some minimal prolongation of survival compared with supportive care alone (Yagoda 1979).

Cisplatin combination chemotherapy regimens have been utilized for the past five to seven years. In the late 1970s, combination chemotherapy with cisplatin, doxorubicin, and cyclophosphamide was quite popular. However, several random prospective studies done by the major U.S. cooperative groups failed to reveal any obvious response rate or survival advantage over cisplatin alone. However, recent studies have been considerably more encouraging, and these have been based upon combining cisplatin with methotrexate. Perhaps the most promising of these is the M-VAC (methotrexate, vinblastine, doxorubicin, and cisplatin) regimen (Sternberg et al. 1985). Another promising regimen has been a combination of cisplatin, methotrexate, and vinblastine (Harker et al. 1985). With both of these treatment regimens, not only is a high partial remission rate being achieved, but for the first time a substantial complete remission rate has been attained as well. Several of these complete remissions, especially with M-VAC, have been durable (over two years), and there is some optimism that perhaps a very small minority of these patients with metastatic bladder cancer may enjoy long-term survival and even cure. At the present time, at Indiana University in conjunction with the Southeastern Cancer Study Group, the Southwest Oncology Group, the National Cancer Institute of Canada, and an Australian group headed by Doctors Derek Raghavan and Brian Hillcoat, we are currently involved in a phase III randomized prospective study comparing the M-VAC regimen to single-agent cisplatin in patients with metastatic bladder cancer. This important phase III study will determine whether there is or is not benefit both in terms of response rate and, more important, in terms of survival with this promising new combination chemotherapy regimen.

Ovarian Cancer

Cisplatin is reported to yield an overall response rate of approximately 30% in ovarian cancer (Katz et al. 1981). Usually these patients have had previous therapy with an alkylating agent, but cisplatin is one of the few agents able to achieve partial remissions for patients who have progressive disease on alkylating agent therapy. Cisplatin combination chemotherapy has been studied, and probably the most widely used regimen is a combination of cyclophosphamide, doxorubicin, and cisplatin. In addition, malignant ovarian germ cell tumors appear to respond to PVB chemotherapy as their testicular germ cell neoplasm counterparts do, making it the standard therapy for this disease.

Head and Neck Cancer

Cisplatin is clearly active in metastatic head and neck cancer, achieving approximately a 30% response rate in recurrent head and neck cancer in patients treated with cisplatin alone. This makes this drug as active as any single agent, including methotrexate and bleomycin, the other commonly used single agents.

Probably the most widely used treatment regimen in head and neck cancer is a combination of cisplatin and continuous infusion 5-FU (Kish et al. 1982). This regimen has been widely used as initial therapy in patients with stage III or stage IV head and neck cancer followed by surgery or surgery and radiotherapy. The chemotherapy itself produces a very high complete remission rate, and some of the surgical specimens have been sterile with no viable tumor found after the chemotherapy. Part of the enthusiasm for cisplatin and 5-FU once again may be based upon the synergism of these two drugs (Schabel et al. 1979). However, it remains to be determined in a random prospective study whether these apparently active regimens are better in treating metastatic disease than methotrexate alone and whether cisplatin and 5-FU initial therapy confers any survival advantage over surgery or radiotherapy alone in patients with stage III or stage IV disease who have had no prior therapy.

Lung Cancer

The prospects for successful chemotherapeutic management of non–small cell lung cancer continue to be dismal. There are many reported single-institution, nonrandomized studies of various cisplatin combination chemotherapy regimens demonstrating relatively high response rates and survival advantage compared with those of historical controls. However, all random prospective studies, especially those done by the cooperative groups, have failed to show one type of treatment regimen is superior to another or, indeed, superior to supportive care alone. There is no evidence that any cisplatin-based chemotherapy regimen or, for that matter, any type of chemotherapy can produce any improvement in survival over supportive care alone. Nevertheless, cisplatin combination chemotherapy regimens certainly may be capable of offering some mental or physical palliation, and in this setting perhaps one of the most widely used regimens is a combination of cisplatin and etoposide.

The prospects in small cell lung cancer are different. Unlike non–small cell lung cancer, there are chemotherapeutic agents that have significant single-agent activity. One of the most commonly used regimens in small cell lung cancer is cyclophosphamide, doxorubicin, and vincristine (CAV). Second-line chemotherapy after progression on these drugs had largely been unsuccessful until cisplatin and etoposide were combined. This combination regularly produces a 40% to 50% objective response rate. In one study of refractory disease, the response rate with single-agent cisplatin was only 13% (15 of 116 patients). However, this rate is comparable with that of etoposide in similar patients. Furthermore, the platinum analogue carboplatinum has recently been evaluated in patients with no prior chemotherapy: 14 of 21 with extensive disease responded, 4 of 9 with limited disease responded, and all 11 patients with Karnofsky performance status scores 80–100 responded (median survival, 8 months) (Smith 1985).

Perhaps the major value of cisplatin and etoposide is as first-line therapy. Several studies are comparing CAV with cisplatin and etoposide combined as initial therapy or alternating the two drug regimens and comparing them with CAV alone. A recently completed study by the Southeastern Cancer Study Group compared six courses of CAV with or without chest radiotherapy with the identical chemotherapy followed by two consolidation courses of cisplatin and etoposide for patients with limited small cell lung cancer who achieved a complete remission or partial remission. One hundred thirty-three patients were randomized, and preliminary analysis shows that there is a statistically significant survival advantage for patients who received the consolidation courses of cisplatin and etoposide.

Gastrointestinal Neoplasms

Cisplatin appears to be marginally effective as a single agent in esophageal cancer. The Southeast Cancer Study Group found that 4 of 26 patients (15%) responded to 90 mg/m^2 of cisplatin. In contrast, the Southwest Oncology Group study, utilizing 50 mg/m^2 on day 1 and day 8 every 28 days, found that 9 of 35 patients (26%) responded to single-agent cisplatin. One of the problems in esophageal cancer is quantitating objectively a partial remission. But despite limitations, it does appear that cisplatin has a modest benefit. Recently, cisplatin has been used either in combination with continuous infusion 5-FU or with other agents such as the combination of vindesine and bleomycin with promising preliminary results as initial therapy. These are patients who have had no prior surgery and radiotherapy, so several courses of cisplatin combination chemotherapy have often been followed by surgery. These findings are analogous to those in head and neck cancer in patients with no prior therapy, and only a well-designed, well-stratified phase III prospective study will determine the ultimate role of initial cisplatin combination chemotherapy in the management of esophageal cancer.

In gastric cancer, cisplatin has enjoyed a resurgence of interest in the last several years. In eight published studies, 26 of 132 (20%) responded. This is all the more impressive when one realizes that a significant number of these patients had undergone prior chemotherapy, including prior chemotherapy with 5-fluorouracil, doxorubicin, and mitomycin C. These data are not only from single institutions but also from cooperative group studies that include the European Organization for Research and Treatment of Cancer, the Eastern Cooperative Oncology Group, and the Cancer and Leukemia Group B, all with results demonstrating definite single-agent activity. Based upon this single-agent activity, several studies have looked at 5-FU, doxorubicin, and cisplatin combination chemotherapy in gastric cancer. In six published studies, 48 of 112 (43%) responded. The response rates range from 29% to 50%, and responders included several patients with complete remissions. The North Central Cancer Treatment Group is currently comparing this three-drug regimen to single-agent 5-FU in a phase II randomized study in metastatic gastric cancer.

At Indiana University, we began studies with cisplatin and 5-FU in colorectal cancer because of their synergism (Schabel et al. 1979) and cisplatin's demonstration as one of the most active agents against the colon carcinoma LoVo cell line. Patients were treated with 60 mg/m^2 cisplatin every three weeks for six courses and 15 mg/kg 5-FU i.v. push weekly during the six courses of cisplatin. We saw 11 partial remissions and 1 complete remission in 41 patients for response rates of 29%

for eligible patients and 32% for evaluable patients. Thirteen additional patients had stable disease, which was defined as no progression for a minimum of three months. Thirty-three patients had elevated carcinoembryonic antigen (CEA) levels, including 15 with levels over 100 ng/ml and 7 with levels over 1000 ng/ml. Seventy-five percent of these patients had a greater than 50% decrease in elevated CEA levels after two courses of chemotherapy. A decrease in CEA level was not a criterion for objective response. Now we are in the process of completing a phase III randomized prospective study comparing this 5-FU and cisplatin regimen to single-agent 5-FU in colorectal cancer to determine whether there is any response or survival benefit. Including the Indiana study, there are eight separate studies evaluating cisplatin and 5-FU in colorectal cancer, in which 55 of 190 patients responded (29%). Once again, whether this translates to any patient benefit will best be determined by the ongoing randomized study comparing it to 5-FU alone.

Miscellaneous Tumors

Cisplatin has been found to have activity in a variety of other diseases, including adrenal carcinoma, thymoma, neuroblastoma, carcinoma of the anus, thyroid cancer, osteogenic sarcoma, and other bone sarcomas. Perhaps one of the more interesting diseases in which cisplatin has recently been studied is metastatic breast cancer. In patients with prior combination chemotherapy, the response rate with cisplatin is usually 10% or lower. However, a study from Yugoslavia revealed a 70% response rate when cisplatin was used as initial single-agent chemotherapy for patients with metastatic breast cancer (Kolaric and Roth 1983). Because of these results, we have begun evaluating cisplatin in patients who are not candidates for hormonal therapy and have had no prior chemotherapy for metastatic disease (prior chemotherapy as an adjuvant was permitted). We have enrolled 21 patients in this study, and our results are confirming the very high level of activity of cisplatin as a single agent. This is somewhat analogous to the results with etoposide and cisplatin as single agents in small cell lung cancer in patients with prior combination chemotherapy. The response rates are relatively low in heavily pretreated patients but exceedingly high in patients with no prior chemotherapy. The ultimate role of cisplatin as part of a combination chemotherapy regimen in breast cancer remains to be determined.

Platinum Analogues

The initial impetus for platinum analogues such as carboplatinum and CHIP was the need for an analogue that would have less nephrotoxicity. However, that was the strategy of the 1970s. In the 1980s, nephrotoxicity is not the dose-limiting problem that we earlier believed it would be. Certainly, carboplatinum and CHIP do have less nephrotoxicity and they are of value in that less hydration is required, simplifying administration. Carboplatinum and, to a lesser degree, CHIP are probably also associated with less nausea and vomiting. Carboplatinum excites special interest because it appears to have little, if any, neuromuscular toxicity, and its dose-limiting toxicity is myelosuppression. That makes it an intriguing candidate for very high dose therapy with autologous bone marrow transplantation rescue in diseases such as refractory testicular cancer.

CONCLUSIONS

From the important observation of the inhibition of *E. coli* replication near a platinum electrode to the subsequent incorporation of cisplatin in human chemotherapeutic trials, cisplatin has become one of the most important agents used in clinical oncology today. This drug is responsible for revolutionizing the cure rate in testicular cancer, improving in stage III disease from 10% or less to 80% and from 50% for all stages to 95% for stages I, II, and III combined. It also has as wide a spectrum of activity of any currently available antineoplastic agent and is as active, if not more active, than any single agent in ovarian cancer, bladder cancer, and head and neck cancer. It also has significant activity in a variety of other tumors. Being the first heavy metal ever to be evaluated as an antineoplastic agent, this agent represents a brand new class of drugs. As we approach the second decade of cisplatin's use, we are continuing to find increasing clinical utility for this intriguing and clinically useful cancer chemotherapeutic agent.

ACKNOWLEDGMENTS

This work was supported in part by U.S. Public Health Service Grant R35 CA 39844-02 and U.S. Public Health Service GCRC Grant MO1 RROO 750-06.

REFERENCES

Drasga RE, Einhorn LH, Williams SD, et al. 1983. Fertility after chemotherapy for testicular cancer. *J Clin Oncol* 1:179–183.

Einhorn LH. 1981. Testicular cancer as model for curable neoplasia: The Richard and Hinda Rosenthal Foundation Award Lecture. *Cancer Res* 41:3275–3280.

Einhorn LH, Donohue JP. 1977. Cisdiamminedichloroplatinum, vinblastine, and bleomycin combination chemotherapy in disseminated testicular cancer. *Ann Intern Med* 87:293–298.

Einhorn LH, Williams SD. 1980. Chemotherapy of disseminated testicular cancer. *Cancer* 46:1339–1344.

Einhorn LH, Williams SD, Mandelbaum I, et al. 1981. Surgical resection in disseminated testicular cancer following chemotherapeutic cytoreduction. *Cancer* 48:904–908.

Einhorn LH, Williams SD, Troner M, et al. 1981. The role of maintenance therapy in disseminated testicular cancer. *N Engl J Med* 305:727–731.

Gralla RJ, Itri LM, Pisko SE, et al. 1981. Antiemetic efficacy of high dose metoclopramide: Randomized trials with placebo in prochlorperazine in patients with chemotherapy induced nausea and vomiting. *N Engl J Med* 305:905–909.

Hainsworth JD, Williams SD, Einhorn LH, et al. 1985. Successful treatment of resistant germinal neoplasms with VP-16 and cisplatin: Results of Southeastern Cancer Study Group Trial. *J Clin Oncol* 3:666–671.

Harker WG, Meyers FJ, Freiha FS, et al. 1985. Cisplatin, methotrexate, and vinblastine (CMV): An effective chemotherapy regimen for metastatic transitional cell carcinoma of the urinary tract. *J Clin Oncol* 3:1463–1470.

Higby DJ, Wallace HJ, Albert DJ, et al. 1974. Diamminedichloroplatinum: A phase I study of responses in testicular and other tumors. *Cancer* 33:1219–1225.

Katz ME, Schwartz PE, Kapp DS, et al. 1981. Epithelial carcinoma of ovary: Current strategies. *Ann Intern Med* 95:98–111.

Kish J, Drelichman A, Jacobs J, et al. 1982. Clinical trials of cisplatin and 5-FU infusion as initial therapy for advanced squamous cell carcinoma of head and neck. *Cancer Treat Rep* 66:471–474.

Kolaric K, Roth A. 1983. Phase II clinical trial of cisdichlorodiammineplatinum for anti-tumorigenic activity in previously untreated patients with metastatic breast cancer. *Cancer Chemother Pharmacol* 11:108–112.

Lippard SJ. 1982. New chemistry of an old molecule, cisplatin. *Science* 218:1075–1082.

Qazi R, Chang A, Borch R, et al. 1986. Phase I trial of DDTC as a chemoprotector of cisplatin toxicity (abstract). *Proceedings of the American Society of Clinical Oncology* 5:31.

Rosenberg B, VanCamp L, Krigas T. 1965. Inhibiton of cell division in *Escherichia coli* by electrolysis products from a platinum electrode. *Nature* 205:698–699.

Schabel FM Jr, Trader MW, Laster WR, et al. 1979. *Cis*-dichlorodiammineplatinum (II): Combination chemotherapy in cross-resistance studies with tumors of mice. *Cancer Treat Rep* 63:1459–1473.

Schilsky RL, Anderson T. 1979. Hypomagnesemia and renal magnesium wasting in patients receiving cisplatin. *Ann Intern Med* 90:929–931.

Seigel LJ, Longo DL. 1981. The control of chemotherapy induced emesis. *Ann Intern Med* 95:352–359.

Smith I. 1985. CBDCA in small cell lung cancer. *Cancer Treat Rep* 69:43–46.

Sternberg CN, Yagoda A, Scher HI, et al. 1985. Preliminary results of M-VAC (methotrexate, vinblastine, doxorubicin, and cisplatin) for transitional cell carcinoma of the urothelium. *J Urol* 133:403–407.

Vincent BJ, McQuisten DJ, Einhorn LH, et al. 1983. Review of cannabinoids and their anti-emetic effectiveness. *Drugs* 25:52–62.

Williams SD, Einhorn LH, Greco FA, et al. 1980. VP-16-213 salvage therapy for refractory germinal neoplasms. *Cancer* 46:2154–2158.

Yagoda A. 1979. Phase II trials with cisdichlorodiammineplatinum in the treatment of urothelial cancer. *Cancer Treat Rep* 63:1565–1572.

Contributors

David A. Ahlquist, M.D.
Consultant in Gastroenterology
Mayo Clinic
Rochester, Minnesota

Jaffer A. Ajani, M.D.
Assistant Professor of Medicine
Department of Medical Oncology
The University of Texas M. D. Anderson
    Hospital and Tumor Institute at Houston
Houston, Texas

George F. Babcock, Ph.D.
Assistant Professor of Surgery
    (Immunology)
Department of General Surgery
The University of Texas M. D. Anderson
    Hospital and Tumor Institute at Houston
Houston, Texas

**Robert W. Baldwin, Ph.D.,
F.R.C., Path.**
Professor of Tumor Biology
and Director, Cancer Research Campaign
    Laboratories
University of Nottingham
Nottingham, England

Robert W. Beart, Jr., M.D.
Associate Professor of Surgery
Department of Surgery
Mayo Clinic
Rochester, Minnesota

Roxann Blackburn, R.N.
Research Nurse
Department of Medical Oncology
The University of Texas M. D. Anderson
    Hospital and Tumor Institute at Houston
Houston, Texas

Bruce M. Boman, M.D., Ph.D.
Assistant Professor of Medicine and
Assistant Professor of Tumor Biology
Section of Gastrointestinal Oncology and
    Digestive Diseases
Department of Medical Oncology
The University of Texas M. D. Anderson
    Hospital and Tumor Institute at Houston
Houston, Texas

Vera S. Byers, M.D., Ph.D.
Project Director, Colorectal Cancer Program
Xoma Corporation
Berkeley, California

C. Humberto Carrasco, M.D.
Assistant Professor of Radiology
Department of Diagnostic Radiology
The University of Texas M. D. Anderson
    Hospital and Tumor Institute at Houston
Houston, Texas

Eric Chang-Tung, M.D.
Faculty Associate
Department of Thoracic Surgery
The University of Texas M. D. Anderson
    Hospital and Tumor Institute at Houston
Houston, Texas

Chusilp Charnsangavej, M.D.
Associate Professor of Radiology
Associate Radiologist
Department of Diagnostic Radiology
The University of Texas M. D. Anderson
    Hospital and Tumor Institute at Houston
Houston, Texas

Churnfang A. Chen, M.S.
Computer Programmer
Department of Preventive Medicine
and Public Health
Creighton University School of Medicine
and the Hereditary Cancer Institute
Omaha, Nebraska

Laura Claghorn, B.A.
Assistant Epidemiologist
Department of Medical Oncology
The University of Texas M. D. Anderson
Hospital and Tumor Institute at Houston
Houston, Texas

Deborah Coody, R.N., M.S.
Clinical Nurse Specialist
Department of Medical Oncology
The University of Texas M. D. Anderson
Hospital and Tumor Institute at Houston
Houston, Texas

Robert E. Davis, M.D.
Assistant Clinical Professor of Medicine
Baylor College of Medicine
Houston, Texas

Eugene P. DiMagno, M.D.
Professor of Medicine
Mayo Medical School
and Consultant in Gastroenterology and
Internal Medicine, Mayo Clinic
Rochester, Minnesota

Lawrence H. Einhorn, M.D.
Walther-American Cancer Society Clinical
Professor in Oncology
Department of Medicine
Indiana University Medical Center
Indianapolis, Indiana

Jack S. Faintuch, M.D.
Assistant Professor of Medicine
Section of Gastrointestinal Oncology and
Digestive Diseases
The University of Texas M. D. Anderson
Hospital and Tumor Institute at Houston
Houston, Texas

Isaiah J. Fidler, D.V.M., Ph.D.
R. E. "Bob" Smith Chair in Cell Biology
Professor and Chairman
Department of Cell Biology
The University of Texas M. D. Anderson
Hospital and Tumor Institute at Houston
Houston, Texas

Jennifer Fieck
Study Assistant, Cancer Center Statistics
Mayo Clinic
Rochester, Minnesota

Robert J. Fitzgibbons, Jr., M.D.
Assistant Professor
Department of Surgery
Creighton University School of Medicine
and the Hereditary Cancer Institute
Omaha, Nebraska

**Margaret M. Flanagan, R.N.,
M.S.N.**
Surgery Branch, National Cancer Institute
National Institutes of Health
Bethesda, Maryland

Eileen A. Friedman, Ph.D.
Assistant Cell Biologist
Department of Gastrointestinal Cancer
Research
Memorial Sloan-Kettering Cancer Center
New York, New York

Raffaella Giavazzi, Ph.D.
Assistant Professor of Cell Biology
Assistant Biologist
Department of Cell Biology
The University of Texas M. D. Anderson
Hospital and Tumor Institute at Houston
Houston, Texas

Geoffrey M. Graeber, M.D.
Division of Surgery
Walter Reed Army Medical Center
Washington, D.C.

Leonard L. Gunderson, M.D., M.S.
Professor of Oncology, Mayo Medical School
and Vice Chairman and Consultant
in Radiation Oncology
Mayo Clinic
Rochester, Minnesota

J. Milburn Jessup, M.D.
Associate Professor of Surgery and
Immunology
Associate Surgeon
Department of General Surgery
The University of Texas M. D. Anderson
Hospital and Tumor Institute at Houston
Houston, Texas

Michael C. Kew, M.D.
Senior Physician and Professor of Medicine
University of the Witwatersrand Medical
School
and Johannesburg and Baragwanath
Hospitals
Johannesburg, South Africa

Mary Kriegler, R.N., B.S.N.
Research Assistant
Department of Preventive Medicine
and Public Health
Creighton University School of Medicine
and the Hereditary Cancer Institute
Omaha, Nebraska

Stephen J. Lanspa, M.D.
Assistant Professor
Department of Medicine (Gastroenterology)
Creighton University School of Medicine
and the Hereditary Cancer Institute
Omaha, Nebraska

Bernard Levin, M.D.
Robert R. Herring Professor of Clinical
Research
Professor of Medicine
and Chief, Section of Gastrointestinal
Oncology and Digestive Diseases
The University of Texas M. D. Anderson
Hospital and Tumor Institute at Houston
Houston, Texas

Martin Lipkin, M.D.
Member and Attending Physician
Memorial Sloan-Kettering Cancer Center
New York, New York

Patrice Lointier, M.D.
Visiting Scientist
Section of Gastrointestinal Oncology and
Digestive Diseases
Department of Medical Oncology
The University of Texas M. D. Anderson
Hospital and Tumor Institute at Houston
Houston, Texas

Henry T. Lynch, M.D.
Professor and Chairman
and Professor of Medicine
Department of Preventive Medicine
and Public Health
Creighton University School of Medicine
and the Hereditary Cancer Institute
Omaha, Nebraska

Jane F. Lynch, B.S.N.
Instructor
Department of Preventive Medicine
and Public Health
Creighton University School of Medicine
and the Hereditary Cancer Institute
Omaha, Nebraska

Patrick M. Lynch, J.D., M.D.
Gastroenterology Fellow
Department of Medicine
Baylor College of Medicine
Houston, Texas

Donald McIlrath, M.D.
Professor of Surgery
Mayo Medical School
and Consultant in Surgery
Mayo Clinic
Rochester, Minnesota

Marion J. McMurtrey, M.D.
Professor of Thoracic Surgery
Department of Thoracic Surgery
The University of Texas M. D. Anderson
Hospital and Tumor Institute at Houston
Houston, Texas

Joseph N. Marcus, Ph.D.
Assistant Professor
Department of Pathology
Creighton University School of Medicine
and the Hereditary Cancer Institute
Omaha, Nebraska

James A. Martenson, M.D.
Assistant Professor of Oncology
Mayo Medical School
Senior Associate Consultant in Radiation
Oncology and Consultant in Surgery
Mayo Clinic
Rochester, Minnesota

J. Kirk Martin, Jr., M.D.
Assistant Professor of Surgery
Mayo Medical School
and Consultant in Surgery, Mayo Clinic
Rochester, Minnesota

Robert J. Mayer, M.D.
Associate Professor of Medicine
Dana-Farber Cancer Institute
Harvard Medical School
Boston, Massachusetts

Charles G. Moertel, M.D.
Purvis and Roberta Tabor Professor of
Oncology
Mayo Clinic and Mayo Medical School
Rochester, Minnesota

Kiyoshi Morikawa, M.D.
Visiting Scientist
Department of Cell Biology
The University of Texas M. D. Anderson
Hospital and Tumor Institute at Houston
Houston, Texas

Clifton F. Mountain, M.D.
Professor of Thoracic Surgery
Department of Thoracic Surgery
The University of Texas M. D. Anderson
Hospital and Tumor Institute at Houston
Houston, Texas

David M. Nagorney, M.D.
Consultant in Surgery
Mayo Clinic
Rochester, Minnesota

Guy Newell, M.D.
Chairman
Departments of Cancer Prevention and
Control
The University of Texas M. D. Anderson
Hospital and Tumor Institute at Houston
Houston, Texas

Michael J. O'Connell, M.D.
Professor of Oncology
Department of Oncology
Mayo Clinic
Rochester, Minnesota

Harvey I. Pass, M.D.
Surgery Branch, National Cancer Institute
National Institutes of Health
Bethesda, Maryland

Sen Pathak, Ph.D.
Professor of Genetics
Department of Cell Biology
The University of Texas M. D. Anderson
Hospital and Tumor Institute at Houston
Houston, Texas

Yehuda Z. Patt, M.D.
Associate Professor of Medicine
Associate Internist
and Chief, Regional Therapy Section
Department of Medical Oncology
The University of Texas M. D. Anderson
Hospital and Tumor Institute at Houston
Houston, Texas

Tyvin A. Rich, M.D.
Associate Professor of Radiotherapy
Department of Clinical Radiotherapy
The University of Texas M. D. Anderson
Hospital and Tumor Institute at Houston
Houston, Texas

Robert H. Riddell, M.D., F.R.C., Path., F.R.C.P.(C)
Professor of Pathology
McMaster University Medical Centre
Hamilton, Ontario
Canada

Jerry C. Rosenberg, M.D.
Division of Surgery
Hutzel Hospital
Detroit, Michigan

Jack A. Roth, M.D.
Professor of Thoracic Surgery
and Chairman, Department of Thoracic
   Surgery
The University of Texas M. D. Anderson
   Hospital and Tumor Institute at Houston
Houston, Texas

Naguib A. Samaan, M.D., Ph.D.
Chief, Section of Endocrinology
Department of Medicine
The University of Texas M. D. Anderson
   Hospital and Tumor Institute at Houston
Houston, Texas

Tom E. Smyrk, M.D.
Assistant Professor
Department of Pathology
Creighton University School of Medicine
   and the Hereditary Cancer Institute
Omaha, Nebraska

Marilyn Soski, R.N., B.S.
Research Nurse
Department of Medical Oncology
The University of Texas M. D. Anderson
   Hospital and Tumor Institute at Houston
Houston, Texas

Stuart Jon Spechler, M.D.
Associate Chief of Gastroenterology
Boston Veterans Administration Medical
   Center
and Associate Professor of Medicine
Boston University School of Medicine
Boston, Massachusetts

Margaret Spitz, M.D.
Associate Professor of Cancer Prevention
Departments of Cancer Prevention
   and Control
The University of Texas M. D. Anderson
   Hospital and Tumor Institute at Houston
Houston, Texas

Glenn Steele, Jr., M.D.
William McDermott Professor of Surgery
and Chairman, Department of Surgery
New England Deaconess Hospital
Harvard Medical School
Boston, Massachusetts

Seth M. Steinberg, Ph.D.
Biostatistics and Data Management Section,
National Cancer Institute
National Institutes of Health
Bethesda, Maryland

Grant N. Stemmermann, M.D.
Pathology Consultant
Japan-Hawaii Cancer Study
Kuakini Medical Center
Honolulu, Hawaii

John R. Stroehlein, M.D.
Associate Professor of Medicine
Gastroenterology Section
Baylor College of Medicine
Houston, Texas

Peter Thomas, Ph.D.
Assistant Professor and Director
Laboratory of Cancer Biology of the
   Department of Surgery
New England Deaconess Hospital
Harvard Medical School
Boston, Massachusetts

Victor Vogel, M.D.
Assistant Professor of Medicine and
   Epidemiology
Department of Medical Oncology
The University of Texas M. D. Anderson
   Hospital and Tumor Institute at Houston
Houston, Texas

Sidney Wallace, M.D.
Professor of Radiology
Deputy Department Chairman
Division of Diagnostic Imaging
The University of Texas M. D. Anderson
  Hospital and Tumor Institute at Houston
Houston, Texas

Michael J. Wargovich, Ph.D.
Assistant Professor of Cell Biology
and Assistant Cell Biologist
Section of Gastrointestinal Oncology and
  Digestive Diseases
Department of Medical Oncology
The University of Texas M. D. Anderson
  Hospital and Tumor Institute at Houston
Houston, Texas

Patrice Watson, Ph.D.
Assistant Professor
Department of Preventive Medicine
  and Public Health
Creighton University School of Medicine
  and the Hereditary Cancer Institute
Omaha, Nebraska

David M. Wildrick, Ph.D.
Project Investigator
Section of Gastrointestinal Oncology and
  Digestive Diseases
Department of Medical Oncology
The University of Texas M. D. Anderson
  Hospital and Tumor Institute at Houston
Houston, Texas

Sidney J. Winawer, M.D.
Chief, Gastroenterology Service
Co-Head, Laboratory for Gastrointestinal
  Cancer Research
Memorial Sloan-Kettering Cancer Center
and Professor of Clinical Medicine
Cornell University Medical College
New York, New York

Rodger J. Winn, M.D.
Director, Community Oncology Program
Department of Medical Oncology
Division of Medicine
The University of Texas M. D. Anderson
  Hospital and Tumor Institute at Houston
Houston, Texas

Index